Retina Atlas

Series Editors

Sandeep Saxena, MS, FRCSEd, FRCS, FRCOphth
Department of Ophthalmology,
King George's Medical University,
Lucknow, Uttar Pradesh, India

Richard F. Spaide, MD
Vitreous Retina Macula Consultants of New York,
New York, NY, USA

Eric H. Souied, MD
Department of Ophthalmology,
University Paris-Est Créteil,
Créteil Cedex, France

Timothy Y.Y. Lai, MD, FRCS, FRCOphth
Department of Ophthalmology and Visual Sciences,
Chinese University of Hong Kong,
Hong Kong, Hong Kong

The 9-volume atlas covers validated and comprehensive information on retinal imaging, retinal vascular disorders, macular disorders, vitreoretinal surgical diseases, infectious and inflammatory disorders, retinal degenerations and dystrophies, pediatric retinal diseases, oncology, and trauma. This atlas with over 100 chapters is well supported with hundreds of high-quality images and text notes providing in-depth details and information in a well-organized manner.

The editors Sandeep Saxena (India), Richard F. Spaide (USA), Eric H. Souied (France) and Timothy Y.Y. Lai (Hong Kong), volume editors and contributing authors are reputed eye physicians in their field with vast clinical experience.

This series has a full dedicated volume on imaging and includes various imaging technologies like optical coherence tomography, fluorescein angiography, etc. It provides global perspective of vitreoretinal diseases extensively covering medical and surgical aspects of the disease. Uncommon retinal findings in diseases such as Dengue hemorrhagic fever, malaria etc. are also covered well.

Retina Atlas is a useful go-to series meant for ophthalmology residents, retina fellows, and retina specialists as well as general ophthalmologists.

'Retina Atlas' series includes the following 9 Volumes:

1. Retinal Imaging
2. Retinal Vascular Disorders
3. Macular Disorders
4. Surgical Retina
5. Inflammatory and Infectious Ocular Disorders
6. Hereditary Chorioretinal Disorders
7. Pediatric Retinal Diseases
8. Ocular Oncology
9. Trauma and Miscellaneous Disorders in Retina

More information about this series at http://www.springer.com/series/16451

Gemmy Cheung
Editor

Hereditary Chorioretinal Disorders

Springer

Editor
Gemmy Cheung
Singapore National Eye Center
Singapore

ISSN 2662-5741 ISSN 2662-575X (electronic)
Retina Atlas
ISBN 978-981-15-0413-6 ISBN 978-981-15-0414-3 (eBook)
https://doi.org/10.1007/978-981-15-0414-3

This Springer imprint is published by the registered company Springer Nature Singapore Pte Ltd.
The registered company address is: 152 Beach Road, #21-01/04 Gateway East, Singapore 189721, Singapore

Contents

About the Editor

Gemmy Cheung is currently Deputy Head and Senior Consultant at the Medical Retina Service, Singapore National Eye Centre. She is also head of the retinal research group at the Singapore Eye Research Institute. Her research interests include the study of risk factors and clinical features of macular diseases that may be unique to Asian populations.

Dr. Cheung has published over 150 articles, mostly on age-related macular degeneration, including polypoidal choroidal vasculopathy. She has conducted several clinical trials on anti-vascular endothelial growth factor therapies. She has been actively involved in training and education and has served as an instructor for APAO and AAO courses and many other educational programs. She is also a volunteer faculty for the ORBIS Flying Eye Hospital program.

Dr. Cheung has received a number of prestigious awards, including the Macula Society Young Investigator Award (2017), APAO Achievement Award (2017), APAO Nakajima Award (2014), APAO Outstanding Service in Prevention of Blindness Award (2013), Bayer Global Ophthalmology Research Award (2012), the Roper-Hall Medal (2005) and the Elizabeth Hunt Medal (Royal College of Ophthalmologists, UK).

Retinitis Pigmentosa

1

Hung-Da Chou, An-Lun Wu, Yu-Chun Cheng, and Nan-Kai Wang

Introduction

Retinitis pigmentosa (RP) is a heterogeneous group of disorders characterized by the degeneration of photoreceptor cells and the retinal pigment epithelium (RPE), leading to profound vision loss or blindness. The prevalence of RP is approximately one in every 4000 individuals worldwide (Hartong et al. 2006). In 1836, Bernhard von Langenbeck used the term *melanosis retinae* to describe the pigmented condition of the retina during a postmortem examination (Langenbeck 1836). Later, in 1838, Friedrich von Ammon published drawings of widespread pigmentation based on pathological studies of the eye but did not correlate the condition to night blindness (Ammon 1838) (Fig. 1.1). After Helmholtz invented the ophthalmoscope in 1851, van Trigt in 1853 and Ruete in 1854 identified this disease in living subjects and linked it to visual symptoms (van Trigt 1853; Ruete 1855) (Fig. 1.2), which was ultimately named *retinitis pigmentosa* in 1857 by Franciscus Donders (Donders 1857). Even though there are no inflammatory processes in RP, the same name is still used today. To date, over a hundred years later, several treatment options have been proposed for patients with RP such as gene therapy, stem cells, and retinal prosthesis. However, long-term outcomes still need further investigation.

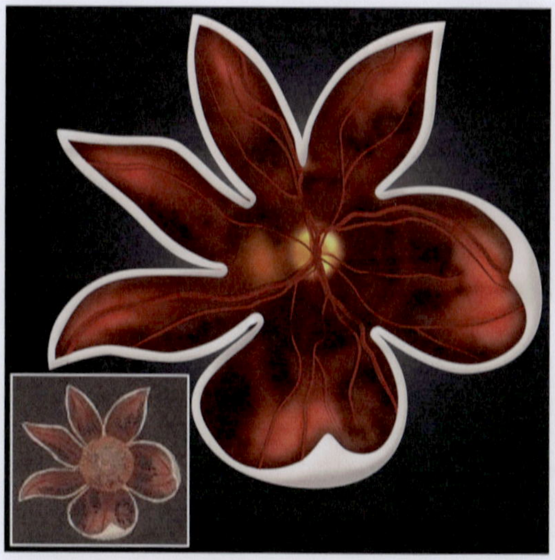

Fig. 1.1 A pathology illustration of retina pigmentation, recreated from the original work by Friedrich von Ammon in 1838 (smaller image). At the time, the condition was not thought to be linked to the clinical symptom of night blindness

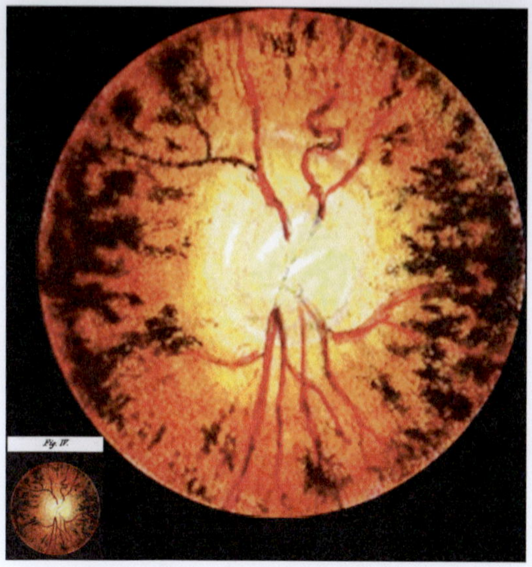

Fig. 1.2 Recreated image of the first illustration of RP under an ophthalmoscope by von Trigt where he described the pigmentation on the upper left blood vessel in 1853 (lower left image)

H.-D. Chou · A.-L. Wu · Y.-C. Cheng
Department of Ophthalmology, Chang Gung Memorial Hospital, Linkou Medical Center, Taoyuan, Taiwan

N.-K. Wang (✉)
Department of Ophthalmology, Chang Gung Memorial Hospital, Linkou Medical Center, Taoyuan, Taiwan

Department of Medicine, Chang Gung University, College of Medicine, Taoyuan, Taiwan

Department of Ophthalmology, Edward S. Harkness Eye Institute, Columbia University, New York, USA

G. Cheung (ed.), *Hereditary Chorioretinal Disorders*, Retina Atlas, https://doi.org/10.1007/978-981-15-0414-3_1

Genetics and Inheritance Patterns

RP can be inherited as an autosomal-dominant (AD) (30–40%), autosomal-recessive (AR) (50–60%), X-linked (XL) (5–15%), or mitochondrial trait (Hartong et al. 2006). It is a highly heterogeneous disorder with more than 50 culprit genes reported (RetNet 2017), and with various phenotypes and variants. One genotype can lead to different phenotypes, and a certain phenotype can be related to several different gene mutations.

RP can be divided into two main categories: *Non-syndromic RP,* where only the eyes are affected, and *syndromic RP,* where other neurosensory or systemic organs are also involved in addition to the eyes.

Non-syndromic Retinitis Pigmentosa

Typical Retinitis Pigmentosa

The initial presentation of RP is most commonly night blindness, which begins before adolescence. Peripheral vision usually starts to be affected from young adulthood, with the visual field gradually constricting as the disease progresses, resulting in central tunnel vision. Depending on the gene involved, some patients may completely lose their vision during their 60s (Hartong et al. 2006).

The classic triad of the fundus's appearance in RP consists of retinal blood vessel attenuation, waxy pallor optic disc, and retinal pigment epithelium (RPE) cell alteration, resulting in bone-spicule intraretinal hyperpigmentation, especially in the mid-peripheral of the retina (Fig. 1.3). It is often a bilateral disease with a highly symmetrical fundus appearance (Fig. 1.4). However, despite the remarkable fundus features, central visual acuity may not be affected due to the preservation of the central retinal function. Several examinations and imaging modalities can help determine and document the severity and progression of RP.

Clinical Assessment

Fundus photography is a basic documentation modality. However, this technique can only capture a limited view of the fundus with one film. Recently, the development of ultrawide field retinal imaging technique has allowed a more convenient way to record a wider view of the fundus without the need of montage. Therefore, it is especially useful in RP (Fig. 1.5).

The Goldmann perimetry is the main functional assessment tool for monitoring RP severity and progression. The classic pattern of visual field (VF) deterioration in RP is concentric VF loss (Fig. 1.6). There are also different patterns, including mid-peripheral arcuate or ring scotoma (Grover et al. 1998) (Fig.1.7). However, all patients eventually end up with a residual central island and finally general depression of the VFs.

The full-field electroretinogram (ERG) demonstrates a reduced rod and cone response amplitude, and a delayed implicit time in RP (Fig. 1.8). ERG aids differential diagnosis and provides objective measurements of visual function and

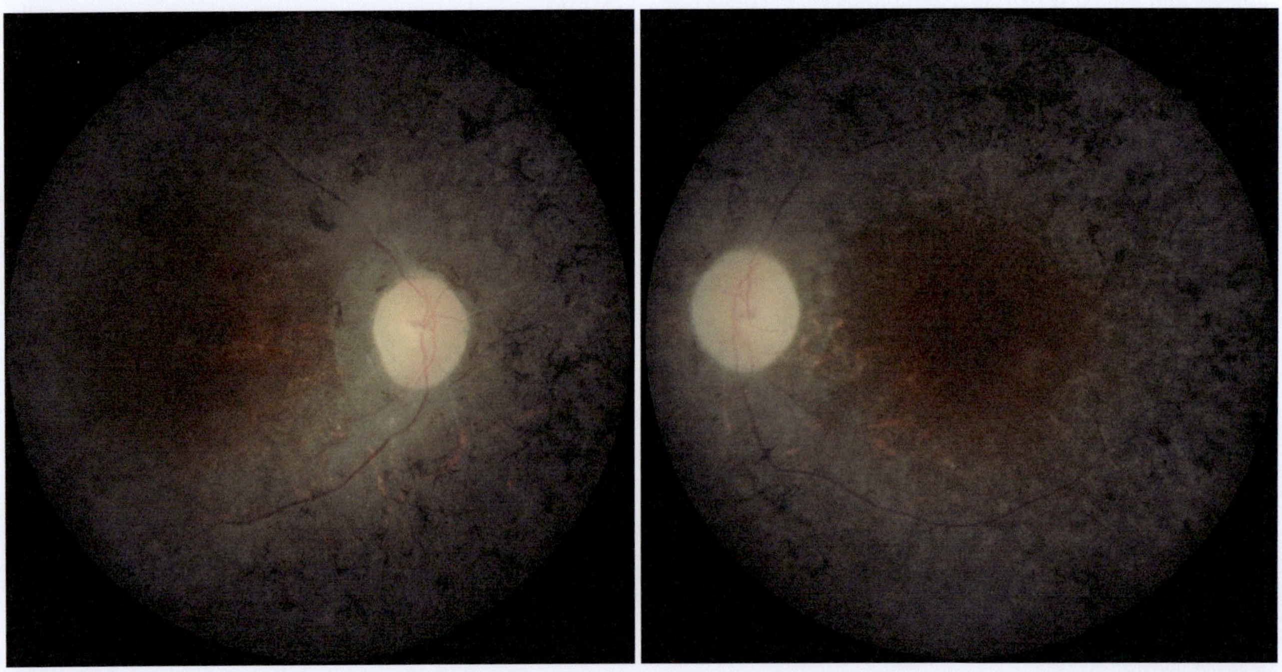

Fig. 1.3 The classic triad of retinitis pigmentosa fundus: waxy pallor disc, attenuated vessels, and mid-peripheral bone-spicule pigmentation. The macula is not yet involved and appears more orange in color

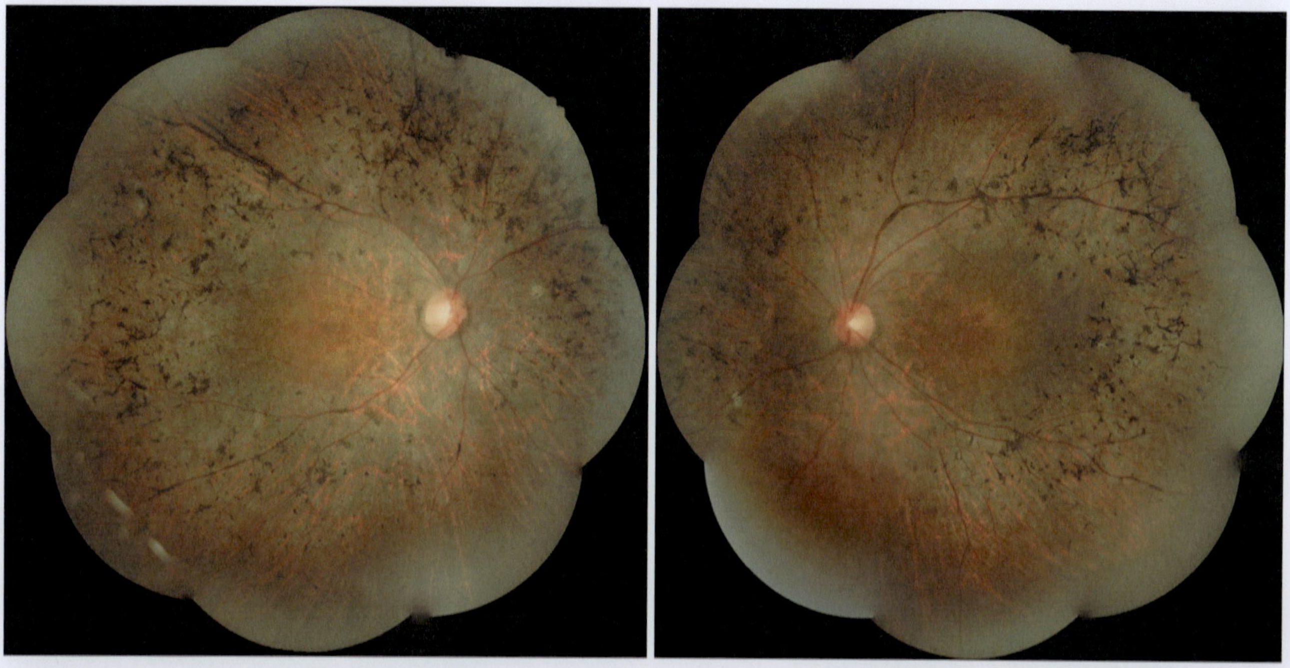

Fig. 1.4 Color fundus photograph showing attenuated retinal vessels and bone-spicule hyperpigmentation in the mid-peripheral of the retina. Note the symmetric fundus appearance between the two eyes

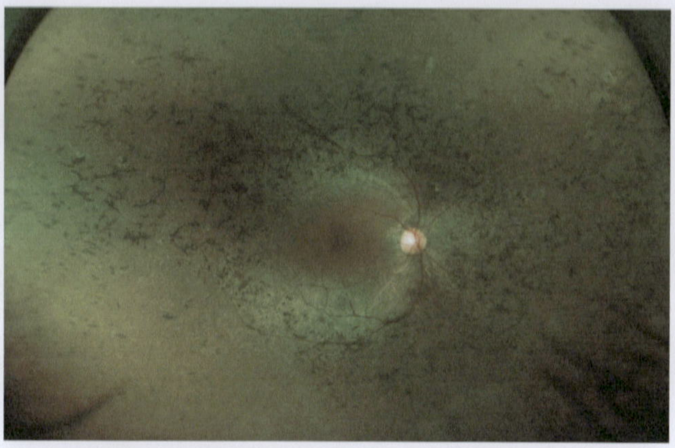

Fig. 1.5 Ultra-wide field retinal image of a patient with retinitis pigmentosa. The image clearly demonstrates the dense accumulation of hyperpigmentation, mainly distributed in the mid-peripheral of the retina. Note the round and patchy atrophic areas of the retina, which is more obvious with fundus autofluorescence imaging (Fig. 1.10). The linear shadow in the inferior were artifacts caused by eyelashes

correlates well with the VF study (Iannaccone et al. 1995; Sandberg et al. 1996).

Optical coherence tomography (OCT) provides structural measurements of the posterior pole. The transitional zone between the reserved central retina and the peripheral abnormal retina show outer retinal structural changes in the OCT (Jacobson et al. 2009; Hood et al. 2011) (Fig. 1.9). Functional studies have found that these structural changes include the thinning of the outer nuclear layer (ONL) and disruption of the ellipsoid zone (EZ) and external limiting membrane (ELM) (Witkin et al. 2006; Sandberg et al. 2005; Matsuo and Morimoto 2007; Jacobson et al. 2010; Wolsley et al. 2009).

Fundus autofluorescence (FAF) imaging is also a useful and non-invasive assessment tool. Excessive accumulation of lipofuscin in RPE cells is related to photoreceptor cell degeneration and can lead to hyper-autofluorescence (AF) (Katz et al. 1986). A hyper-AF ring surrounding the macula was reported as being present in 59% of RP patients (Murakami et al. 2008) (Figs. 1.10 and 1.11). The ring may serve as a precursor of apoptosis of the RPE cells and indicate the transition area between reserved healthy central retina and the degenerated peripheral retina (Lenassi et al. 2012; Greenstein et al. 2012). The hyper-AF ring is related to structural changes of the retina on OCT (Greenstein et al. 2012; Lima et al. 2009), and the diameter of the ring is well correlated with the preserved EZ area (Wakabayashi et al. 2010). The ring diameter is also correlated with functional studies such as perimetry, pattern ERG, and multifocal ERG (Ogura et al. 2014; Oishi et al. 2013; Robson et al. 2003; Robson et al. 2006), representing the size and function of the reserved retina and indicates disease severity. FAF imaging is non-invasive and offers an objective structural parameter, which is ideal for the documentation of progression (Lima et al. 2012; Robson et al. 2006). Together with OCT, it has been proposed that FAF should be performed upon RP patients annually as an assessment and follow-up tool (Sujirakul et al. 2015) (Fig. 1.12).

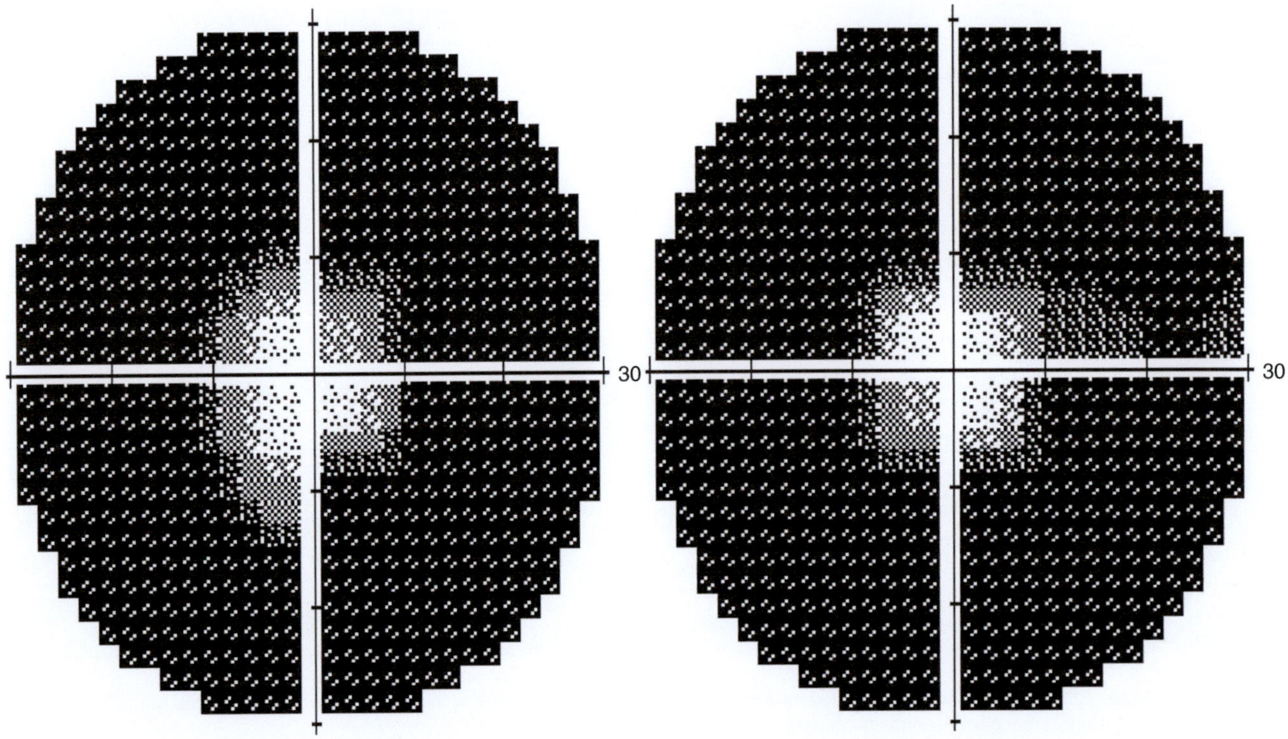

Fig. 1.6 Constricted visual fields in a retinitis pigmentosa patient. The two eyes are symmetric with the macula spared

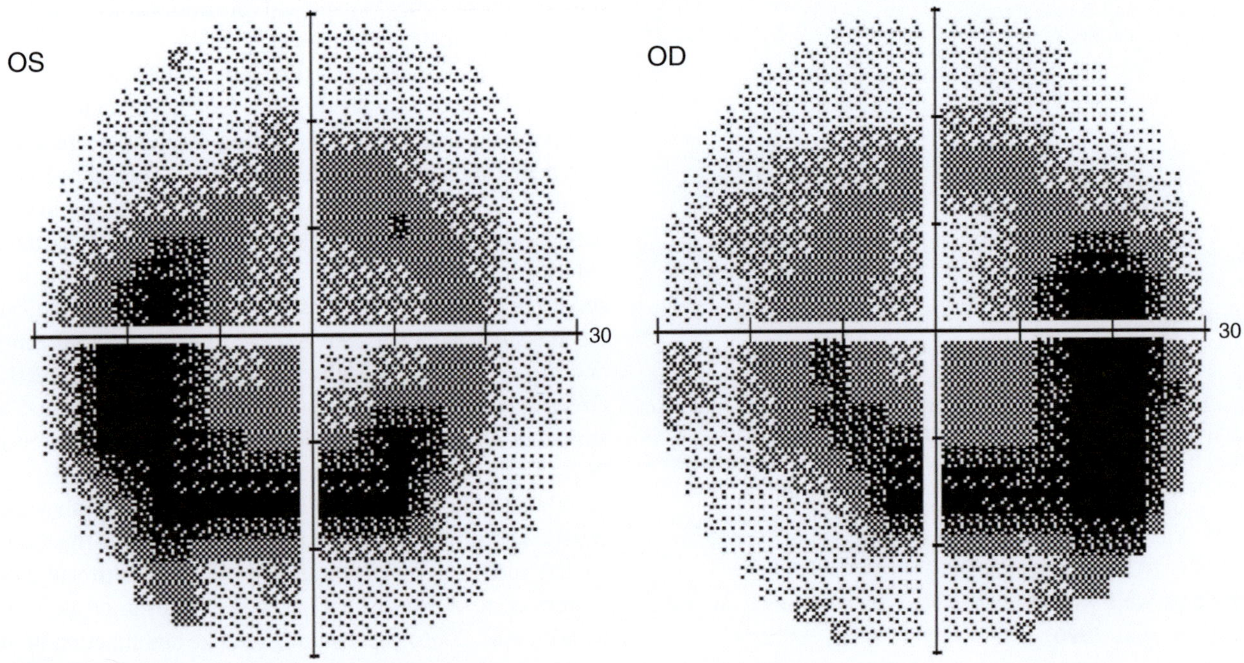

Fig. 1.7 Perifoveal arcuate scotoma is shown in the visual field exam. The arcuate scotoma corresponds well to the hypo-autofluorescent area in the fundus autofluorescence study

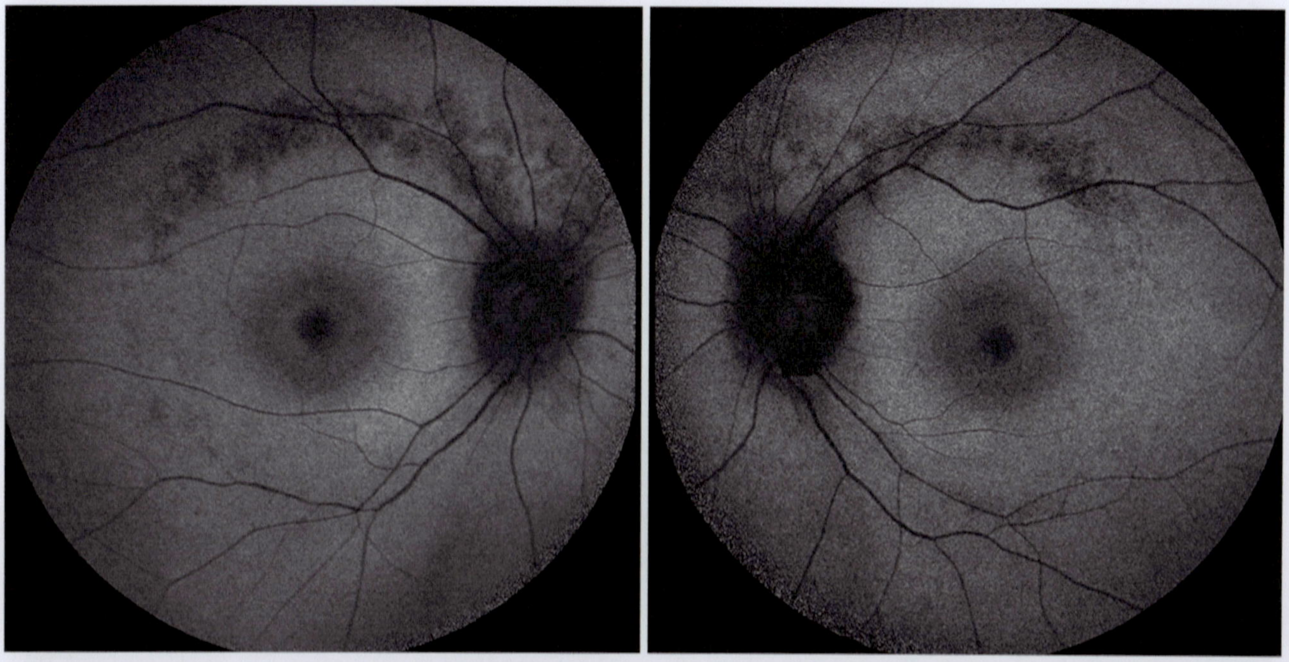

Fig. 1.7 (continued)

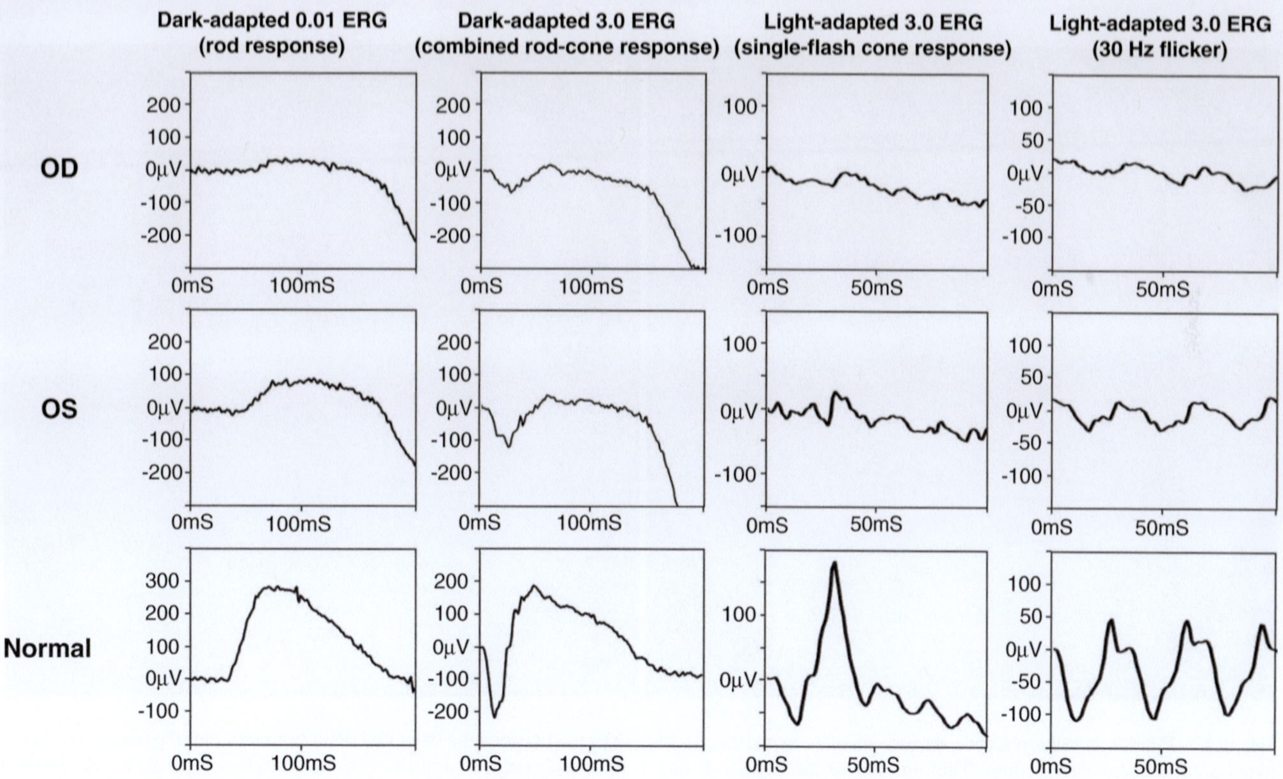

Fig. 1.8 Electroretinogram (ERG) of a patient with retinitis pigmentosa (RP) (upper two rows) compared to a normal subject (lower row). The full-field ERG shows a decrease in rod and cone amplitude in rod response and combined rod-cone response, as well as a delayed implicit time. The single-flash cone response also shows a decreased amplitude. In more advanced RP cases, the ERG is extinguished

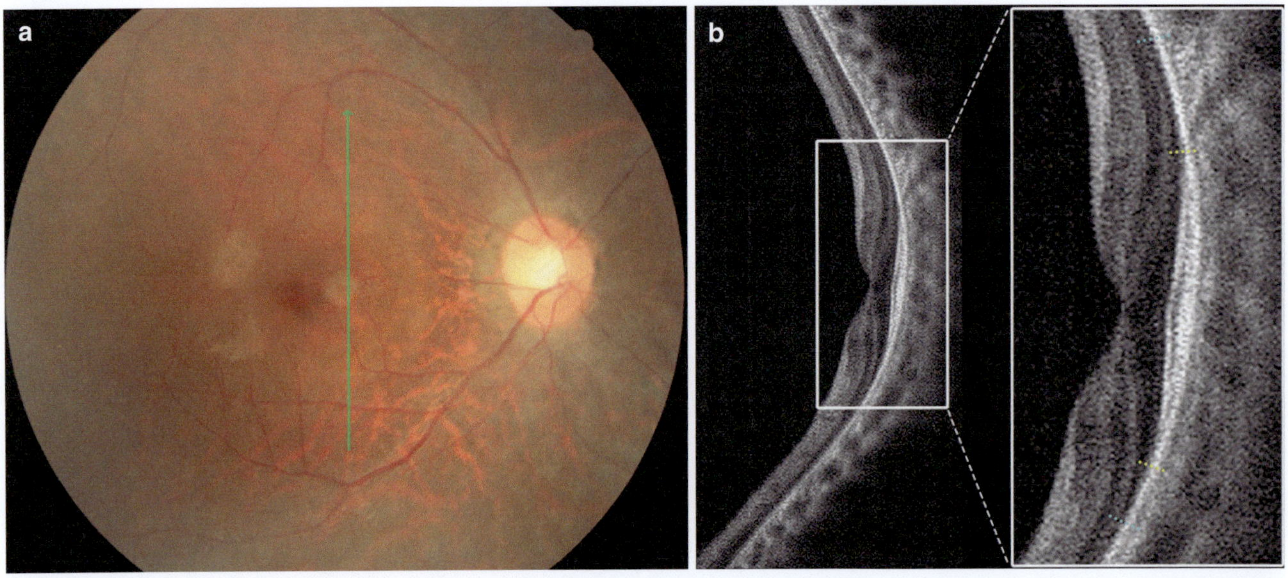

Fig. 1.9 Optical coherence tomography (OCT) images showing structural changes in retinitis pigmentosa. (**a**) The retinal alterations are not obvious in the fundus photograph. The green line indicates the orientation of the OCT. (**b**) The fovea was preserved with normal retinal lamination. The enlarged image demonstrates the transition from a normal retinal lamination in the fovea to a peripheral degenerated retina. These changes include the loss of the external limiting membrane (ELM) and the ellipsoid zone, and the thinning of the outer nuclear layer (ONL). The yellow dotted lines indicate the termination point of the ELM, and the blue dotted lines indicate the termination point of the ONL

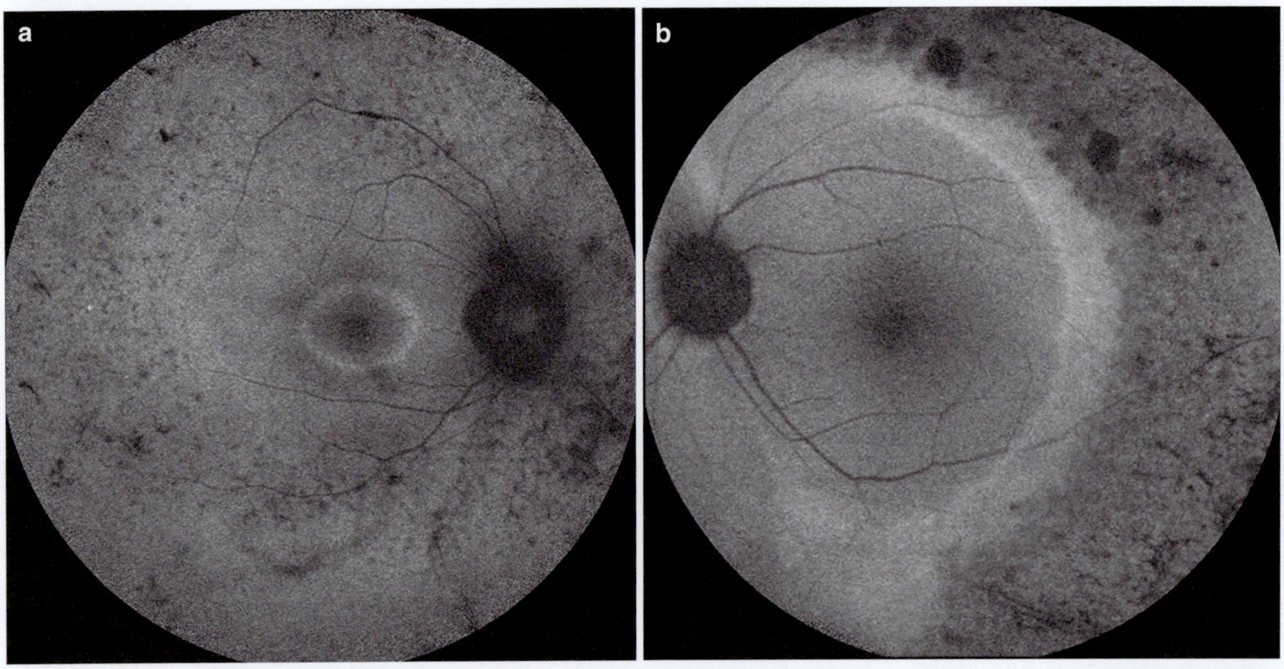

Fig. 1.10 Fundus autofluorescence images displaying variations of hyper-autofluorescent (AF) rings. The diameter of the hyper-AF ring correlated with the size of the preserved retinal structures and also the function of the retina (**a**, **b**). The transitional zone itself (i.e., the hyper-AF area between the inner and outer border of the ring) can be a thin (**a**, **b**) or wide ring (**c**). Some patients have no apparent ring in FAF images (**d**)

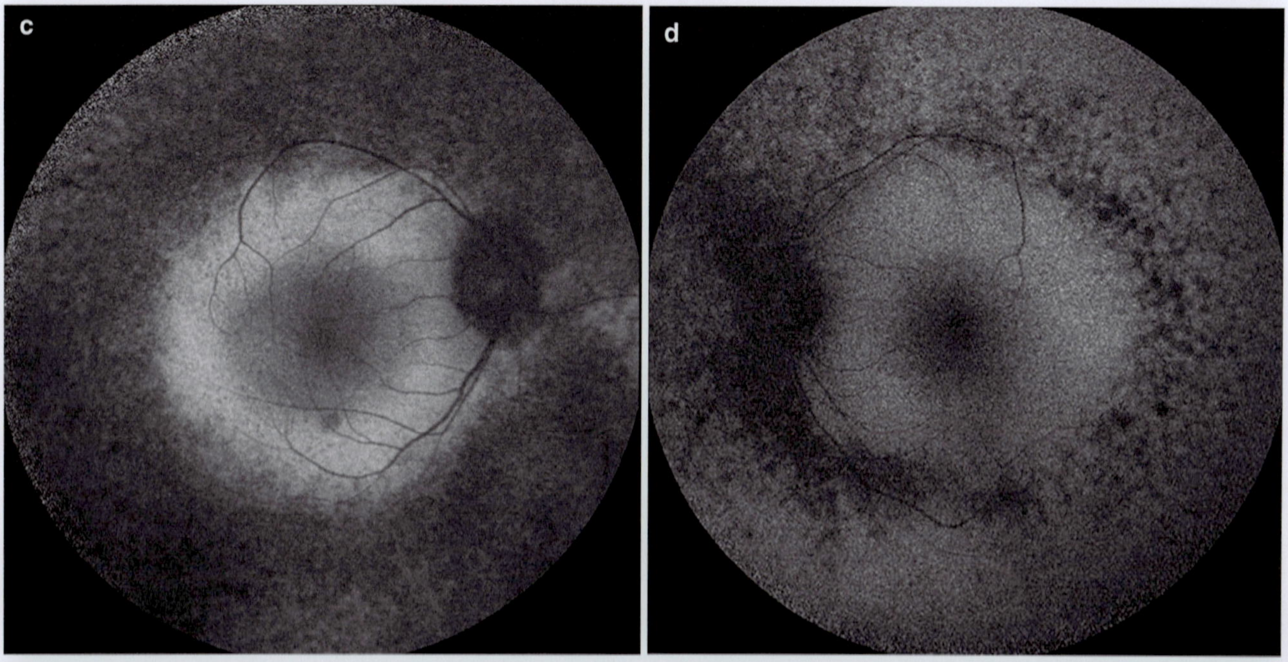

Fig. 1.10 (continued)

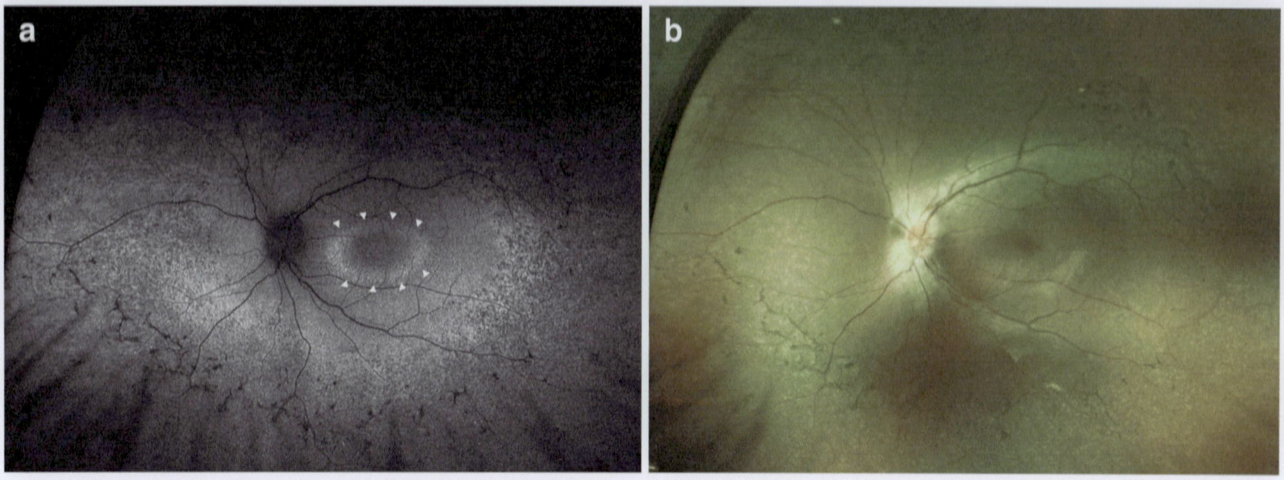

Fig. 1.11 Hyper-autofluorescent ring in retinitis pigmentosa. (**a**) An ultra-wide field fundus autofluorescence (FAF) image showing a hyper-autofluorescent ring surrounding the fovea (white arrowheads). Hyperpigmentation and retinal round or patchy atrophic areas are easily observed by the FAF study. (**b**) The corresponding ultra-wide field color fundus photograph

Macular Abnormalities in Retinitis Pigmentosa

Compared to the general population, macular abnormalities are more frequent in patients with RP (Testa et al. 2014). These abnormalities include cystoid macular edema (CME), epiretinal membrane (ERM), macular hole, macular atrophy, and vitreoretinal interface disorders. An OCT examination is useful for detecting these changes in the posterior pole, and functional studies such as microperimetry offer objective measurements (Lupo et al. 2011; Battu et al. 2015).

CME could compromise the central vision in RP patients earlier in the disease course. CME was reported to be present in approximately 10–50% of RP cases (Strong et al. 2017). Clinical diagnosis of CME is challenging by sole slit-lamp biomicroscopy. In fluorescein angiography (FA) and FAF, CME demonstrates a perifoveal petalloid pattern of hyper-fluorescence and hyper-AF, respectively (McBain et al. 2008) (Fig. 1.13). Various treatment methods have been used. Topical dorzolamide and oral carbonic anhydrase inhibitors (acetazolamide) have been used most widely, but

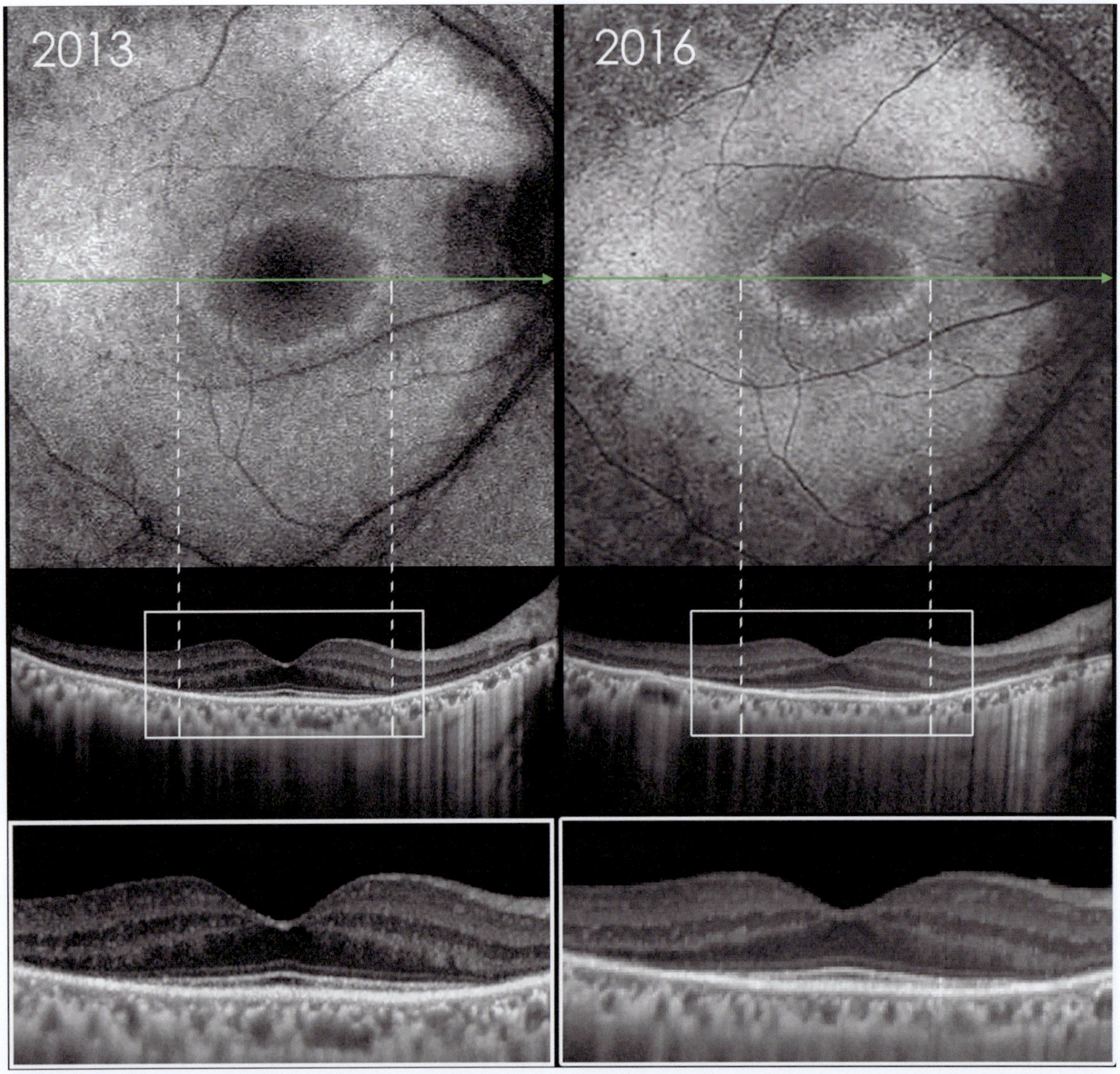

Fig. 1.12 Progression of fundus autofluorescence and optical coherence tomography (OCT) of the same patient 3 years apart. Note the constriction of the ring and the marching of the atrophic areas of retina toward the fovea. The hyper-autofluorescent ring corresponds to the structural alterations on the OCT (white dashed line). The enlarged OCT image showing the disruption of the ellipsoid zone and the external limiting membrane and thinning of the outer nuclear layer. The green lines indicate the orientation of the OCT

the response has been inconsistent. Other options of treating CME have been reported, which include intravitreal injection of anti-vascular endothelial growth factor (anti-VEGF) agents, steroids, and laser photocoagulation (Huckfeldt and Comander 2017).

ERM and macular hole can also interfere with central vision (Figs. 1.14 and 1.15). The prevalence of ERM or vitreomacular traction syndrome was 1.4–20.3%, and 0.5–10% for macular hole (Ikeda et al. 2015). Surgical outcomes for these conditions have been reported, but visual function improvement was limited (Hagiwara et al. 2011; Ikeda et al. 2015).

Macular atrophy and thinning are not rare in RP and have been reported in over 45% of patients (Sayman Muslubas et al. 2017; Thobani et al. 2011; Flynn et al. 2001). Different patterns of macular atrophy can be observed, including bull's eye, cystic, or geographic atrophy (Flynn et al. 2001) (Figs. 1.16, 1.17, and 1.18). Structural assessment by OCT demonstrates a reduction of foveal and ONL thickness, as well as the disruption of the ELM and the EZ (Fig. 1.18).

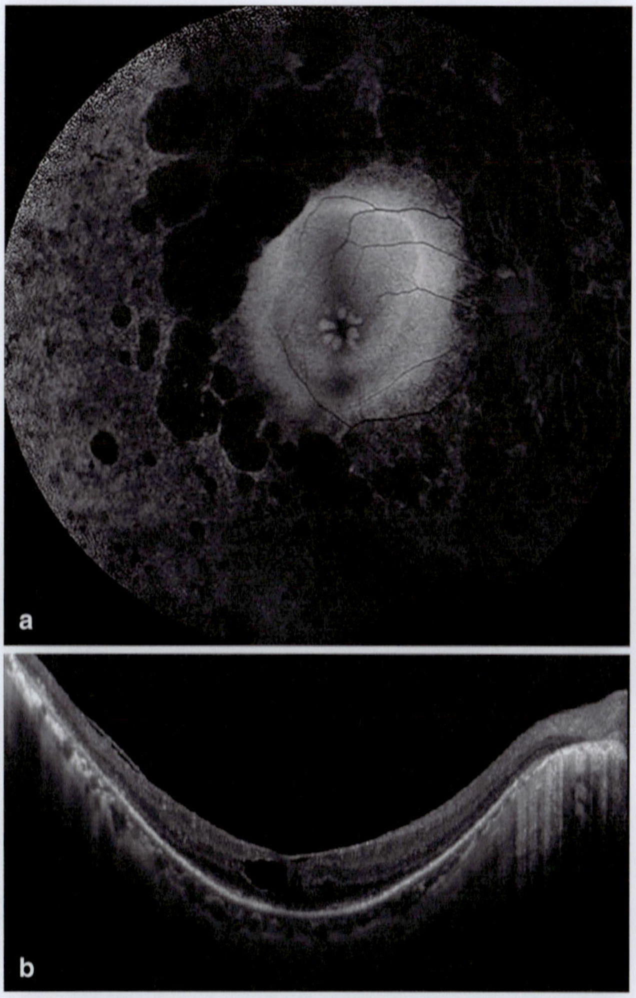

Fig. 1.13 Cystoid macular edema (CME) imaged by fundus autofluorescence (AF). (**a**) The perifoveal petalloid hyper-AF is a characteristic of CME. There are also features of retinitis pigmentosa, including a macula hyper-AF ring and mid-peripheral patchy atrophic areas, which are well demonstrated by hypo-AF. (**b**) The corresponding optical coherence tomography image reveals the thickening and accumulation of cystoid fluid in the fovea

Functional studies such as visual acuity and microperimetry correlated with the above structural alterations (Battu et al. 2015; Aizawa et al. 2009).

A few cases of central serous chorioretinopathy (CSC) have been reported in RP (Dorenboim et al. 2004; Meunier et al. 2008). Fluorescein angiography (FA) study has demonstrated the characteristics of typical CSC including a hyperfluorescent smoke-stack leaking point in the macular area and pooling of fluorescein dye in the subretinal space (Fig. 1.19). Bone-spicule hyperpigmentation blocks fluorescence in both FA and indocyanine green studies. RPE atrophic areas result in window defects in the mid-periphery.

A few other macular abnormalities can be seen in combination with RP, such as macular retinoschisis and posterior staphyloma (Figs. 1.20 and 1.21). These conditions are commonly related to pathological myopia (Steidl and Pruett 1997; Benhamou et al. 2002) but are rarely associated with RP in the literature.

Optic Disc Drusen in Retinitis Pigmentosa

The largest series to date showed that the incidence of nerve fiber layer drusen involving the optic disc or parapapillary regions in RP was approximately 10% (Grover et al. 1997), which is higher than the incidence of 0.34–2.4% in the general population (Auw-Haedrich et al. 2002). In a specific subgroup of RP with preserved para-arteriolar RPE, the incidence was even higher (39%) (van den Born et al. 1994). Optic disc drusen (ODD) was also found in some syndromic RP such as Usher syndrome and nanophthalmos-retinitis pigmentosa-foveoschisis-ODD syndrome (Edwards et al. 1996; Ayala-Ramirez et al. 2006) and was related to mutations in the membrane-type frizzled-related protein (*MFRP*) gene and the crumbs homolog 1 (*CRB1*) gene (Crespi et al. 2008; Paun et al. 2012).

Differentiating ODD from papilledema via funduscopic examination can be difficult, because both situations appear as swollen optic discs. B-scan echography can readily detect ODD, but only if the drusen become calcified. On FAF imaging, if the ODD is superficially located, it appears as a marked hyper-AF spot in the optic disc (Fig. 1.22). On FA imaging, ODD displays staining without leakage, whereas true papilledema shows leakage in the early or late phases (Chang and Pineles 2016).

Other Abnormalities in Retinitis Pigmentosa

Although rare, retinal exudation, retinal hemorrhage, telangiectasia, retinal angioma, and exudative retinal detachment can also be found in RP. These retinal changes have a resemblance with Coats' disease and are referred to as *Coats-like RP* (see Coats-like Retinitis Pigmentosa). The condition is related to the *CRB1* gene mutation (de Hollander et al. 2001; Bujakowska et al. 2012) but has been also reported in Usher syndrome and other RP variants (Fig. 1.23) (Murthy and Honavar 2009; Kiratli and Ozturkmen 2004; Osman et al. 2007). Retinal angioma is a secondary vasoproliferative tumor caused by benign vascular and glia proliferations. It is usually small, remains stable, and requires no treatment.

Differential Diagnosis

Many retinopathies with pigmentary changes can mimic RP and lead to misdiagnosis or diagnostic confusion. We should be especially aware of the three treatable RP-like conditions: abetalipoproteinemia (Bassen–Kornzweig syndrome), phytanic acid oxidase deficiency (Refsum disease), and familial isolated vitamin E deficiency (Grant and Berson 2001). Early diagnosis and treatment of these abnormalities could reverse the disease's impact on vision.

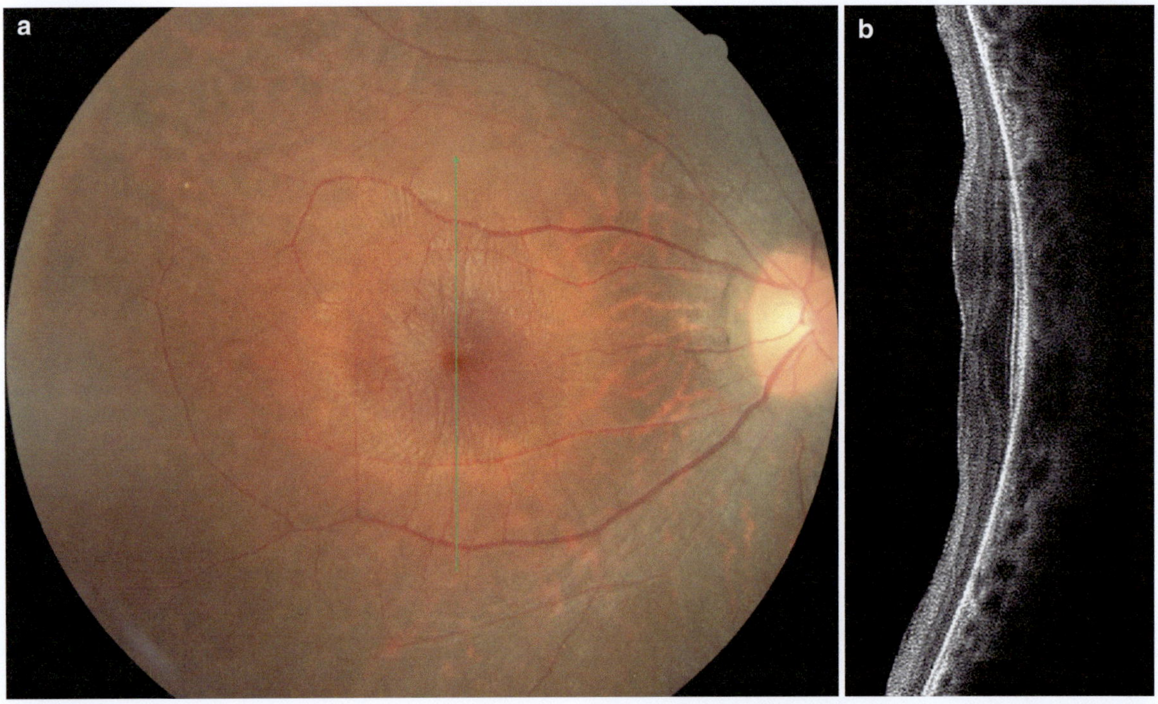

Fig. 1.14 Retinitis pigmentosa with epiretinal membrane (ERM). (**a**) The color fundus photography shows puckering of the macula. There are some atrophic areas outside the macular area, but the typical pigmentary changes in the mid-peripheral retina are not well demonstrated in this picture. The more recent technique of ultra-wide field retinal imaging can more readily document changes outside the posterior pole (Fig. 1.5). The green line indicates the orientation of the OCT. (**b**) An optical coherence tomography examination was used to detect macular changes, revealing a thin whitish epiretinal membrane

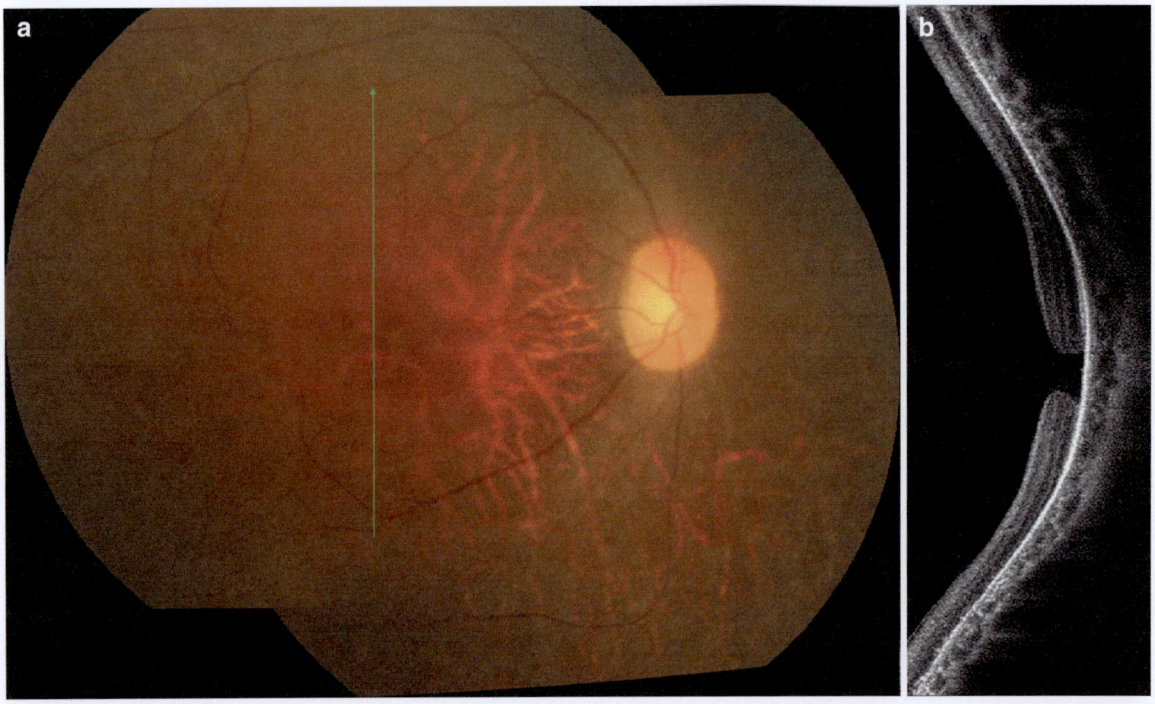

Fig. 1.15 Usher syndrome with macular hole. (**a**) A middle-aged woman had attenuated retinal vessels, mid-peripheral hyperpigmentation (not visible on this posterior pole picture), macular hole, and hearing impairment. The green line indicates the orientation of the OCT. (**b**) Optical coherence tomography image shows a full-thickness macular hole formation. Her older brother had similar fundus appearance except for the macular hole and had hearing problems. Their parents were first cousins without similar ocular or hearing abnormalities. Based on the symptoms and family history, the impression was Usher Syndrome with macular hole formation

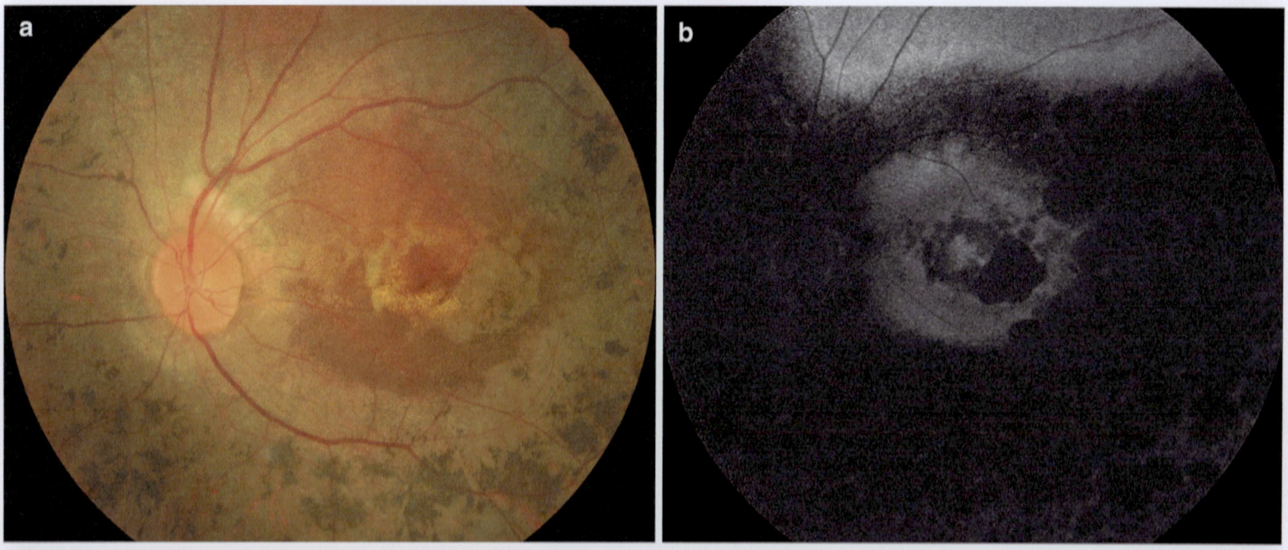

Fig. 1.16 "Bull's eye" macular atrophy in retinitis pigmentosa (RP). There are typical changes of RP in the mid-periphery (**a**) with the superior sector spared. (**b**) The macular atrophy is apparent with a remaining perifoveal ring and a foveal island, forming a "bull's eye" configuration

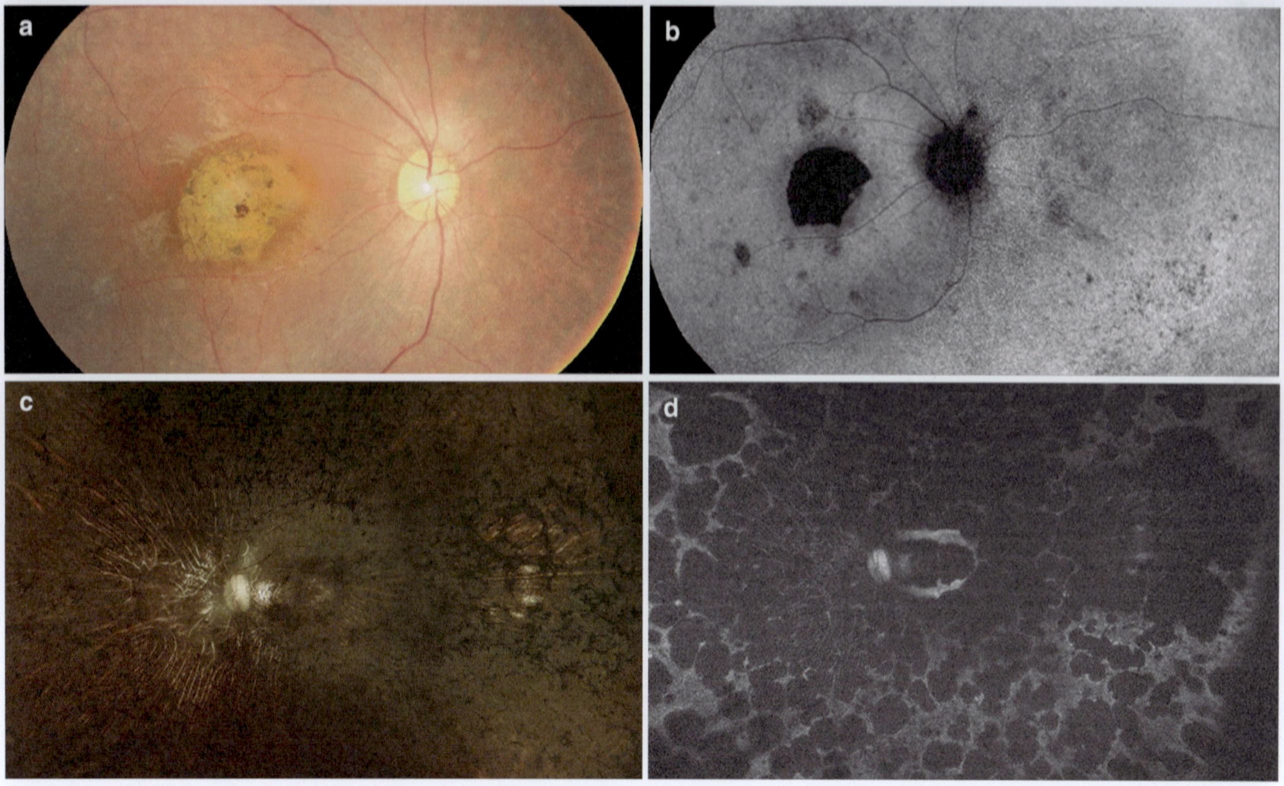

Fig. 1.17 Geographic macular atrophy in retinitis pigmentosa. The well-demarcated macular atrophic area is seen in the fundus photos (**a**, **c**) and is more apparent in the fundus autofluorescence images (**b**, **d**). The fovea was affected

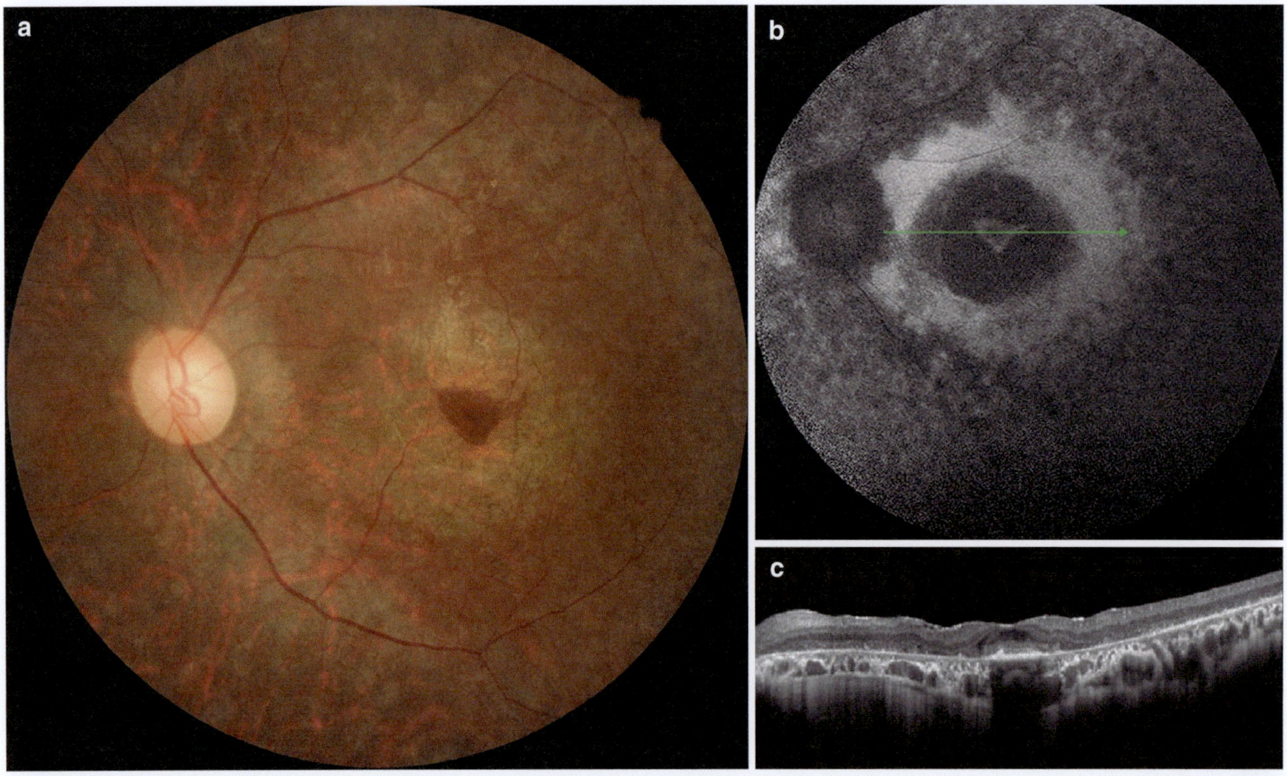

Fig. 1.18 A 32-year-old patient with retinitis pigmentosa with "bull's eye" macular atrophy and peripapillary atrophy. (**a**) Only a perifoveal ring and a small central foveal island are left. (**b**) However, the perifoveal ring and the foveal island both show hyper-autofluorescence, indicating that retinal pigment epithelial cell function was already altered in these areas. The green line indicates the orientation of the optical coherence tomography cross section. (**c**) Outside the central island, the outer retinal structures are lost. The vision was counting fingers

Many inherited retinal diseases can also be difficult to distinguish from RP. Cone/cone-rod dystrophy (CRD) is a form of retinal dystrophy, involving macular cone cells initially, and can have RP-like peripheral bone-spicule pigmentation in later stages. Leber's congenital amaurosis (LCA) is featured by severe visual impairment since infancy, often accompanied with nystagmus and oculo-digital sign. The fundus appearance in LCA could range anywhere from normal to RP-like. Other conditions such as Bietti's crystalline dystrophy, choroideremia, Sorsby fundus dystrophy, and Stargardt macular dystrophy can also be confused with RP in advanced stages.

Some acquired conditions can cause diffuse chorioretinal atrophy and *pseudoretintis pigmentosa*. Syphilis, congenital rubella, drug toxicity (thioridazine, chloroquine, hydroxychloroquine, quinine, chlorpromazine), acute zonal occult outer retinopathy (AZOOR), or cancer-associated retinopathy (CAR) should all be listed as RP differentials. Traumatic retinopathy and diffuse unilateral subacute neuroretinitis (DUSN) cause unilateral pigment clumping and *unilateral RP*. Careful ophthalmic examinations and systemic investigations in the patient and family members are the key to a final diagnosis.

Treatment

Although a definitive cure for RP has not yet been discovered, ophthalmologists, armed with new knowledge regarding the disease, are now even more able to offer aid to patients. These *treatments* include careful refraction, low vision aids, and genetic consultations. Managing RP complications, such as cataract and CME, is also an important measure.

Whether to use nutritional supplements is a question frequently asked in clinics. These supplements include vitamin A, vitamin E, docosahexaenoic acid (DHA), lutein, and β-carotene, but the effectiveness of these drugs remain controversial (Rayapudi et al. 2013; Brito-Garcia et al. 2017; Berson et al. 1993, 2004, 2010).

Several new treatment approaches are under investigation in clinical trials or animal studies (Jacobson and Cideciyan 2010). Electronic retinal implants are already available commercially and could offer limited vision for end-stage RP patients (Luo and da Cruz 2016; Chuang et al. 2014). An innovative method for LCA, which is caused by an *RPE65* gene mutation, is gene therapy (see Treatment section in Leber's Congenital Amaurosis). Inspired by success in LCA, *optogenetic therapy* involves the introduction of genetically encoded light sensors via adeno-associated viral (AAV)

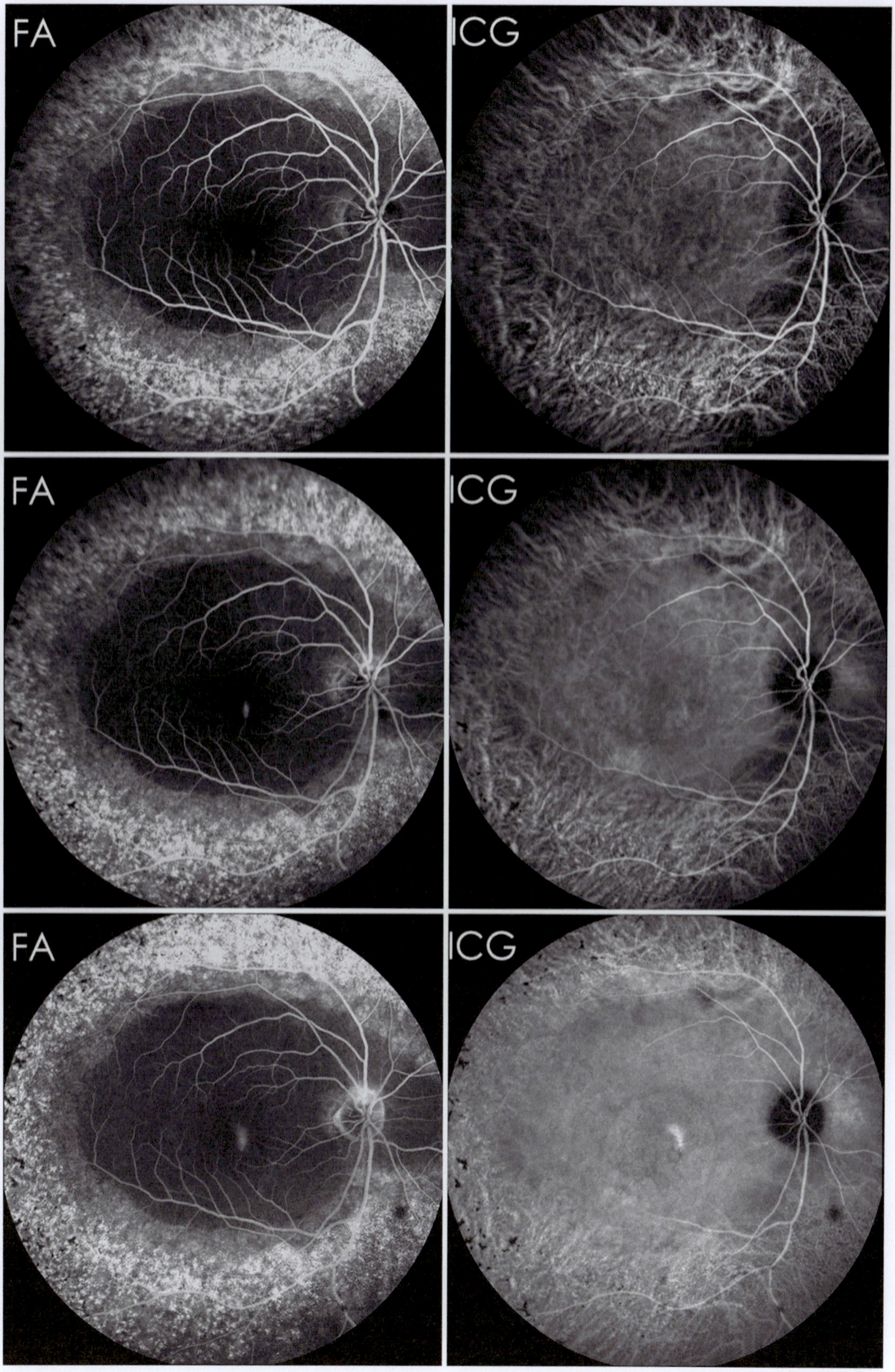

Fig. 1.19 Retinitis pigmentosa with central serous chorioretinopathy. The typical smoke-stack leakage is well demonstrated by the serial fluorescein angiography (FA) images. In the mid-periphery, bone-spicule hyperpigmentation blocks fluorescence in both FA and indocyanine green (ICG) images, and the hyperfluorescent spots clearly demarcate the atrophic areas

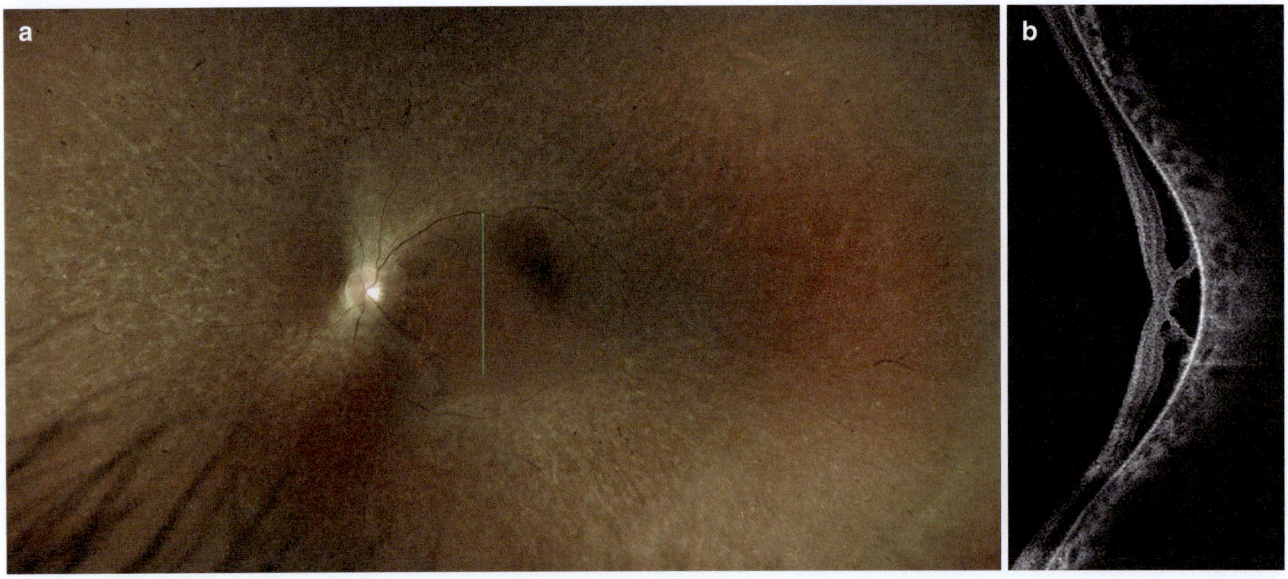

Fig. 1.20 Macular retinoschisis in retinitis pigmentosa. The 31-year-old woman has myopia −3.0 diopter in the left eye, and she reported to have distorted vision. (**a**) It is hard to appreciate the schisis change in the macula in the ultra-wide field fundus photograph. Some scattered pigmentation and atrophic areas are seen in the periphery. The green line marks the orientation of the optical coherence tomography (OCT). (**b**) The OCT image reveals schisis in the outer plexiform layer, compatible with outer retinoschisis

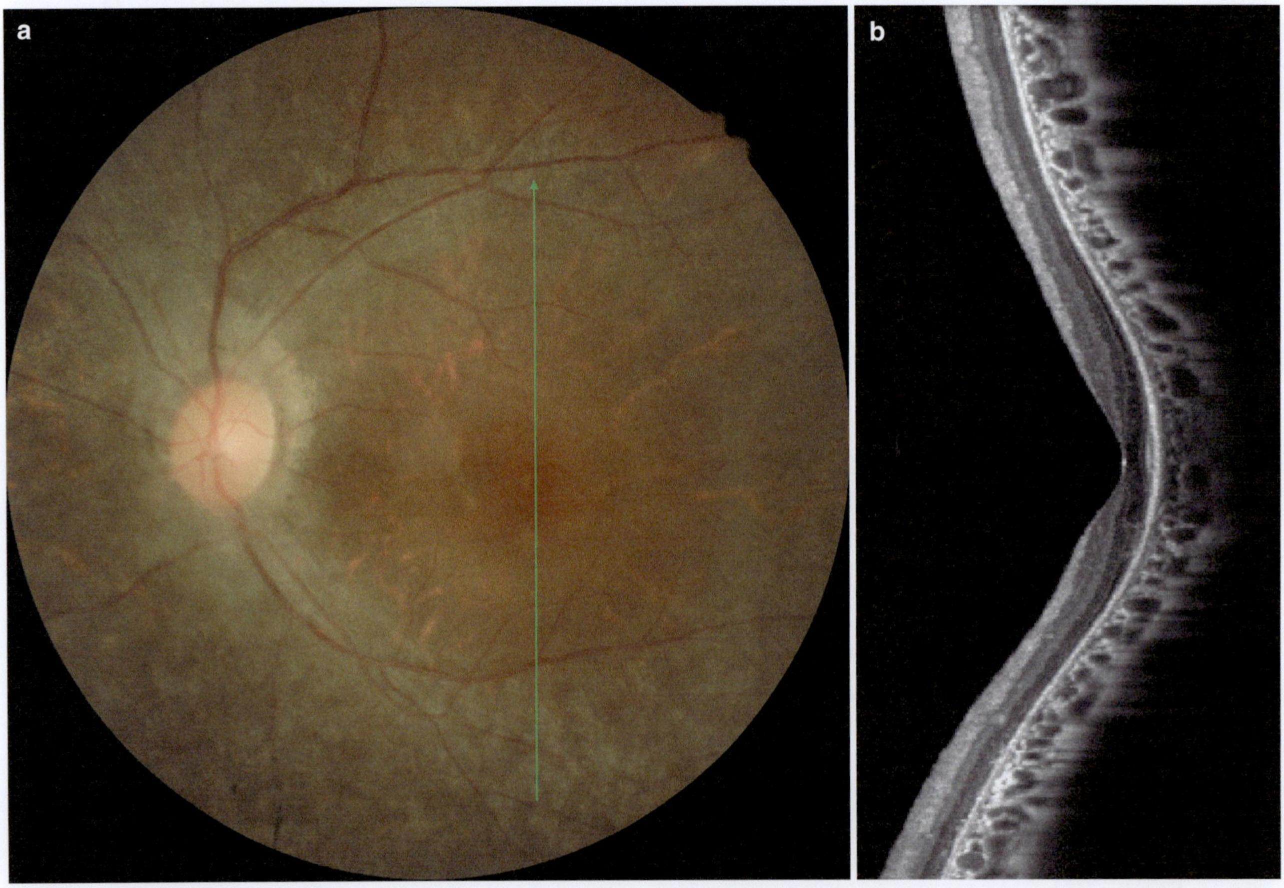

Fig. 1.21 A 28-year-old woman with retinitis pigmentosa and posterior staphyloma. She has no myopia (+0.25 diopter by both autorefraction and subjective refraction). (**a**) The fundus photography shows chorioretinal atrophy with macular sparing. The green line marks the orientation of the SD-optical coherence tomography (OCT). (**b**) The SD-OCT image displays posterior staphyloma at the macular area. There are also outer retinal structural changes, including thinning of the outer retinal layer and disrupted external limiting membrane and ellipsoid zone

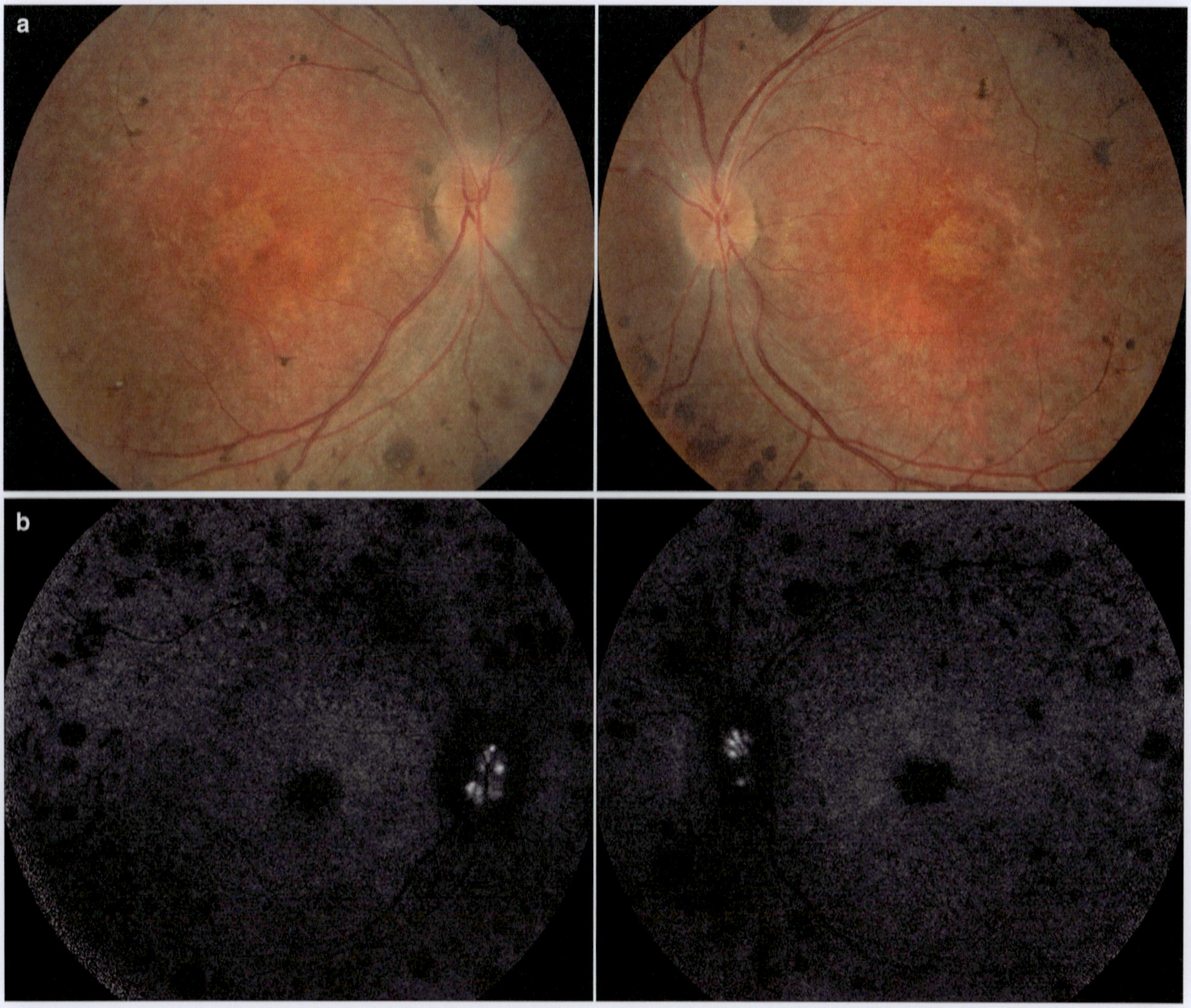

Fig. 1.22 Bilateral optic disc drusen (ODD) in a patient with retinitis pigmentosa (RP). The ODD could be an isolated feature or found in some syndromic RP such as Usher syndrome and nanophthalmos-RP-foveoschisis-optic disc drusen syndrome. (**a**) Fundus images display blurred optic disc margins. (**b**) ODD appears as a well-defined hyper-autofluorescent lesion on the fundus autofluorescence examination

vectors, making retinal cells responsive to light stimuli in animal studies (Busskamp et al. 2010; Bi et al. 2006; Lagali et al. 2008). It is hoped that these experimental approaches could assist RP patients, as well as patients with other inherited retinal dystrophy, in the near future.

X-Linked Retinitis Pigmentosa

Introduction

X-linked retinitis pigmentosa (XLRP) is an inherited condition that accounts for 6~17% of RP cases, but generally results in more severe phenotypes (Boughman et al. 1980; Boughman and Fishman 1983; Fishman 1978; Haim 1993). Although several XLRP pedigrees were reported in the early 1900s, Usher was recognized as the first author who described an X-linked recessive RP pedigree in 1935 (Usher 1935). Affected men (Fig. 1.24) show early onset of visual symptoms with night blindness followed by progressive constriction of the field of vision before the first two decades of life, which often leads to legal blindness in the fourth or fifth decade (Fishman et al. 1988). XLRP is a genetically heterogeneous disorder. Mutations in the genes *RP GTPase regulator* (*RPGR*) located at Xp21.1 and *RP2* located at Xp11.23 are responsible for most cases of XLRP (Breuer et al. 2002). The *RPGR* gene sequence variants account for more than 70% of XLRP (Pelletier et al. 2007; Sharon et al. 2003) and the *RP2* gene mutation is responsible for a further 5–20% (Breuer et al. 2002; Pelletier et al. 2007; Sharon et al. 2003).

In contrast, female carriers are usually asymptomatic, and their fundus appearance is variable (Wu et al. 2018). The

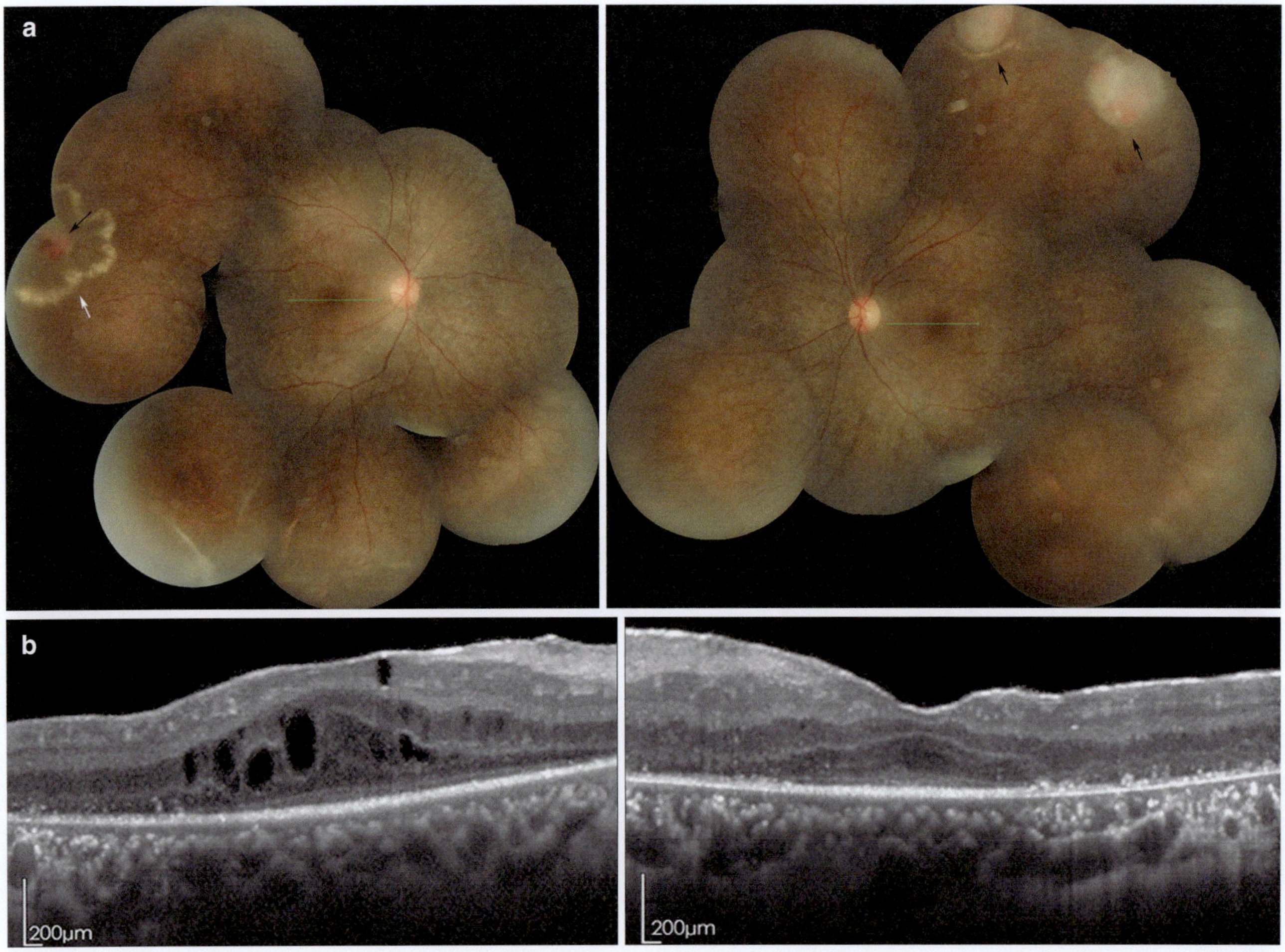

Fig. 1.23 A 25-year-old man with retinitis pigmentosa and Coats-like exudative vasculopathy. (**a**) Fundus examination showed peripheral multiple macroaneurysms (black arrows) with exudations (white arrow). His visual fields were severely constricted and electroretinogram was extinguished. The green lines indicate the orientation of the OCT. (**b**) SD-OCT revealed "thickened" and abnormally laminated retina. The foveal thickness was 446 μm in the right eye and 428 μm in the left eye. The patient also had hearing impairment since adolescence. *USH2A* mutation was confirmed and the final diagnosis was Usher syndrome with Coats-like exudative vasculopathy

pathogenic mechanisms of XLRP carriers are not well understood. However, histopathological studies in affected female carriers with different mutations in *RPGR* genes have shown some loss of photoreceptor cell nuclei and RPE abnormalities (Ben-Arie-Weintrob et al. 2005). A combination of adaptive optics with scanning laser ophthalmoscopy was used to demonstrate the mosaic pattern of cone disruption, although carriers had normal visual acuity and no visual symptoms (Pyo Park et al. 2013). Furthermore, the radial pattern of locally increased FAF was described as a bright radial reflex extending to the periphery against a dark background and was further investigated in carriers of XLRP (Wegscheider et al. 2004; Wu et al. 2018) (Fig. 1.30). These results suggested that in XLRP carriers, random X-inactivation may aid in early embryogenesis during clonal expansion in photoreceptor cell differentiation and peripheral migration in the developing retina. Correct identification of XLRP in female carriers can lead to an accurate diagnosis and confirm the nature of an unrecognizable entity in an affected male relative. Early diagnosis of XLRP carriers and their sons is essential for genetic counseling and for identifying patients who may benefit from future experimental therapy.

Clinical Features

Fundus appearance of affected men with XLRP may often show typical RP with or without the early onset of macular atrophy, including the characteristic bone-spicule clumping of intraretinal pigment located in the mid-periphery (Fig. 1.25), retinal arteriolar attenuation and a generalized hypopigmentation of RPE (Fig. 1.26). Waxy pallor of the disc and macular atrophy are usually signs of a more advanced disease (Fig. 1.27). FAF may show the presence of variably sized perifoveal rings and an arc of hyper-AF, which is not apparent on funduscopic photography, representing an area of an abnormal accumulation of lipofuscin in the RPE around a preserved sub-foveal region (Figs. 1.24, 1.25, and

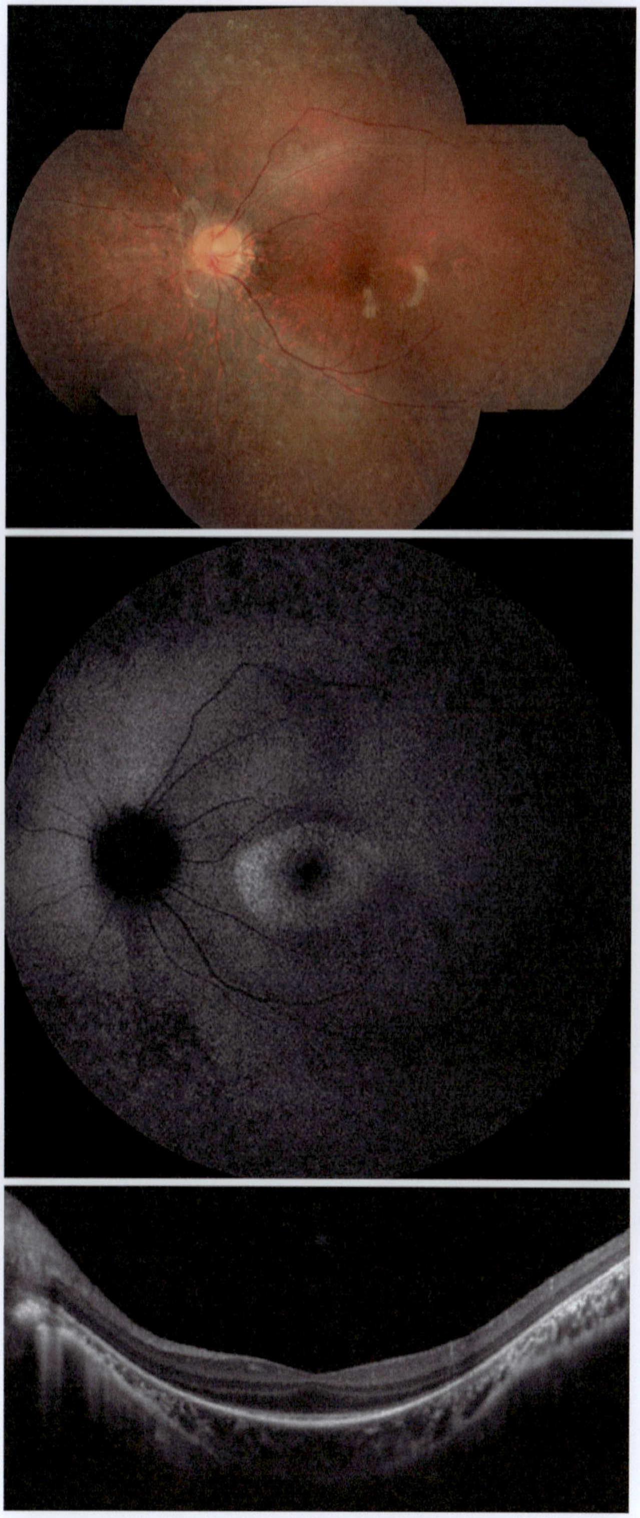

Fig. 1.24 This 11-year-old boy with X-linked retinitis pigmentosa had a history of poor visual acuity since his childhood. The visual acuity was 20/60 in the right eye and 20/30 in the left eye. The fundus is remarkable for hypopigmentation over the mid and extending into the far peripheral of the fundus. The fundus autofluorescence shows the presence of the perifoveal hyper-autofluorescence ring, which cannot be seen when using funduscopic photography. The optical coherence tomography illustrates the preserved ellipsoid layer in the fovea

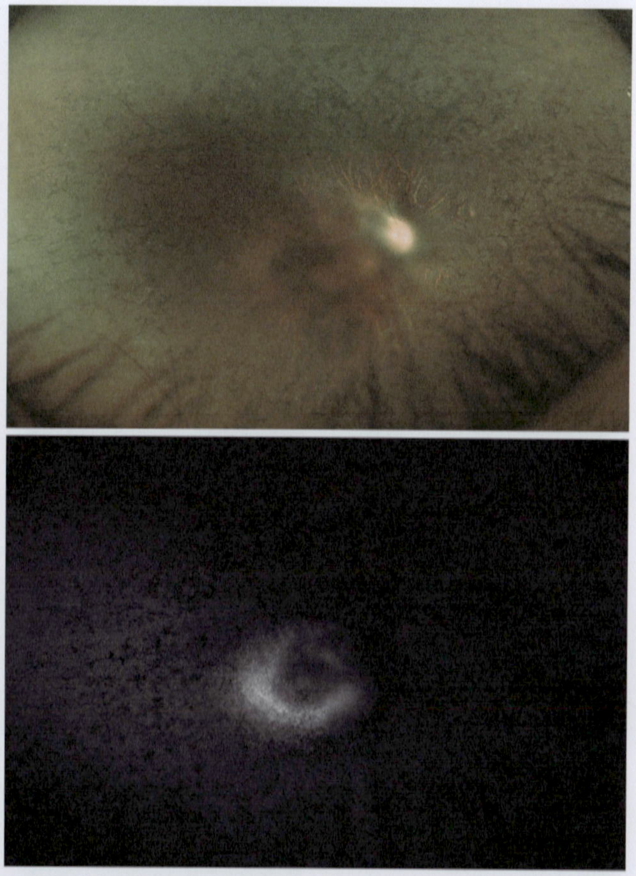

Fig. 1.25 An ultra-wide field color fundus photograph of a patient with X-linked retinitis pigmentosa (XLRP), confirmed by genetic testing for mutation in *RP2*, which showed lacy-like spicules of pigment epithelial hyperplasia over the mid and far peripheral fundus. The fundus autofluorescence image shows the presence of the perifoveal hyper-autofluorescence ring. We differentiated the correct diagnosis from a typical diagnosis of retinitis pigmentosa clinically by identifying the presence of XLRP in the female carrier of his sister in Fig. 1.30

1.26). The increased central hyper-AF ring is associated with the disruption of the EZ and a decrease in outer retinal thickness on OCT (Figs. 1.26 and 1.27) (Lima et al. 2009). EZ width might be considered a structural surrogate for the VF in RP (Birch et al. 2013). An ERG result may reveal absent or subnormal amplitudes.

In carriers of XLRP, fundus appearance is variable, ranging from unremarkable (Fig. 1.29) to the presence of pigmentary change and tapetal-like reflex (TLR), which is a golden metallic-luster sheen on the retinal surface, usually within the perimacular area (Fig. 1.28). FAF imaging may show striking findings of TLR with hyper-AF (Figs. 1.28, 1.29, and 1.30), even though TLR was not evident by color fundus examinations (Fig. 1.29). Wide-field AF may exhibit radial hyper-AF-orientated lines extending from the fovea to the periphery, with AF appearing as a characteristic bright reflex against a dark background (Fig. 1.30). Abnormal retinal structure such as EZ irregularities, EZ loss outside

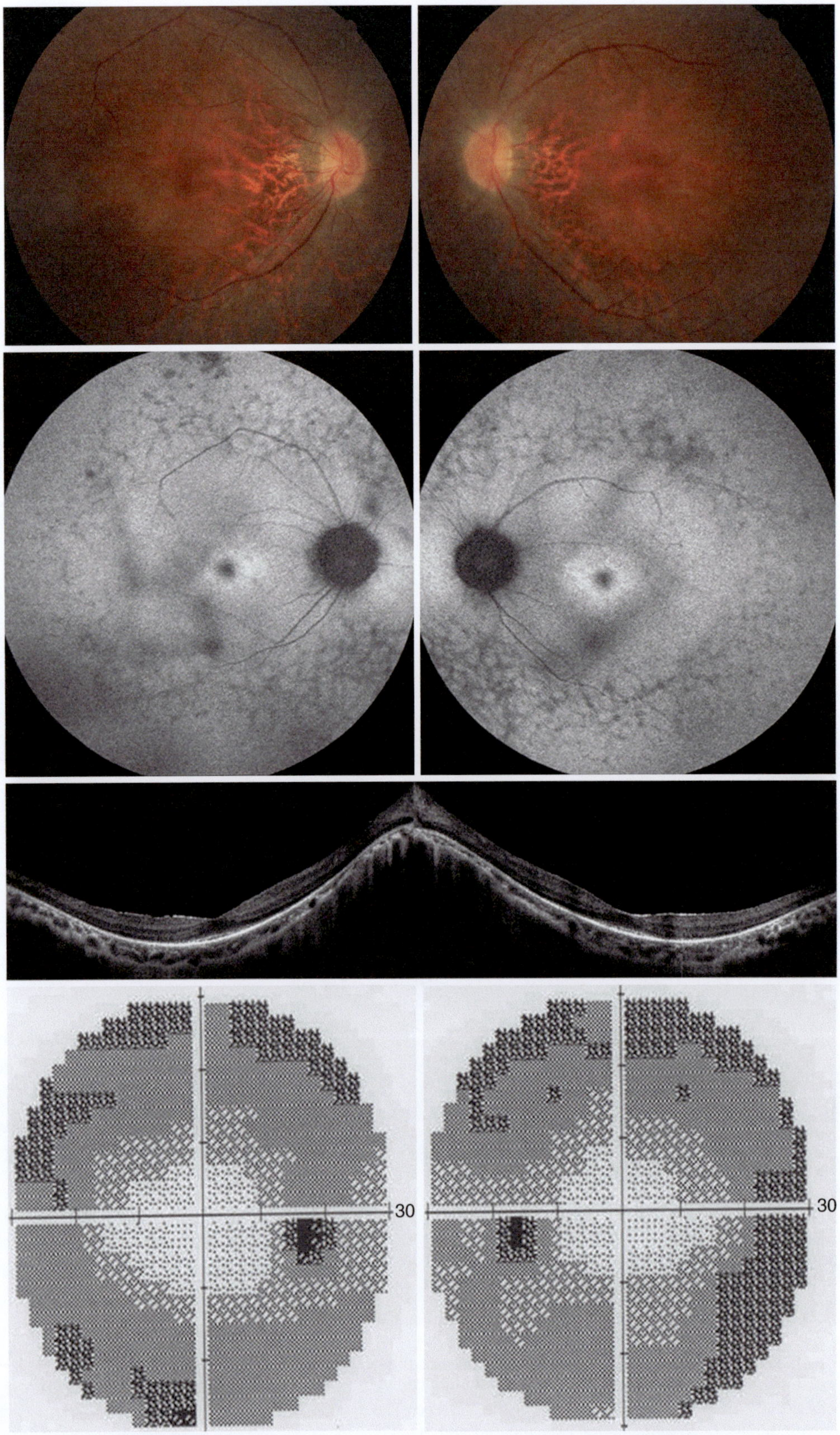

Fig. 1.26 This patient is a 23-year-old man with X-linked retinitis pigmentosa. Note the tessellated fundus change despite the lack of any myopia history. Fundus autofluorescence shows the perifoveal hyper-autofluorescence ring with hypo-fundus autofluorescence flecks. The optical coherence tomography reveals loss of the nerve fiber layer and photoreceptors outside the fovea. A visual field test confirmed peripheral constriction with tunnel vision only. Non-recordable electroretinogram was used to confirm the extinction of all rod and cone responses

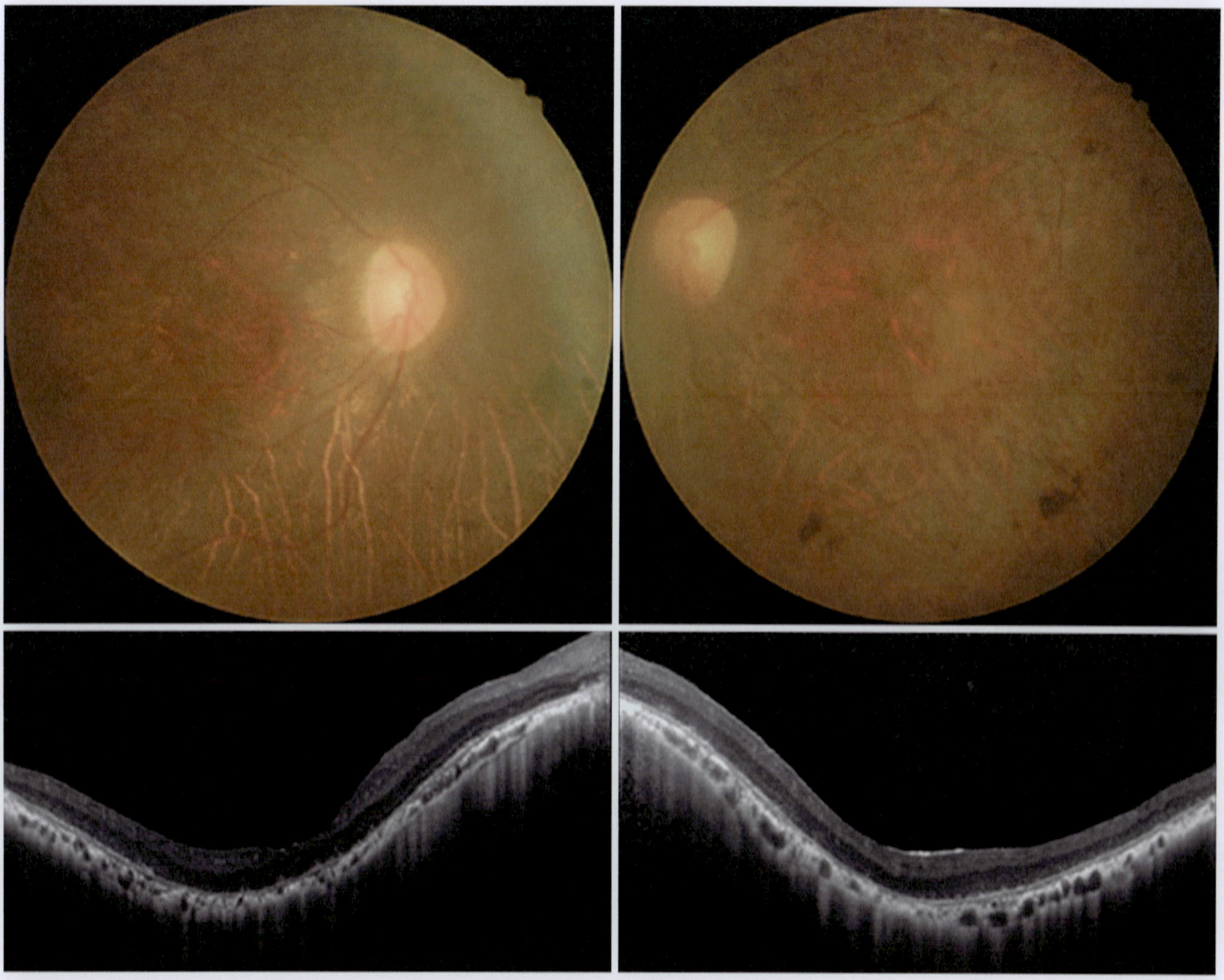

Fig. 1.27 This 59-year-old man with night blindness since high school was found to have retinal arteriolar attenuation and waxy pallor of the disc in both eyes. The optical coherence tomography shows atrophic change of the macula. Genetic testing revealed the presence of the RPGR mutation, confirming the diagnosis of X-linked retinitis pigmentosa

the fovea, increased reflectivity from the RPE–photoreceptor layer complex can be observed (Figs. 1.29 and 1.30). Hyper-AF might be related to the damage of photoreceptor cells, and the abnormal retinal structure with loss of the EZ seen on OCT was localized to areas of enhanced reflectance on FAF images (Fig. 1.30). ERG may show abnormalities of reduced amplitude or delayed cone-wave implicit time. This mosaicism and variability has been ascribed to lyonization (Wuthisiri et al. 2013), a phenomenon characterized by random X-inactivation.

Leber's Congenital Amaurosis

Introduction and Genetics

LCA (Leber congenital tapetoretinal degeneration, heredoretinopathia congenitalis, hereditary retinal aplasia, hereditary epithelial dysplasia of retina, dysgenesis neuroepithelial retinae) is an early onset and severe form of inherited retinal dystrophy responsible for congenital blindness. The estimated prevalence of LCA is 1–3 per 100,000, and it accounts for around 5% of all retinal dystrophies (Alkharashi and Fulton 2017; Chacon-Camacho and Zenteno 2015; Fazzi et al. 2003; Coussa et al. 2017). In 1869, German ophthalmologist Theodor von Leber first described the disease as a disorder characterized by profound visual loss at or near birth, wandering nystagmus, sluggish pupillary response, and a normal appearing fundus that progressed to pigmentary retinopathy (Leber 1869). Franceschetti and Deiterlé later added severely reduced ERG and altered visual evoked potentials (VEP) (Franceschetti 1954). Other associated clinical appearances included oculo-digital sign, cataract, keratoconus, high hyperopia, high myopia, and nyctalopia (Lambert et al. 1989).

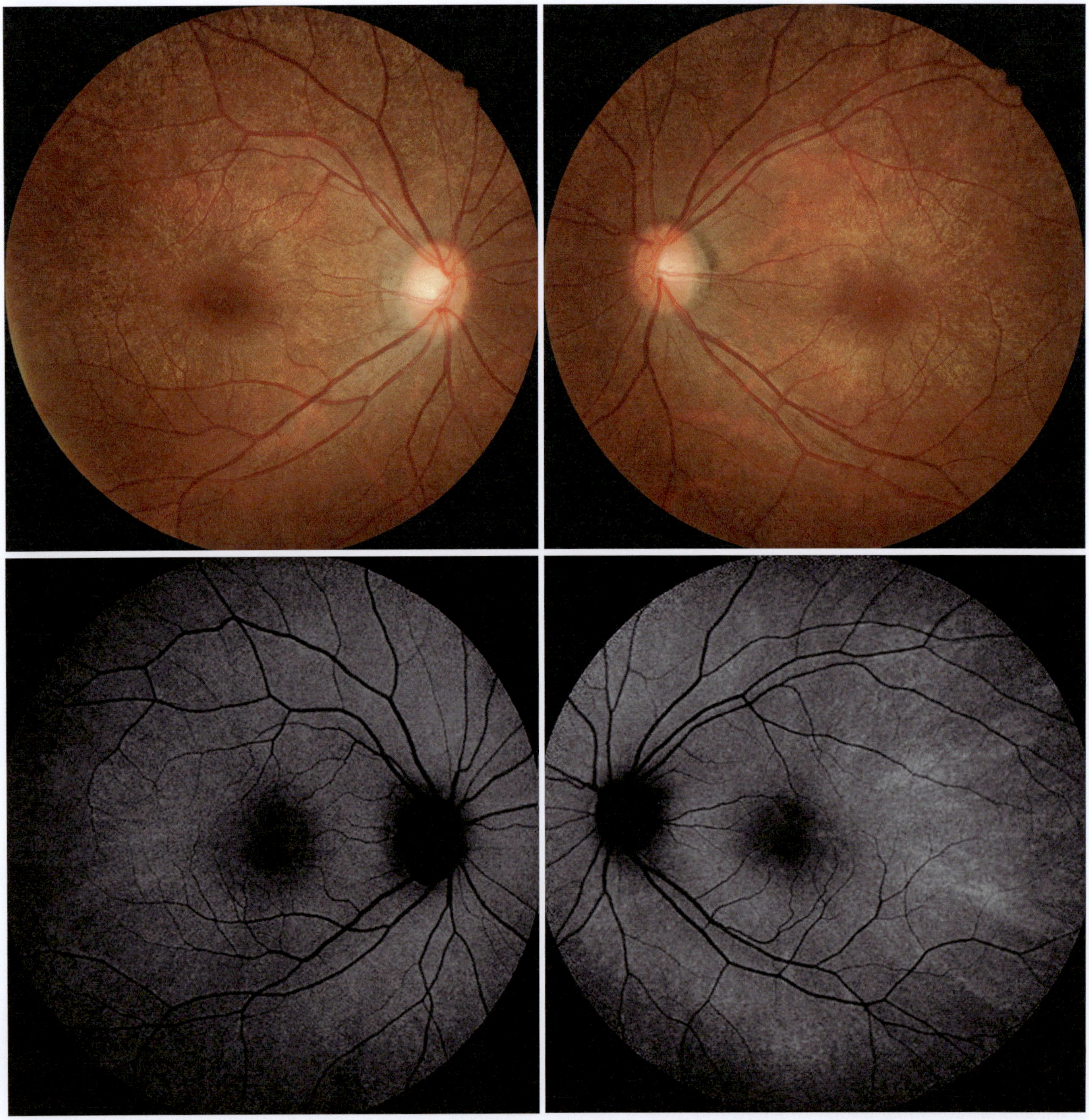

Fig. 1.28 This carrier with X-linked retinitis pigmentosa has a tapetal-like reflex (TLR) and a golden metallic-luster sheen on the retinal surface located within the perimacular area in both eyes. Note that the striking findings of TLR with hyper-autofluorescence are also evident in autofluorescence images

LCA is mostly inherited in an autosomal recessive pattern, with 23 causative genes identified as affecting the developmental and physiological pathway of either photoreceptors or RPE (Chacon-Camacho and Zenteno 2015).

Clinical Features

The diagnosis of LCA is made according to clinical signs. De Laey proposed the diagnostic criteria of LCA in 1991, including (1) early onset of poor vision (mostly before 6 months of age), (2) sluggish pupillary response, (3) nystagmus, (4) oculo-digital sign, (5) extinguished or severely reduced ERG, (6) abnormal VEP, and (7) variable fundus (De Laey 1991).

LCA differs from typical RP in the age of visual impairment and early development of retinopathy. Some inherited retinal dystrophies share similar presentation with LCA. Patients with achromatopsia, congenital stationary night blindness and albinism may all present with nystagmus.

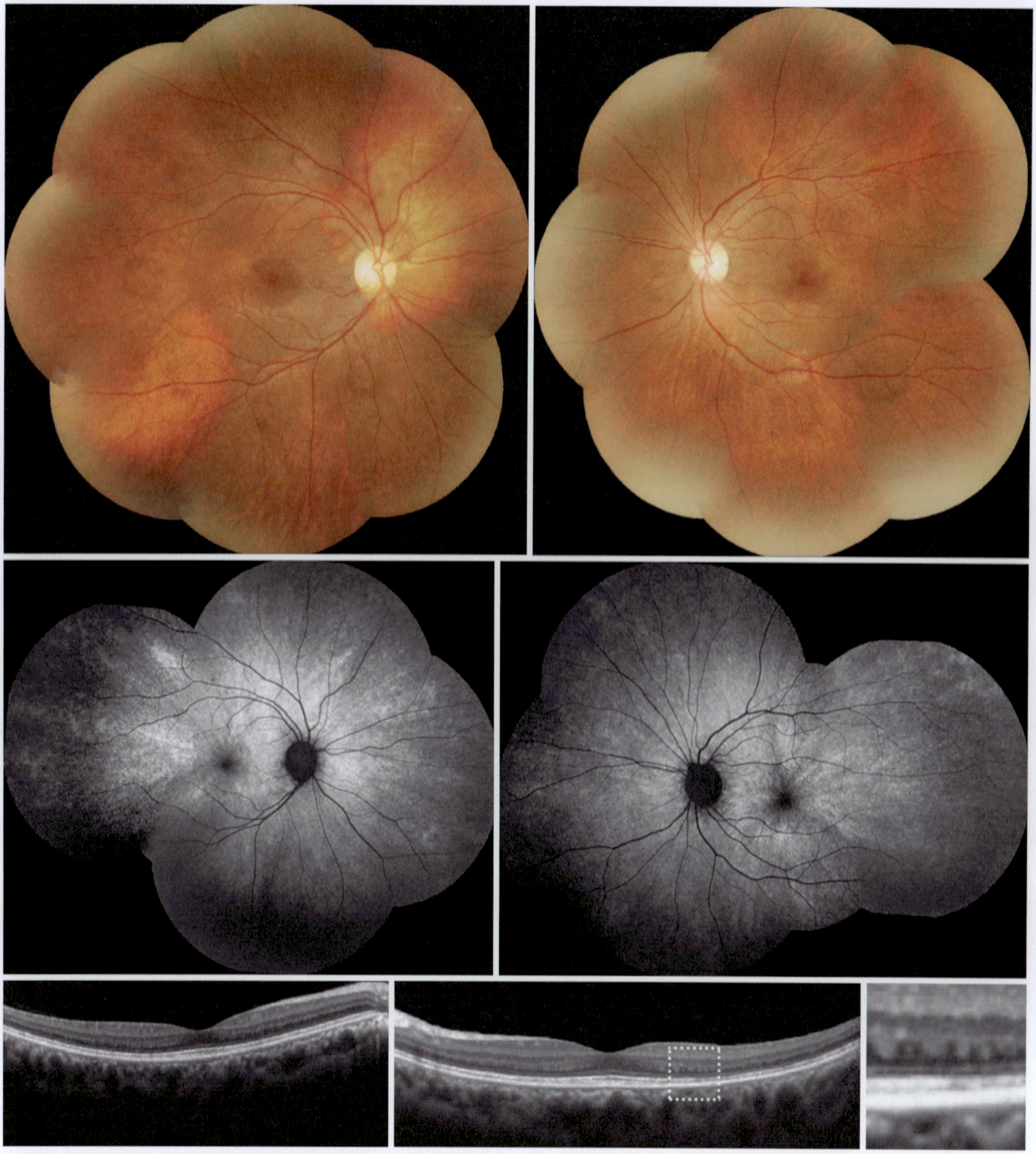

Fig. 1.29 This carrier with X-linked retinitis pigmentosa has a tapetal-like reflex (TLR) with hyper-autofluorescence in the autofluorescence image even though TLR was not evident in the color fundus photo. The optical coherence tomography scan shows irregularities in the ellipsoid zone involving the macula. Higher magnification (right lower) of the area outlined by white dots shows the thinning of the outer nuclear layer (ONL) and a dentate appearance of the outer plexiform layer (OPL)

In comparison, patients with achromatopsia are unable to differentiate between different colors but have an improved contrast sensitivity at dimmer light. In addition, they have an absence of obvious fundus pigmentary changes and abnormal cone but preserved rod function on ERG. On the other hand, patients with congenital stationary night blindness have stationary impaired night vision, a normal fundus appearance, abnormal rod response, and

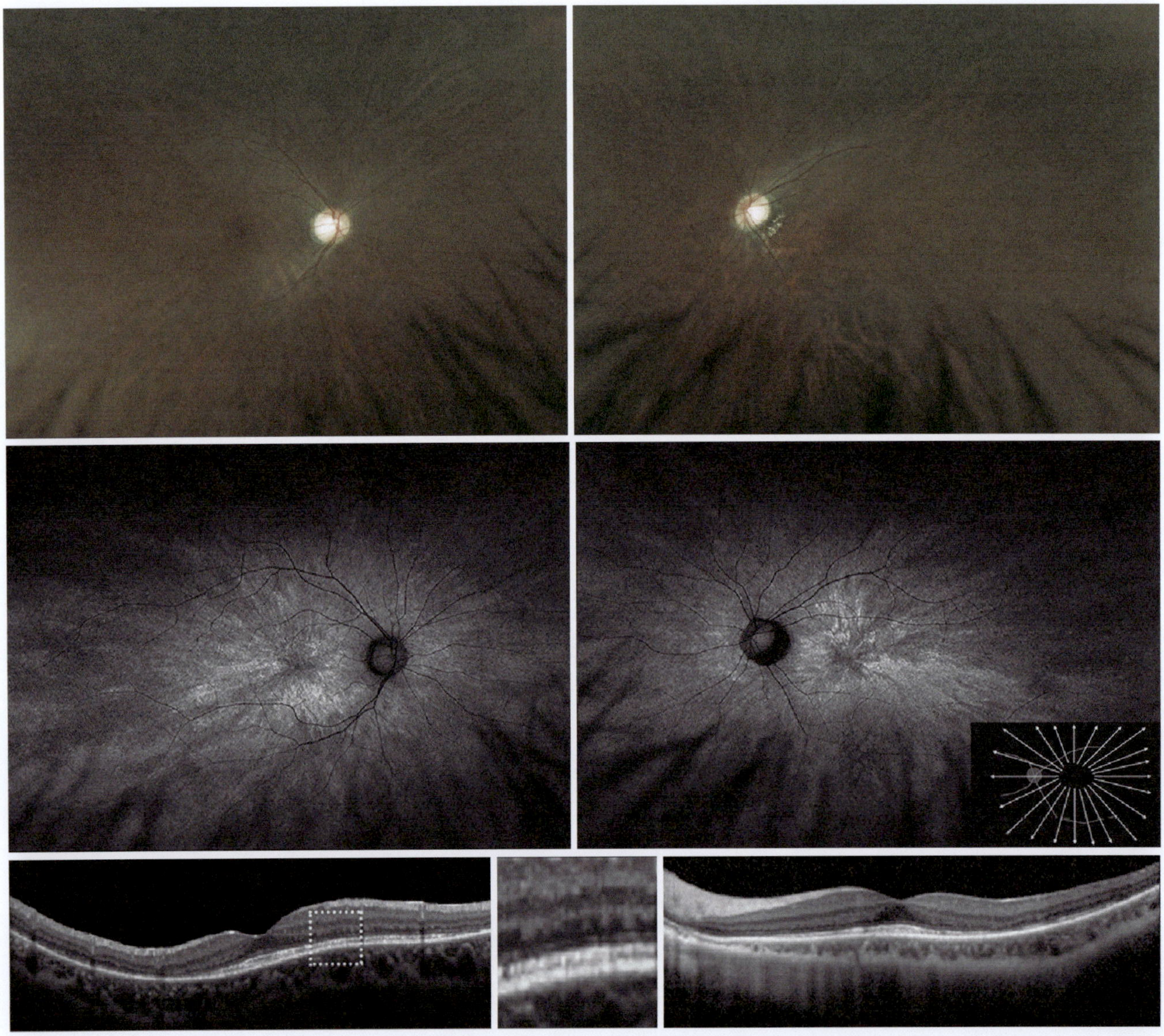

Fig. 1.30 This carrier with X-linked retinitis pigmentosa has tessellated fundus changes of the retina in both eyes. Wide-field fundus autofluorescence exhibit radial hyper-autofluorescence (AF) orientated lines extending from the fovea to the periphery as a characteristic bright reflex against a dark background. The detection of the peripheral radial hyper-AF pattern shown on the ultra-wide field image provided superior visibility. The optical coherence tomography shows ellipsoid zone loss in the macula corresponding to the areas of enhanced reflectance on the autofluorescence image

electronegative ERG. Albinism has generalized fundus depigmentation and foveal hypoplasia (den Hollander et al. 2008; Koenekoop 2004).

The fundus appearance of LCA patients is highly variable, ranging from normal to findings similar to that of typical RP, maculopathy, and macular colobomas (Figs. 1.31 and 1.32). Some genotypes of LCA are associated with certain phenotypes (Table 1.1) (Alkharashi and Fulton 2017; Chacon-Camacho and Zenteno 2015; Coussa et al. 2017). The *RPE65* (LCA2) and *LRAT* (LCA14) genes are both involved in the retinoid cycle, which is responsible for the isomerization of vitamin A and production of lipofuscin (Takahashi et al. 2011). Disruption of the cycle causes a diminished amount of lipofuscin, the source of AF. Therefore, patients with *RPE65* or *LRAT* mutations have a loss of AF (Scholl et al. 2004; Lorenz et al. 2004) (Fig. 1.33). The *CRB1* (LCA8) gene is responsible for the polarization of photoreceptors. The phenotypic particularity of the *CRB1* mutation in LCA patients is an unlaminated thickened retina (Tosi et al. 2009). The *GUCY2D* (LCA1), *AIPL1* (LCA4), and *RD3* (LCA12) genes are part of the photo-transduction cascade (Pasadhika et al. 2010). Mutation in the *AIPL1* (LCA4) and *RD3* (LCA12) genes presents with early maculopathy (Alkharashi and Fulton 2017; Dharmaraj et al.

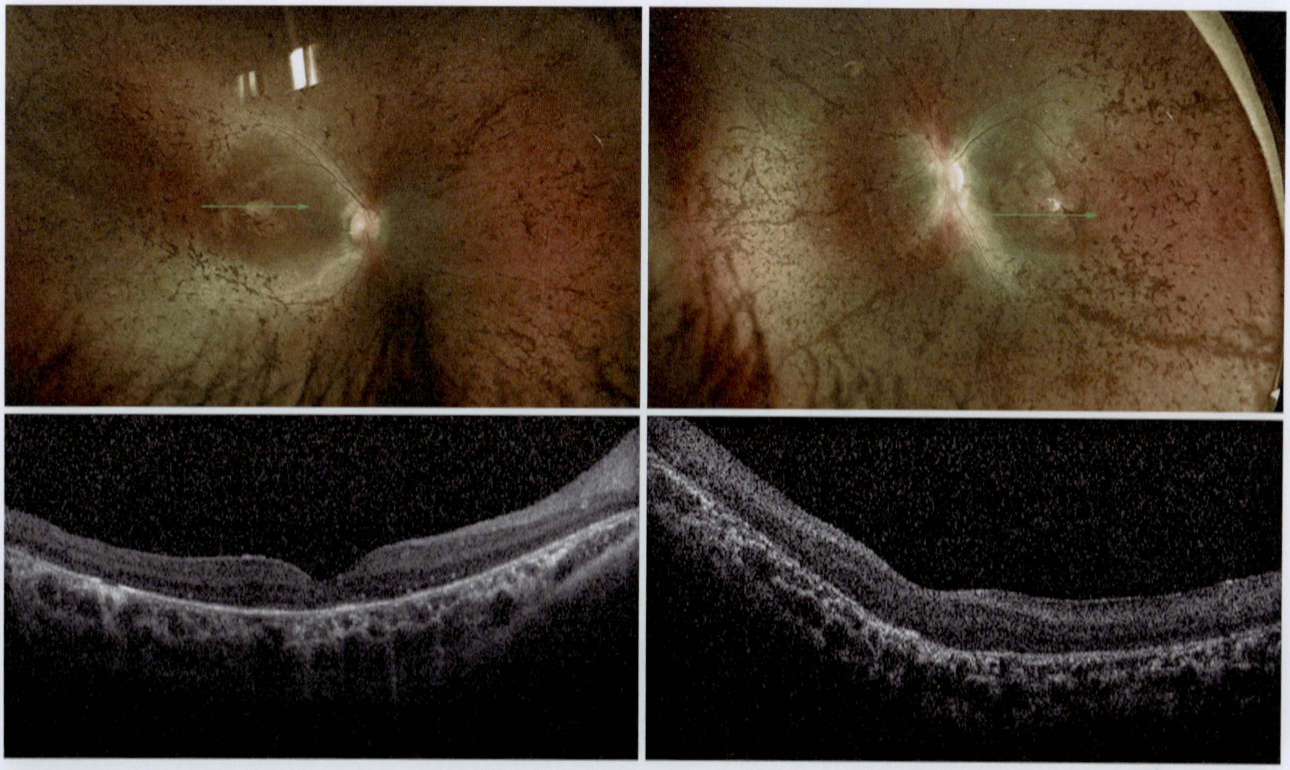

Fig. 1.31 These are the images of a 3-year-old patient with Leber's congenital amaurosis (LCA). The Fundus photo reveals bone-spicule pigmentation at mid-peripheral retina, vessel attenuation, and diffused retinal pigment epithelium (RPE) alteration, which are typical findings of retinitis pigmentosa. Noted the early macula involvement in the LCA and the RPE change are marked. The optical coherence tomography of the macular shows loss of the ellipsoid zone

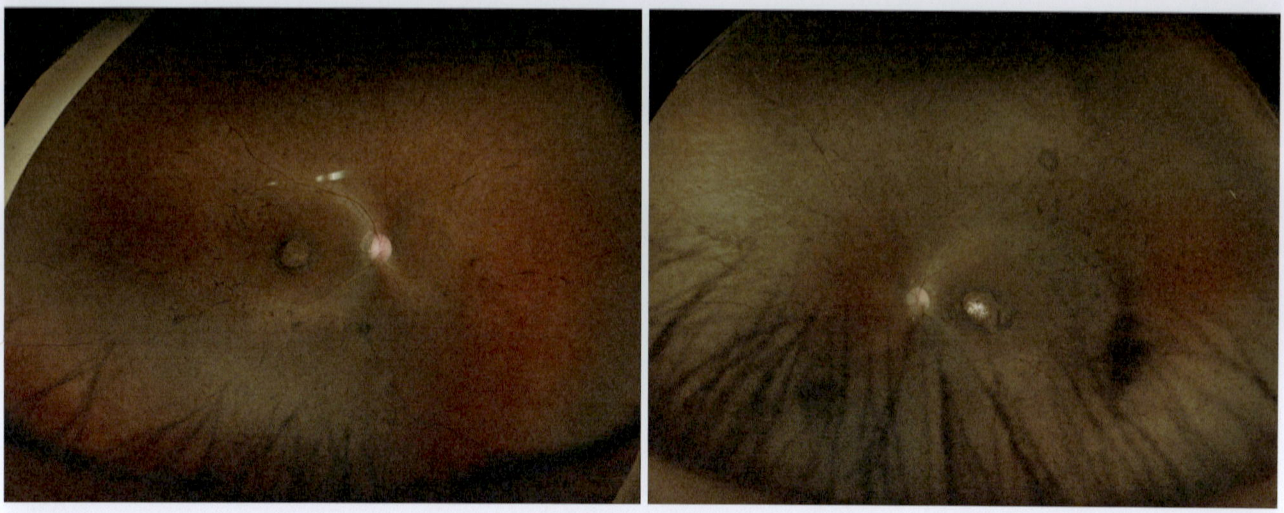

Fig. 1.32 Fundus photo of a 12-year-old boy with Leber's congenital amaurosis, which shows bilateral macula chorioretinal change, and some pigmentation at the mid-peripheral retina. This patient is the elder brother of the patient in Fig. 1.31

2004) (Fig. 1.34). Patients with *CEP290* (LCA10) may present with Coats-like RP (Yzer et al. 2012) (Fig. 1.35). 6q14.1 (LCA5), *CRX* (LCA7), and *NMNAT1* (LCA9) gene mutations are associated with macula-coloboma like fundus (Mohamed et al. 2003; Swaroop et al. 1999; Koenekoop et al. 2012).

Treatment

With notable genetic heterogeneity, LCA was considered incurable previously. Until 2008, with the advances in genome studies, three independent clinical trials have described the phase I-II outcome of gene therapy for RPE65 mutation (LCA 2) (Bainbridge et al. 2008; Maguire et al.

Table 1.1 Reported clinical features of LCA subtypes

Subtype	Gene	Clinical features
LCA1	*GUCY2D*	Normal appearing fundus
LCA2	*RPE65*	Lack of autofluorescence
LCA3	*SPATA7*	Retinal atrophy
LCA4	*AIPL1*	Maculopathy, reduced macula thickness
LCA5	6q 14.1	Macula coloboma-like picture
LCA6	*RPGRIP1*	Normal then pigmentary change
LCA7	*CRX*	Macula coloboma-like picture
LCA8	*CRB1*	Coats-like exudative vasculopathy, thick retina
LCA9	*NMNAT1*	Macula coloboma-like picture
LCA10	*CEP290*	Fundus pigmentation
LCA11	*IMPDH1*	Diffuse RPE mottling
LCA12	*RD3*	Macula atrophy
LCA13	*RDH12*	Bone spicules
LCA14	*LRAT*	Lack of autofluorescence
LCA15	*TULP1*	Salt and pepper retinopathy

2008; Hauswirth et al. 2008). Mutation of RPE65 gene affects vitamin A metabolism, photoreceptor response, and thus vision. In addition, the mutation results in degeneration of RPE and photoreceptor cells. LCA caused by mutated RPE65 has a disproportionately preserved outer retinal structure, giving it a window of opportunity for gene-replacement therapy. The three clinical trials used subretinal delivery of recombinant adeno-associated virus vector during standardized 23 gauge vitrectomy (Wright 2015). The FDA approved 2 potential therapies for RP: a retinal prosthesis, approved only for patients with end-stage RP and RPE65 gene therapy, approved only for patients carrying the RPE65 mutation (Duncan et al. 2018).

All studies have demonstrated an initial improvement with subsequent decline in visual sensitivity after gene therapy, with a possible dose–response effect (Bainbridge

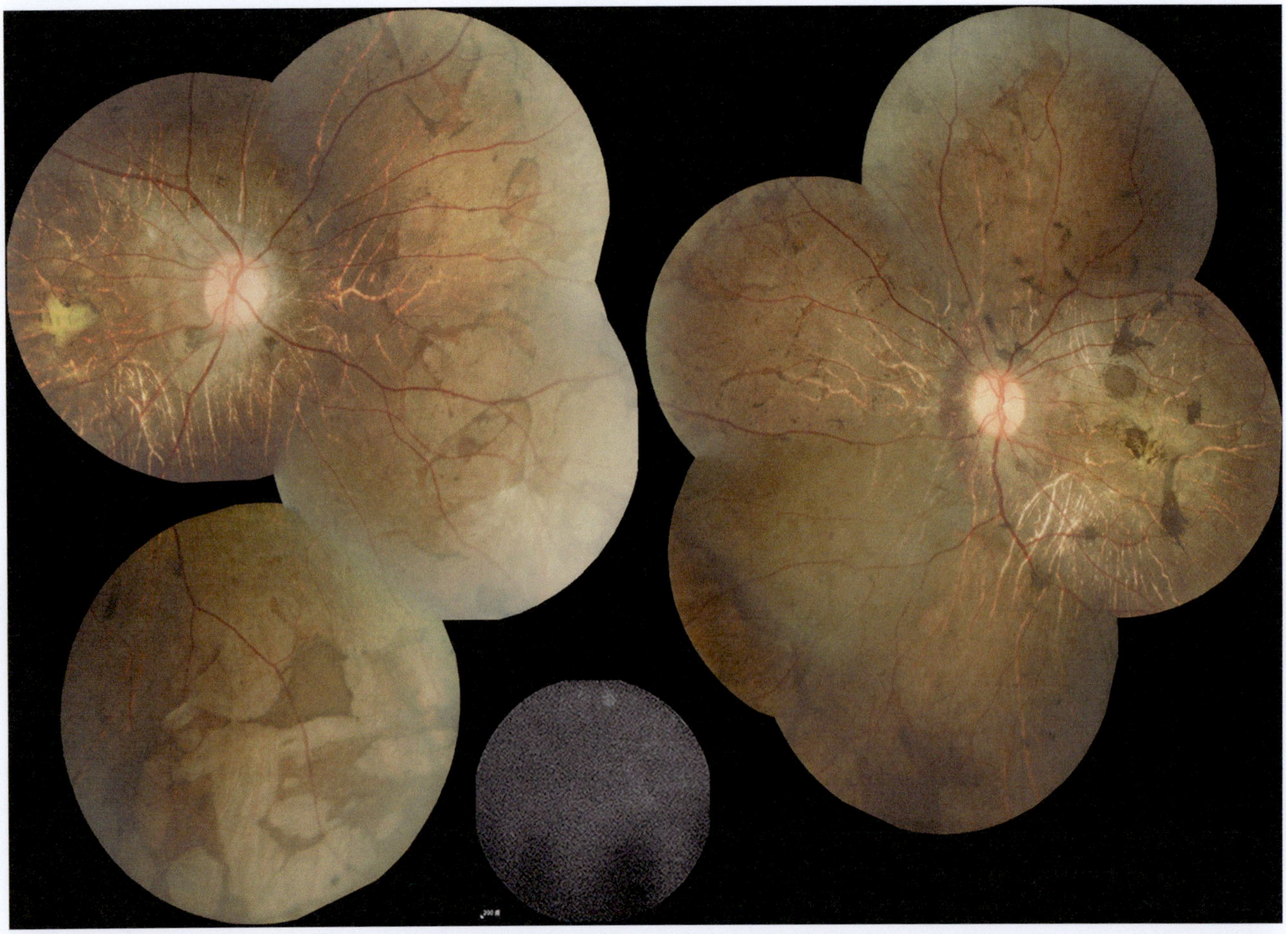

Fig. 1.33 A 9-year-old patient with Leber's congenital amaurosis. The fundus photo reveals diffuse retinal pigment epithelium (RPE) alteration, some bone-spicule pigmentation at the mid-peripheral retina, slight vessel attenuation, and chorioretinal change at the posterior pole. Note the loss of autofluorescence

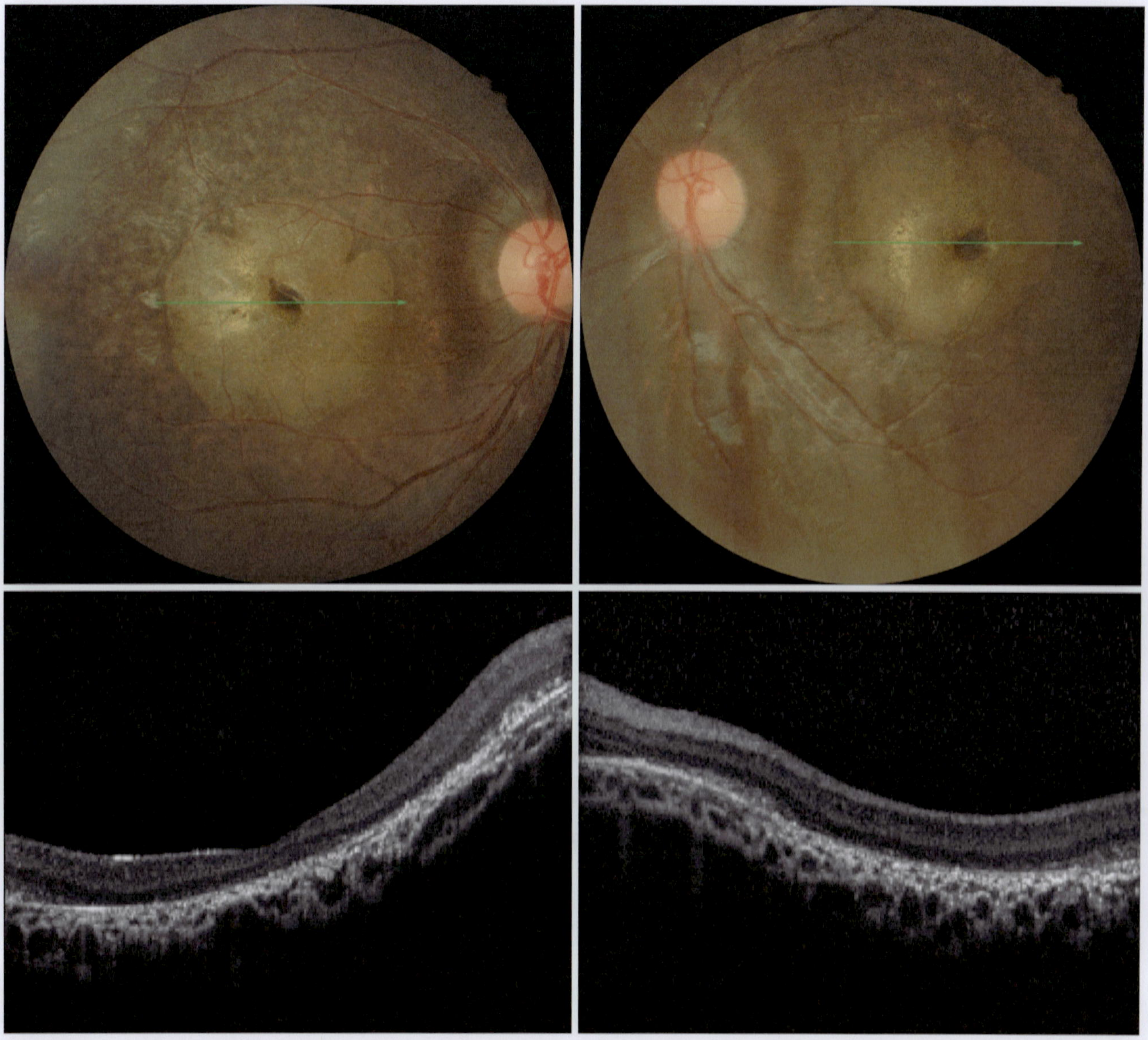

Fig. 1.34 A 2-year-old patient with Leber's congenital amaurosis (LCA) 4 (*AIPL1* gene mutation). The fundus photo demonstrates diffused retinal pigment epithelium (RPE) alteration, especially at the macula with prominent xanthophyll. The optical coherence tomography shows thinning of the macula in the right eye

et al. 2015). Despite functional response, continuous loss of photoreceptors was observed, indicating an ongoing retinal degeneration during the process. The results disclosed that RPE65 gene therapy provided temporary and incomplete restoration of retinal function, prompting further study and the need for a vector delivery system with higher efficiency in the future (Bainbridge et al. 2015; Jacobson et al. 2015).

Sector Retinitis Pigmentosa and Retinitis Pigmentosa Inversa

Sector retinitis pigmentosa is a rare variant of RP, usually involving the inferior nasal quadrant and is often bilaterally symmetric (Omphroy 1984). The affected areas demonstrate the features of typical RP, including retinal vessel attenuation and retinal pigment epithelial cell changes with hyperpigmentation (Figs. 1.36 and 1.37). The central vision is generally maintained, with peripheral VF defects corresponding with the affected areas. The condition is stationary or only slowly progressive. Mutations in the *rhodopsin (RHO)* gene have been associated with sector RP and transmit usually in an AD trait (Krill et al. 1970; Heckenlively et al. 1991).

Retinitis pigmentosa inversa (or inverse RP) is another rare RP variant (Ferrucci et al. 1998; Sheth et al. 2011). Pigmentation and chorioretinal atrophy link this condition to RP, but retinal changes occur in the macula initially and compromise the central vision in the very early phase

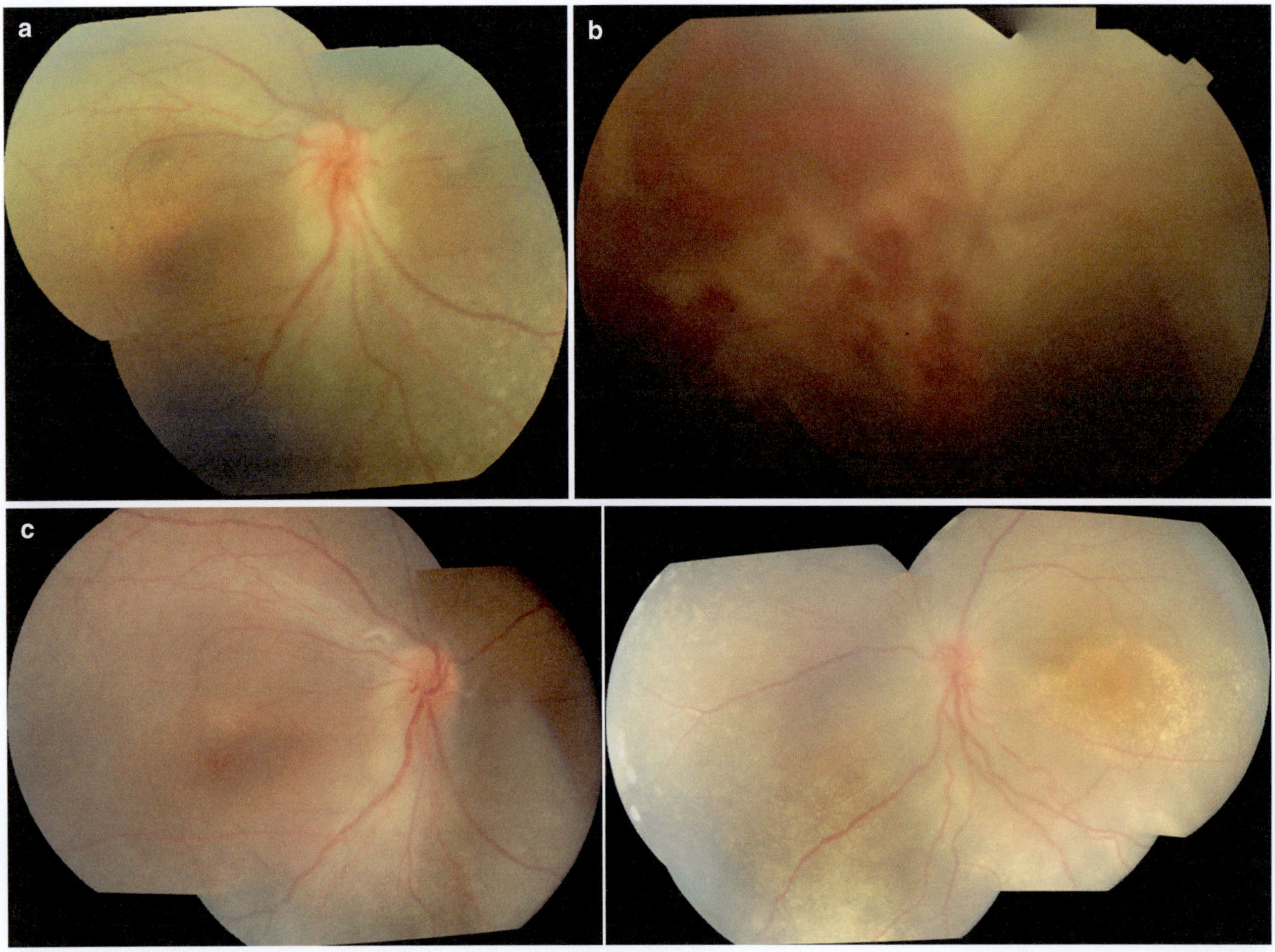

Fig. 1.35 A 9-year-old patient with Leber's congenital amaurosis (LCA) 10 (*CEP290* mutation). (**a**) The fundus photo reveals diffuse white dots in the right eye. (**b**) Coats-like exudation at the inferotemporal and superonasal quadrants with fresh hemorrhage was found in the left eye. The patient underwent cryotherapy and retinal laser photocoagulation. (**c**) Three years later, the fundus photo shows diffuse white dots and marked retinal pigment epithelium (RPE) alteration at the macula

Fig. 1.36 A case with sector retinitis pigmentosa. (**a**) The fundus appearances in the two eyes are highly symmetric. (**b**) Instead of forming a perifoveal hyper-autofluorescent ring, the hyper-autofluorescent area is along the posterior border of the affected retina, designating the area with retinal pigment epithelial cell changes. (**c**) The visual fields corresponded well with the area with hyperpigmentation and chorioretinal atrophy. (**d**) The full-field electroretinogram shows decreased rod and cone response amplitude. The lower row is from a normal subject, for comparison. Despite the ERG changes, the visual acuity was still relatively preserved at 20/30 in both eyes due to macula preservation

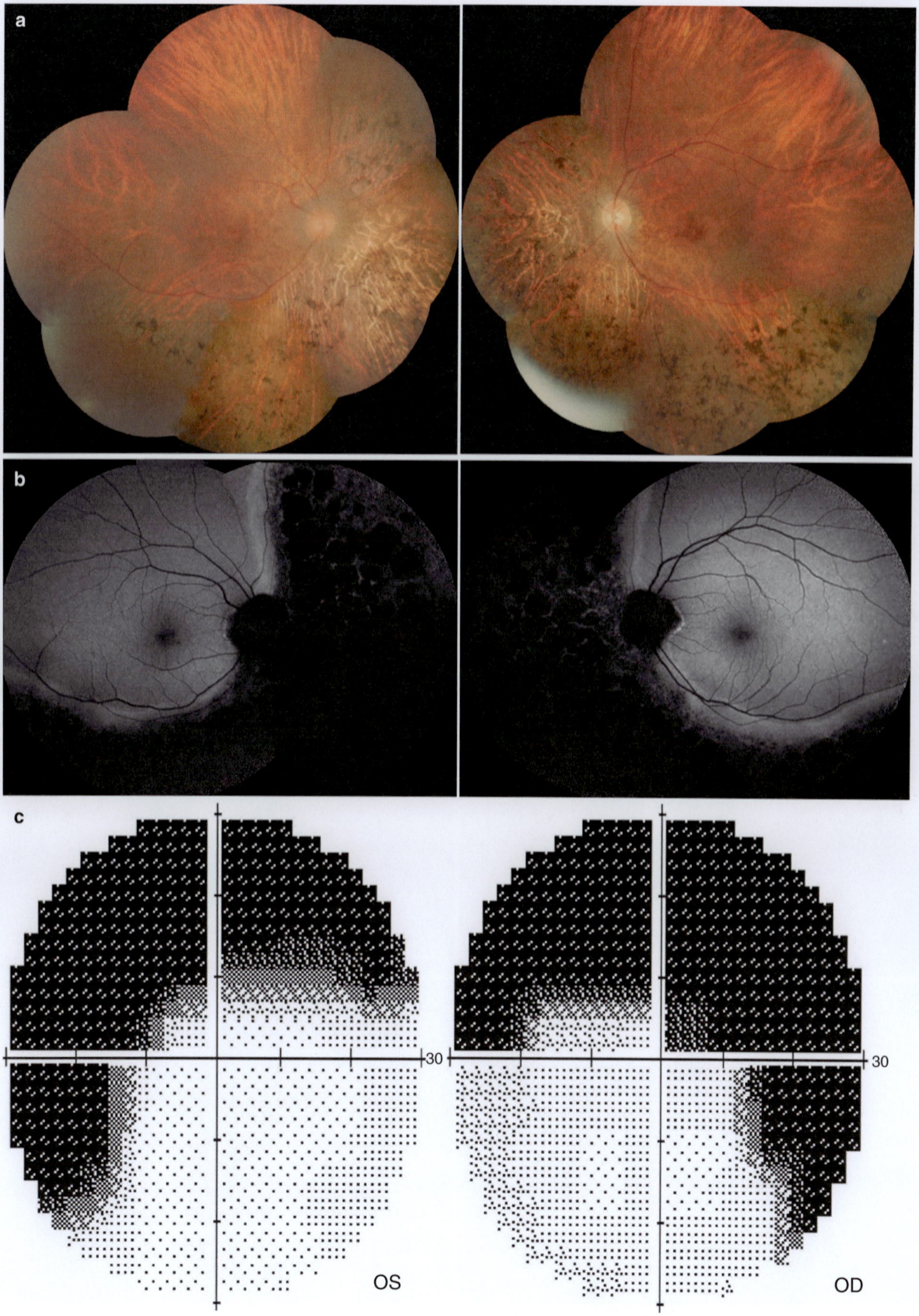
a
b
c
30
30
OS
OD

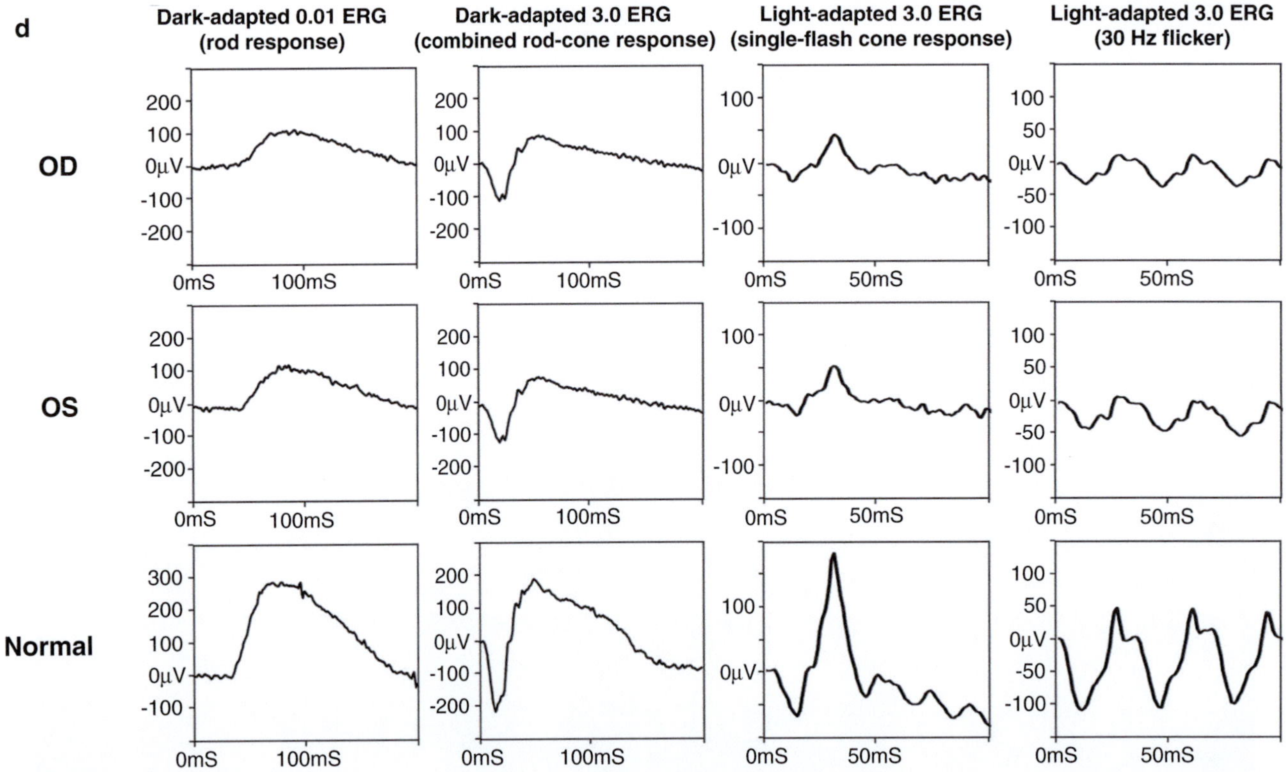

Fig. 1.36 (continued)

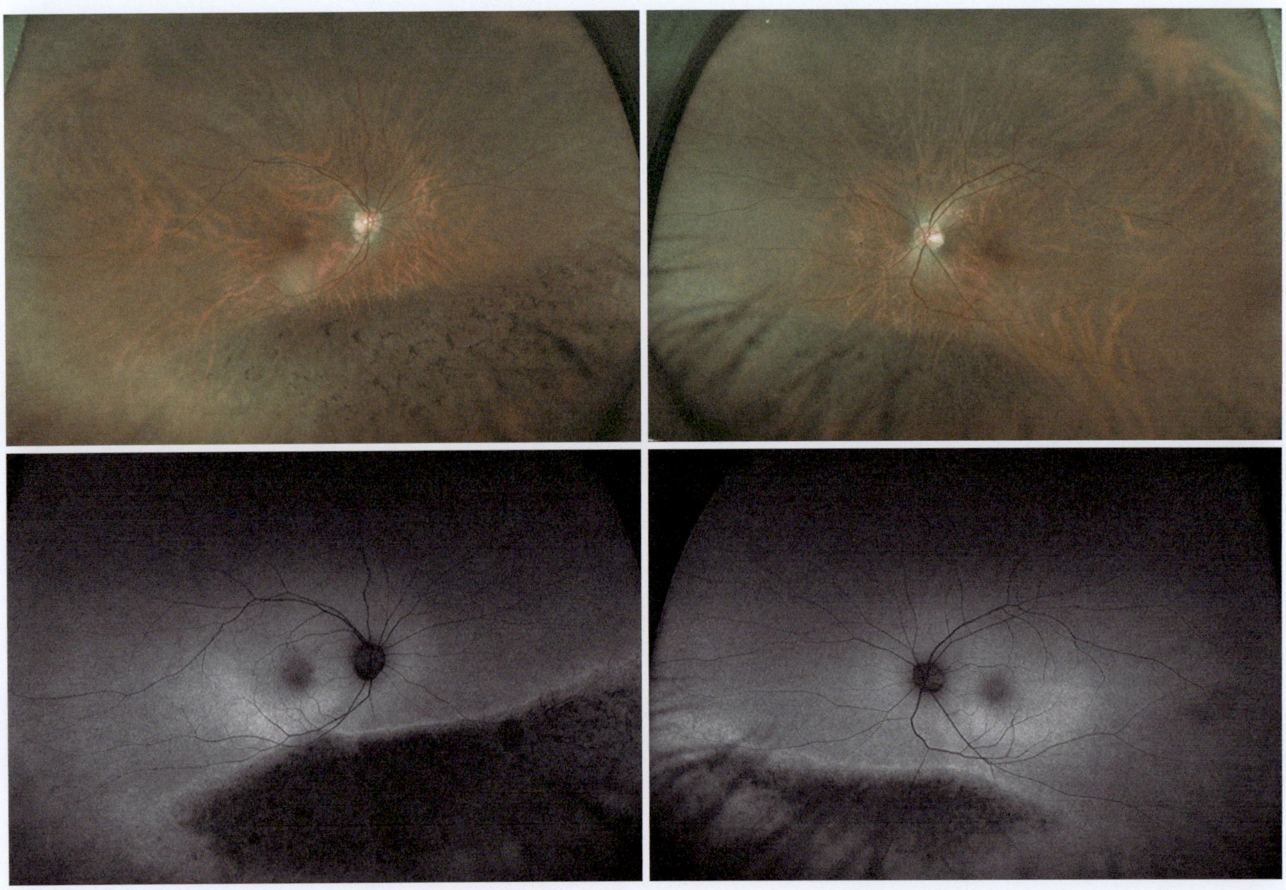

Fig. 1.37 Sector retinitis pigmentosa. The ultra-wide field retinal imaging displays symmetric fundus appearances. Apart from the typical retinitis pigmentosa changes in the inferonasal quadrant, the rest of the unaffected retina appears normal

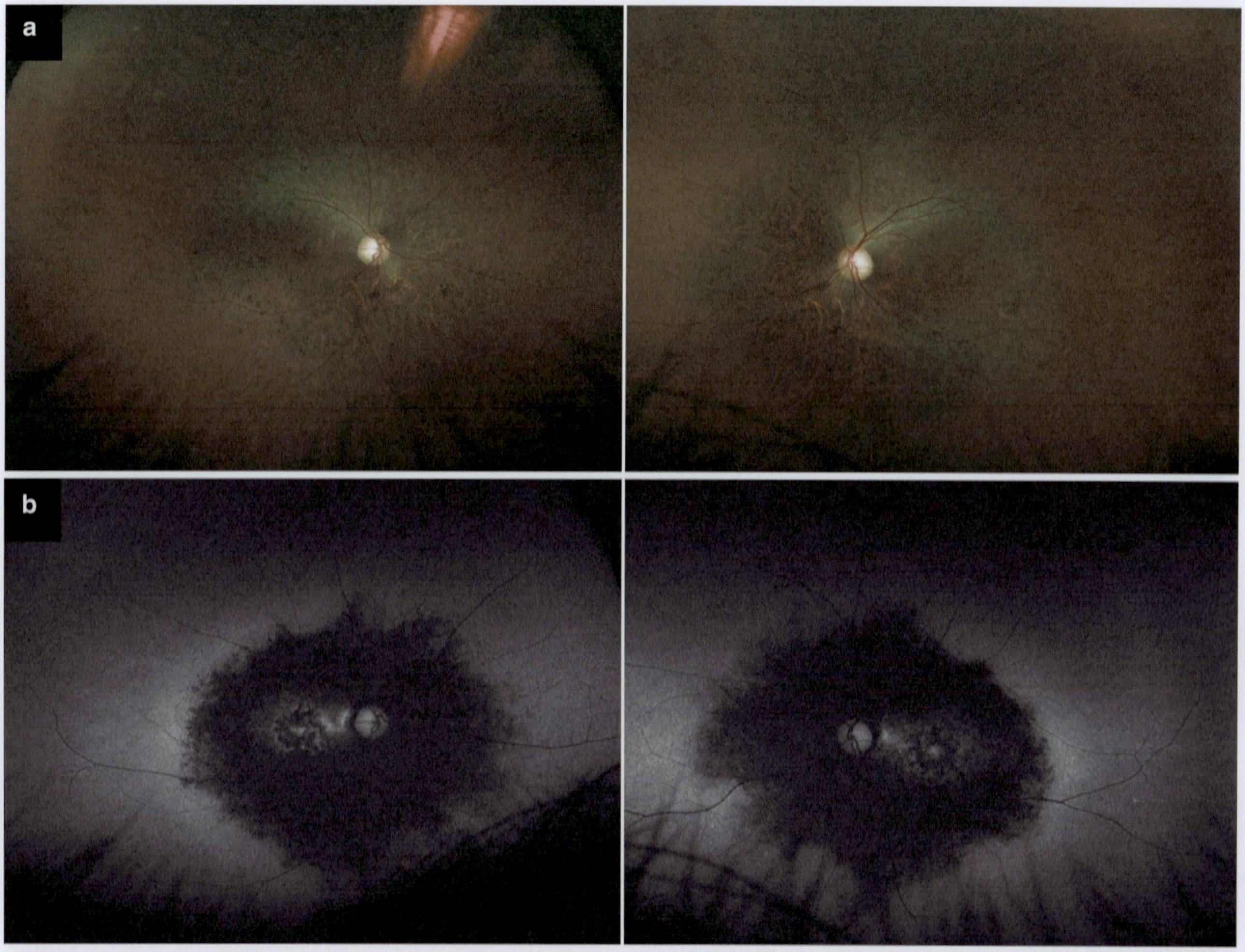

Fig. 1.38 Images of a 59-year-old patient with retinitis pigmentosa inversa. (**a**) Fundus photograph showing accumulated symmetrical pigments and retinal atrophy in the macula. (**b**) The fundus autofluorescence images clearly demonstrate the atrophic area in the posterior pole with some preserved retina in the fovea. The peripheral retina is also intact

(Fig. 1.38). Peripheral vision remains intact. Other differential diagnoses should be ruled out, including LCA, progressive CRD, central areolar choroidal sclerosis, as well as syphilitic retinopathy, retinal toxicity from phenothiazine use, and chloroquine retinopathy.

CRB1 Retinopathy and Related Features

Mutations in the crumbs homolog 1 (*CRB1*) gene have been reported in multiple inherited retinal degeneration (IRD) phenotypes, including LCA8 , early onset rod-cone dystrophy, CRD, autosomal recessive retinitis pigmentosa, retinitis pigmentosa with preserved para-arteriole retinal pigment epithelium (PPRPE), pigmented paravenous chorioretinal atrophy (PPCRA), and retinal telangiectasia with exudation (also referred to as Coats-like vasculopathy or Coats-like RP) (Slavotinek 2016). Other *CRB1*-associated ocular conditions include keratoconus and nanophthalmos. To date, more than 150 mutation variants have been reported on the *CRB1* gene (Slavotinek 2016), but genotype–phenotype correlations are yet difficult to establish.

The *CRB1* gene encodes the CRB1 protein. The CRB1 protein is located in the subapical region of the photoreceptors and abuts the adherens junctions, which form the ELM in the mammalian retina (Bulgakova and Knust 2009). Alterations in the CRB1 protein affect photoreceptor morphogenesis and homeostasis and influence the polarity of epithelial cells (Pocha and Knust 2013).

Unlike in other IRDs, the retina in patients with mutations in *CRB1* is usually thickened and coarsely laminated. The abnormal retinal structure resembles normal human fetal retina and suggests that *CRB1* mutations affect the maturing process of normal retina lamination (Jacobson 2003). This feature is most apparent in OCT studies (Fig. 1.39).

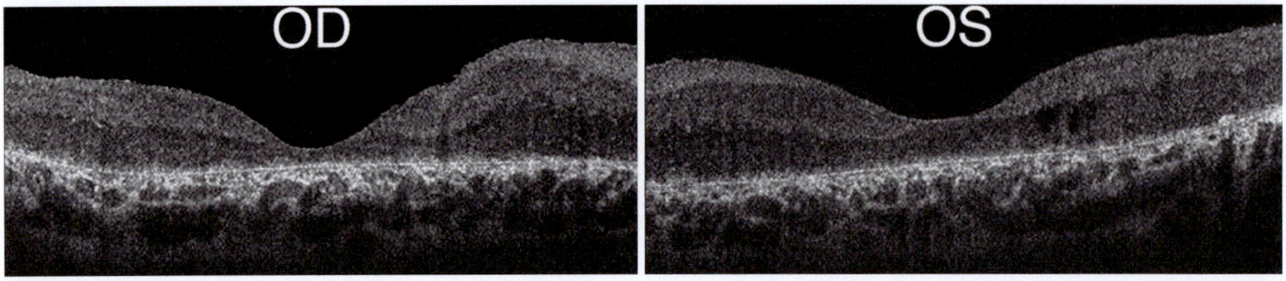

Fig. 1.39 A 17-year-old girl with early-onset retinal dystrophy and confirmed to have the *CRB1* mutation. Fourier domain optical coherence tomography reveals a coarsely laminated and thickened retina, which is a key feature of *CRB1* retinopathy. (Reproduced from Tosi et al. 2009)

Retinitis Pigmentosa with Preserved Para-Arteriole Retinal Pigment Epithelium (PPRPE)

The fundus appearance is unique in RP with PPRPE. Despite diffuse RPE degeneration, the RPE along the retinal arterioles is relatively preserved (Fig. 1.40). *CRB1* mutations have been reported in approximately 74.1% of RP cases with PPRPE (Bujakowska et al. 2012).

Coats-Like Retinitis Pigmentosa (Coats-Like Exudative Vasculopathy)

Coats' disease is a rare idiopathic exudative retinal disease that features by aneurysmal dilation and telangiectatic retinal veins, yellow extravascular lipid depositions, and retinal detachment. It has male predominance and is usually unilateral. The association between RP and exudative retinopathy was first presented by Zamoranin in 1956 and has been termed *Coats-like retinitis pigmentosa* due to the resemblance. It affects 1–4% of RP cases (Pruett 1983) and has been reported to be associated with *CRB1* gene mutations in approximately 53.3% of affected individuals (de Hollander et al. 2001; Bujakowska et al. 2012).

Coats-like RP has different demographic characteristics that relate classic Coats' disease with older age, slight female predominance, and family history. The clinical presentation combines both the features of RP and Coats' disease. Dilated, telangiectatic, or aneurysmal retinal veins are accompanied with lipid depositions and exudative retinal detachment (Fig. 1.41). In the areas not affected by Coats-like changes, typical changes found in RP are displayed (Khan et al. 1988).

Pigmented Paravenous Chorioretinal Atrophy (PPCRA)

RP with PPCRA is a rare phenotype of RP characterized by bilaterally symmetric paravenous distribution of RPE atrophy and pigment clumping. The subjects are often asymptomatic and are diagnosed incidentally during routine eye examination (Fig. 1.42). However, variable clinical presentations do exist, and symptoms of night blindness and ERG abnormalities have been reported (Fig. 1.43). Most documented cases were sporadic, but there was also an association with the *CRB1* gene (McKay et al. 2005). FAF is a useful and noninvasive examination to demonstrate the distribution of RPE alterations (Hashimoto et al. 2012) (Figs. 1.42 and 1.44).

Enhanced S-Cone Syndrome (Goldmann–Favre Syndrome)

Introduction

Enhanced S-cone syndrome (ESCS), also known as Goldmann–Favre syndrome, is a slowly progressive autosomal recessive retinal dystrophy caused by an *NR2E3* (photoreceptor-specific nuclear receptor, PNR) gene mutation. *NR2E3*, located on chromosome 15q23, encodes a ligand-dependent transcription repressor of cone-specific genes in rod photoreceptors and determines the differentiation of retinal progenitor cells. Mutations of *NR2E3* disturb normal photoreceptor differentiation, possibly by encouraging a default from the rod photoreceptor pathway to the S-cone pathway, leading to decreased rod numbers and increased proportion of S-cones (Chen et al. 2005; Bernal et al. 2008; Bumsted O'Brien et al. 2004).

Clinical Features

ESCS was first described by Marmor et al. (1990) as a disease characterized by night blindness, maculopathy, and increased S-cone sensitivity. The fundus appearance is highly variable, with the most classical phenotype being nummular pigment clumping at the level of RPE along the vascular arcades in adult ESCS patients (Yzer et al. 2013; Audo et al. 2008) (Figs. 1.45 and 1.46). Whereas in younger patients, multiple whitish spots, whitish subretinal deposit and maculopathy are found (Wang et al. 2009). Compared to typical RP, the distribution of pigment in ESCS confines to the mid-peripheral retina without peripheral involvement, and in a clumping pattern rather than dispersed. FAF images can present in a similar way to RP or as hyper-AF spots in younger patients. Wang et al. (2013) studied the origin of these hyper-AF spots and found that these hyper-AF spots are not from RPE but microglia cells that phagocytose

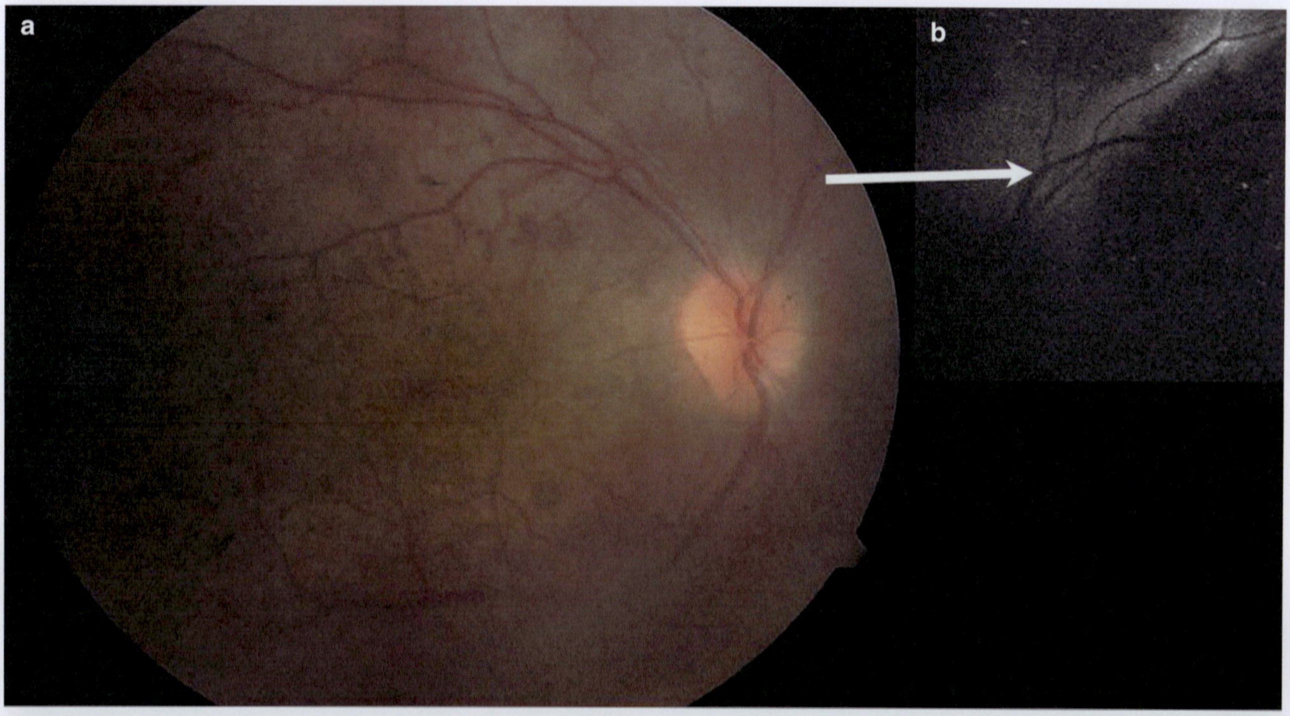

Fig. 1.40 Color fundus photograph and fundus autofluorescence (FAF) image of the same patient in Fig. 1.39. (**a**) There are retinal pigment epithelium (RPE) alterations, RPE atrophy, and hyperpigmentation on color fundus photograph. (**b**) The preserved RPE along the arterioles is easily identified on the FAF study. The diagnosis was *CRB1*-related retinitis pigmentosa with preserved para-arteriole of the retinal pigment epithelium. (Reproduced from Tosi et al. 2009)

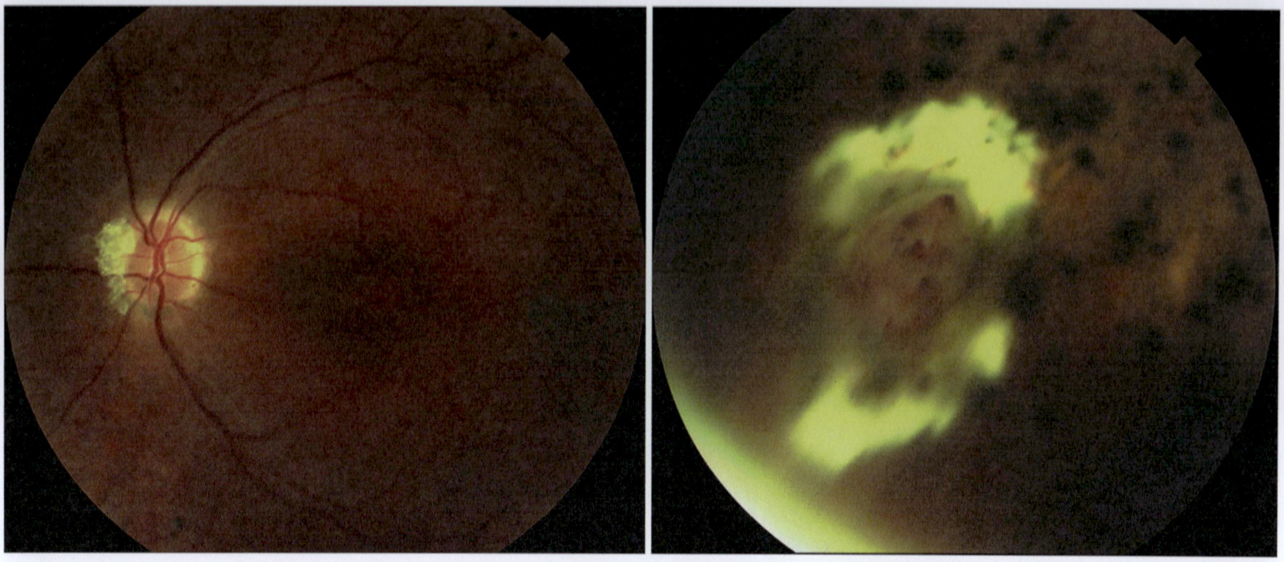

Fig. 1.41 A 23-year-old patient with Coats-like exudative vasculopathy. Fundus photographs showing multiple optic disc drusens, chorioretinal atrophy, lipid depositions, and vessel telangiectasia. (Reproduced from Talib et al. 2017)

photoreceptor outer segments. OCT of macula may show CME, macula scar, or ONL foldings that correspond to the hyper-AF. FA reveals hyper-AF spots corresponding to the white spots, but no fluorescence leakage despite the presence of CME (Wang et al. 2009) (Fig. 1.47). CME without obvious angiographic leakage can also be found in niacin-related maculopathy (Domanico et al. 2013), X-linked retinoschisis, and optic pit (Moisseiev et al. 2015).

ERG plays a key role in diagnosis. Classic ERG findings include (1) no rod response, (2) the waveforms of scotopic maximal response identical to the transient photopic responses except for size, (3) and the amplitude of a wave in

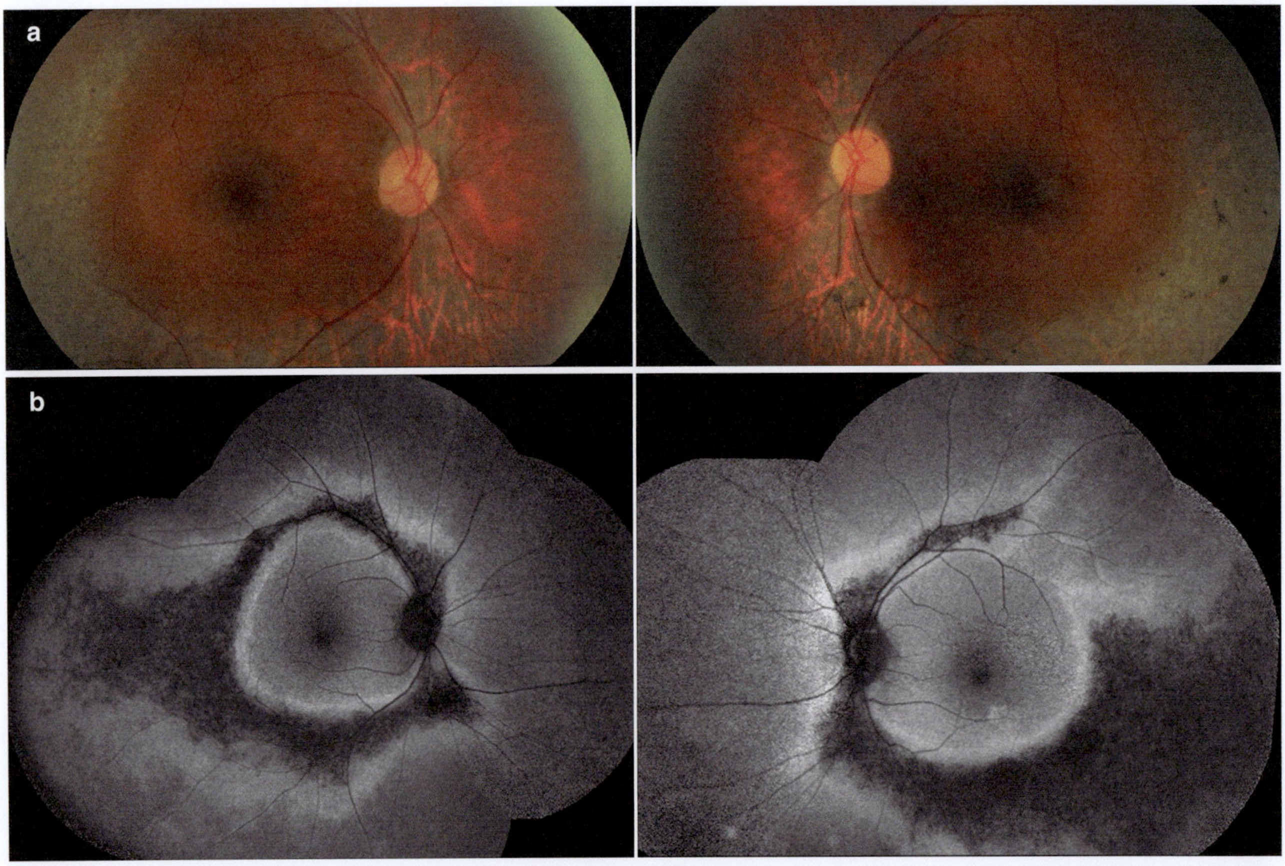

Fig. 1.42 A 59-year-old man with retinitis pigmentosa and pigmented paravenous chorioretinal atrophy. He has ankylosing spondylosis and a history of recurrent acute anterior uveitis in both eyes. He does not have night blindness, and his best-corrected visual acuity was 20/20. (**a**) The fundus appearances are bilaterally symmetric. There is mainly retinal pigment epithelium (RPE) atrophy along the retinal veins, and only some pigment clumping is visible. (**b**) FAF study shows paravenous hypo-autofluorescent areas. Adjacent hyper-autofluorescent borders indicate possible RPE alterations in the future

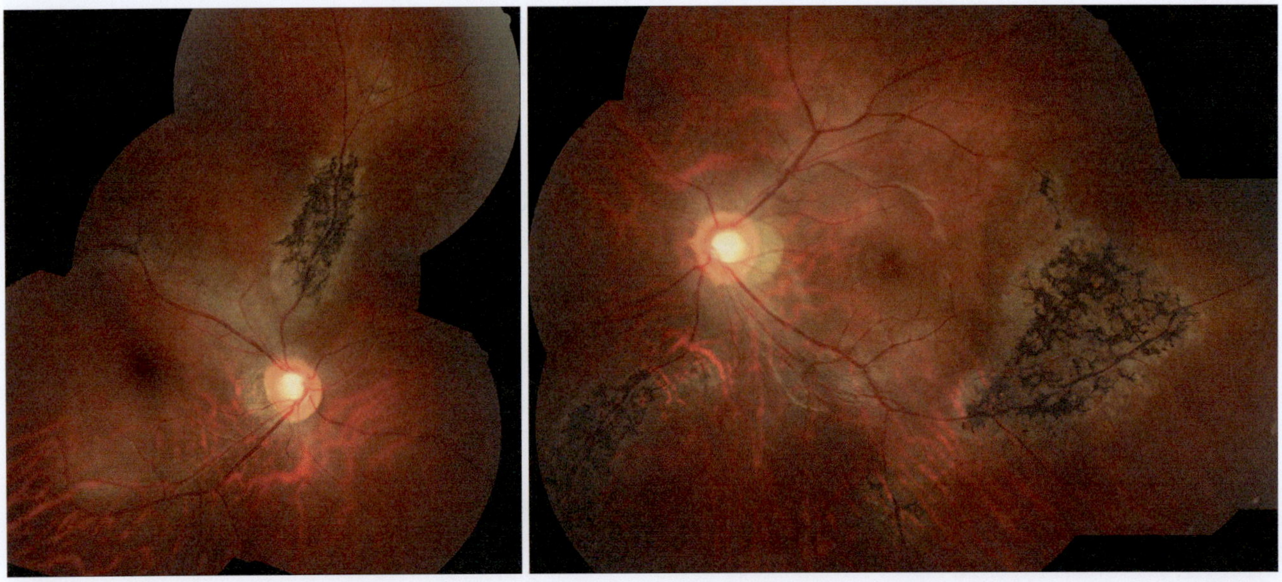

Fig. 1.43 A 26-year-old man with retinitis pigmentosa and pigmented paravenous chorioretinal atrophy. He presented with blurred vision in the right eye. The best-corrected vision was 8/20 in the right eye and 20/20 in the left eye. Both eyes display pigmentation and chorioretinal atrophy along some parts of the retinal veins, but they are not symmetrical. The scotomas on visual field examination corresponded well with the affected areas

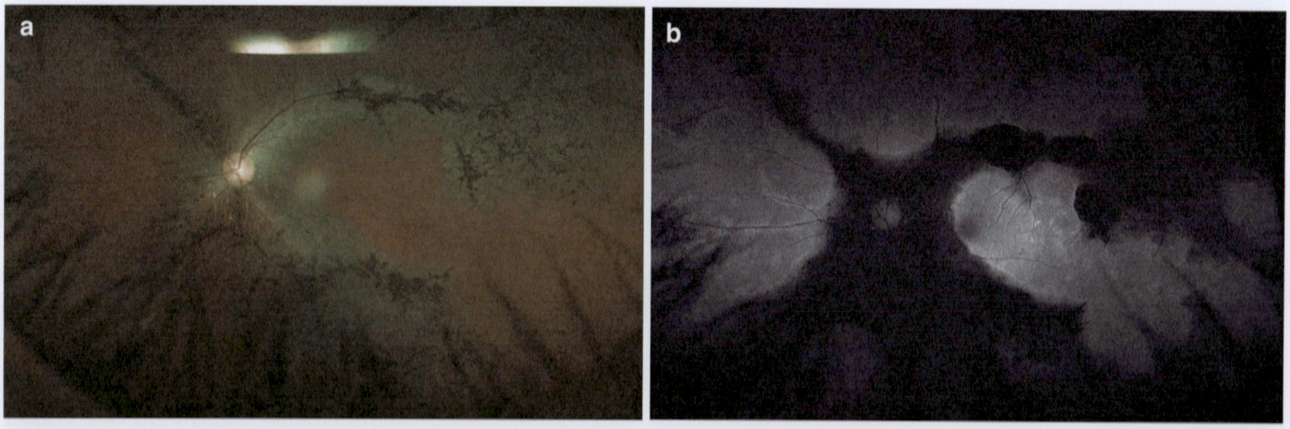

Fig. 1.44 A 52-year-old woman with retinitis pigmentosa and pigmented paravenous chorioretinal atrophy. (**a**) Ultra-wide field color fundus photograph showing pigmentation and retinal pigment epithelium atrophy distributed along the retinal veins. The macula was preserved and she had 8/20 vision in her left eye. (**b**) Ultra-wide field fundus autofluorescence clearly demonstrates the atrophic areas, compatible with the paravenous distribution on the color photograph

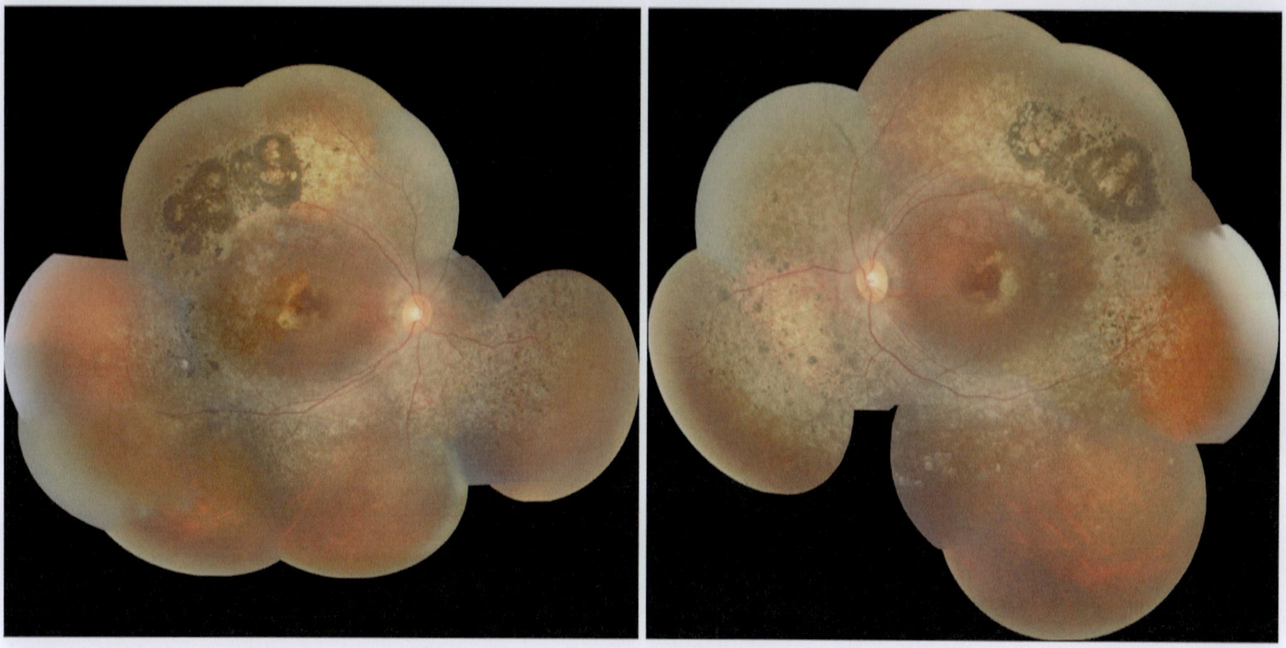

Fig. 1.45 Photograph of the fundus of a 26-year-old patient with enhanced S-cone syndrome (ESCS) revealing multiple white dots with focal hyperpigmentation at mid-peripheral retina and some yellowish pigmentation in the macula

the transient photopic response larger than amplitude of photopic 30 Hz flicker (Wang et al. 2009) (Fig. 1.48).

Syndromic Retinitis Pigmentosa

Usher Syndrome

Usher syndrome (USH) is an autosomal recessive disorder affecting both retina and inner ear. The prevalence is 1–4 per 25,000 people and is the leading cause of deaf-blindness worldwide (Mathur and Yang 2015). Over 10 USH genes have been identified as causative genes. The USH proteins encoded by these genes can be found in several different organs and interact with one another. In the inner ear, USH proteins are related to the functioning and maintenance of inner ear hair cells, whereas the function of these proteins in the retina are still not well understood.

USH has been classified into three subtypes. Each subtype has a variable degree of visual impairment, hearing impairment, or vestibular dysfunction. It is among the most common forms of syndromic RP, and the fundus appearances of USH patients are identical to typical RP (Figs. 1.15 and 1.49).

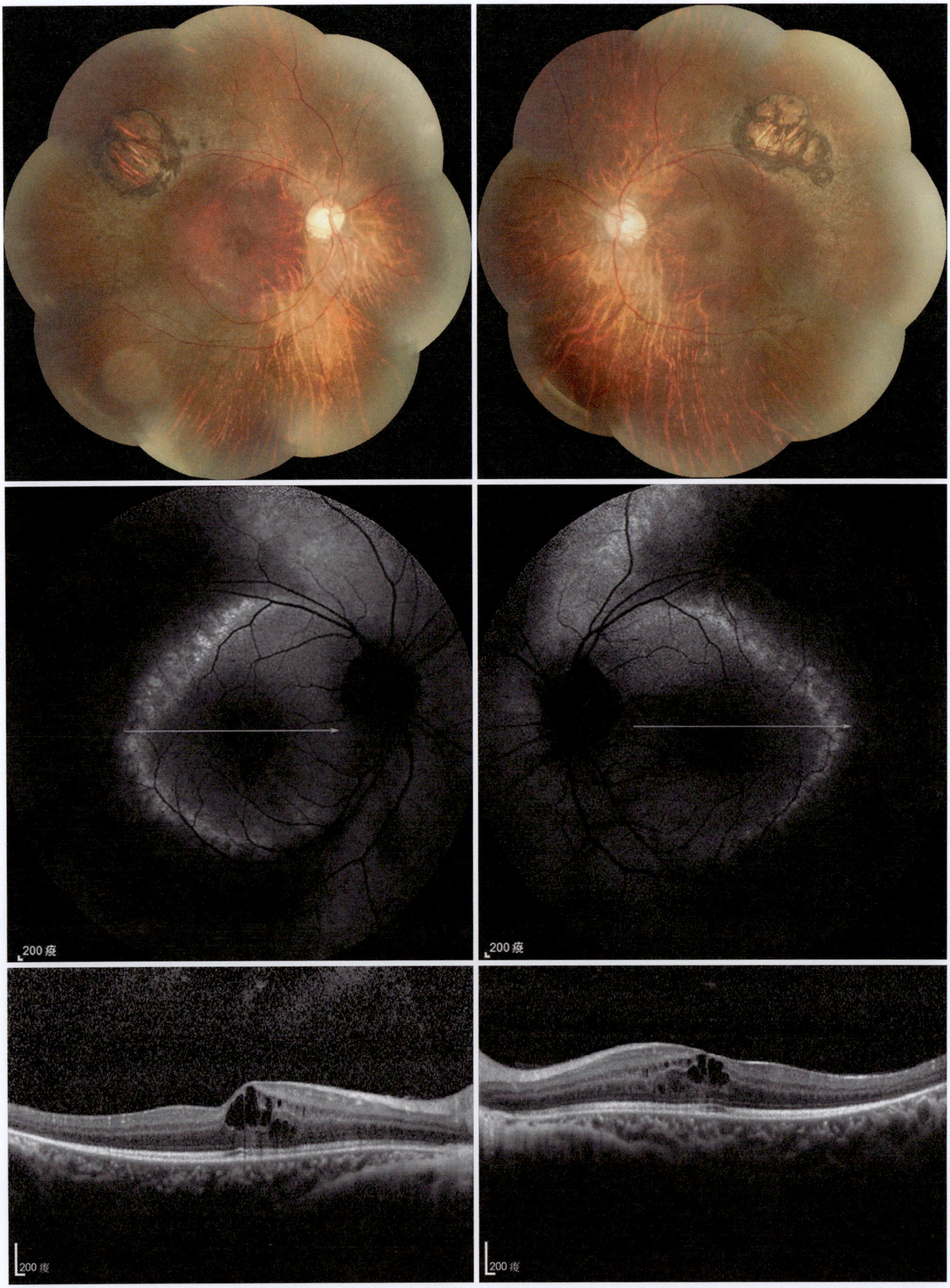

Fig. 1.46 A 22-year-old patient with enhanced S-cone syndrome (ESCS). The photo of the fundus revealed multiple white dots along the vascular arcade with focal hyperpigmentation. Optical coherence tomography revealed the presence of cystoid macula edema. FA found a ring of increased autofluorescence of the white dots

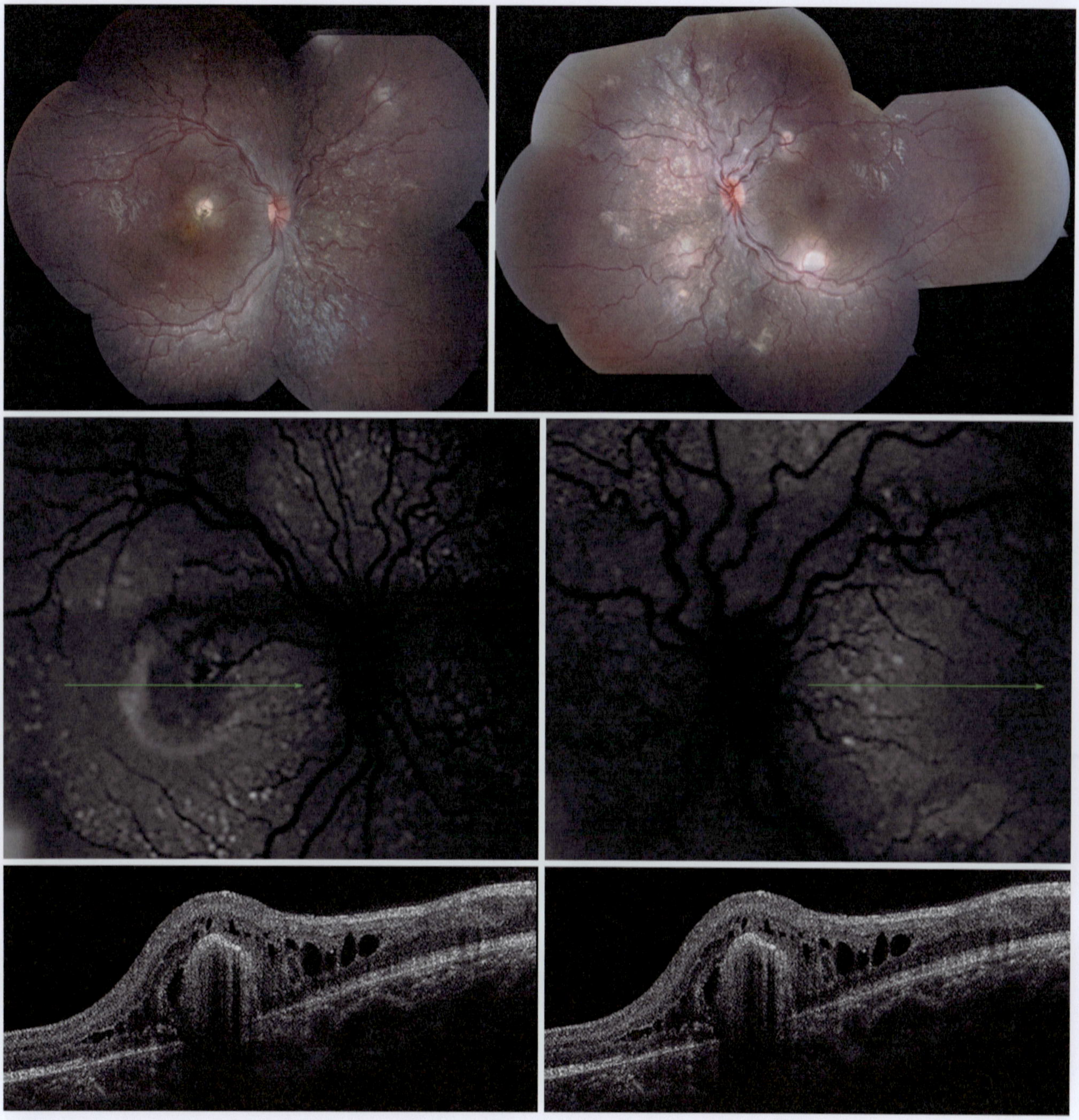

Fig. 1.47 Enhanced S-cone syndrome with cystoid macular edema. Fundus photographs showing multiple white dots at mid-periphery, subretinal whitish deposits at the macula in the right eye, and focal subretinal whitish deposits near the vascular arcade in the left eye. Fundus autofluorescent exam disclosed hyper-autofluorescent spots in the macular and mid-peripheral retina. The hyper-autofluorescence at the mid-periphery corresponds to the whitish spots on the fundus, whereas hyper-autofluorescence within the macula does not. Optical coherence tomography demonstrates intraretinal cystic change at the macula in the right eye. Note the rosette-like intraretinal lesions corresponding to the hyper-autofluorescent spots and loss of retinal lamination

Bardet–Biedl Syndrome

Bardet–Biedl syndrome (BBS) is a rare autosomal recessive multiorgan disorder related to ciliopathy. The cardinal features include retinal degeneration, polydactyly, early obesity, renal dysfunction, genital abnormalities, and learning difficulties (Forsythe and Beales 2013). Rod-cone dystrophy was reported in >90% of cases and is the most common feature (Beales et al. 1999) (Fig. 1.50). RP usually presents in the first decade, and central vision is severely affected before 20 years of age (Klein and Ammann 1969).

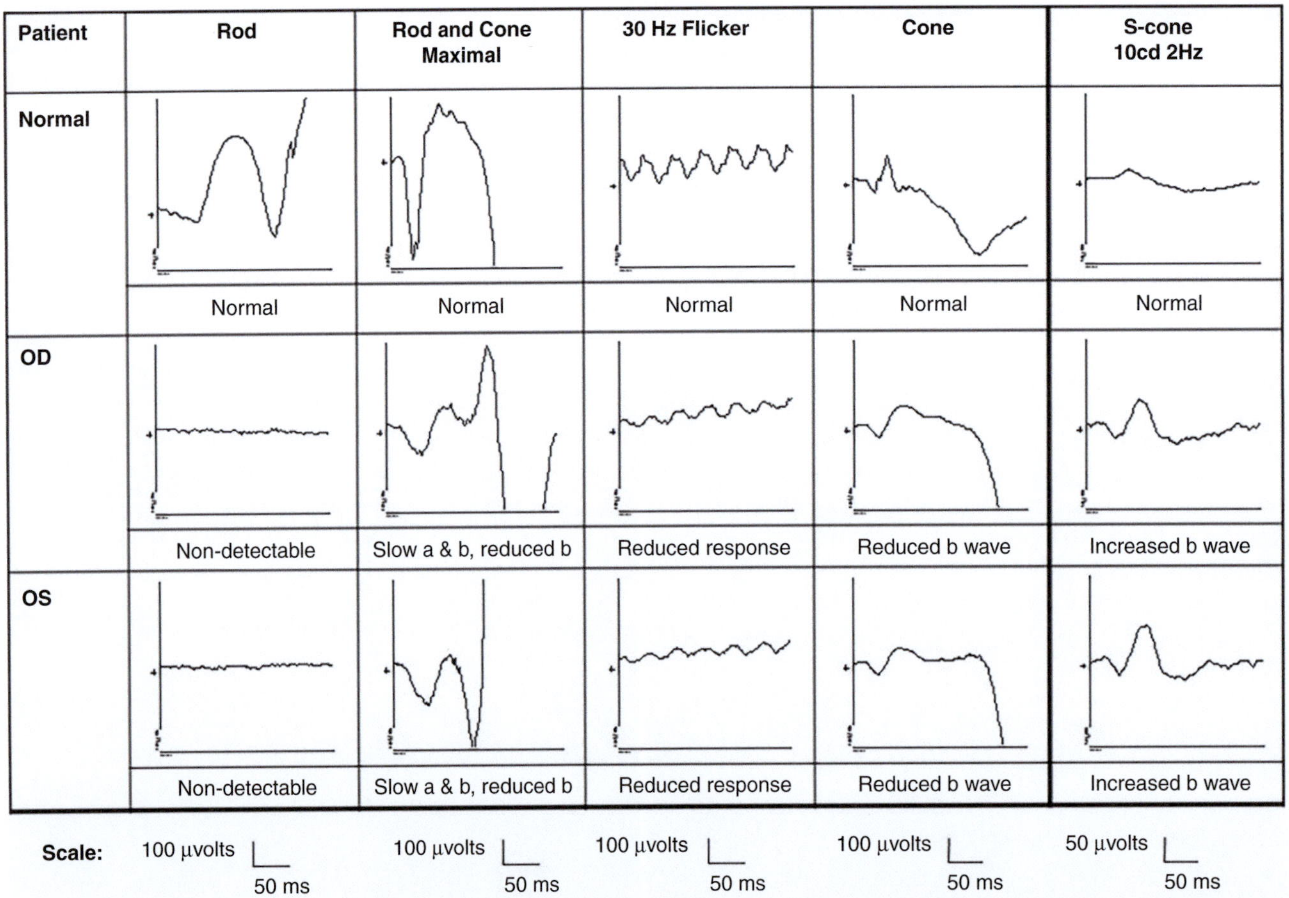

Fig. 1.48 Electroretinogram (ERG) showing classic findings of enhanced S-cone syndrome (ESCS). (1) No rod response, (2) the waveforms of scotopic maximal response identical to the transient photopic responses except for size, and (3) amplitude of a wave in the transient photopic response larger than the amplitude of the photopic 30 Hz flicker. Note the remarkably high amplitude of S-cone specific ERG

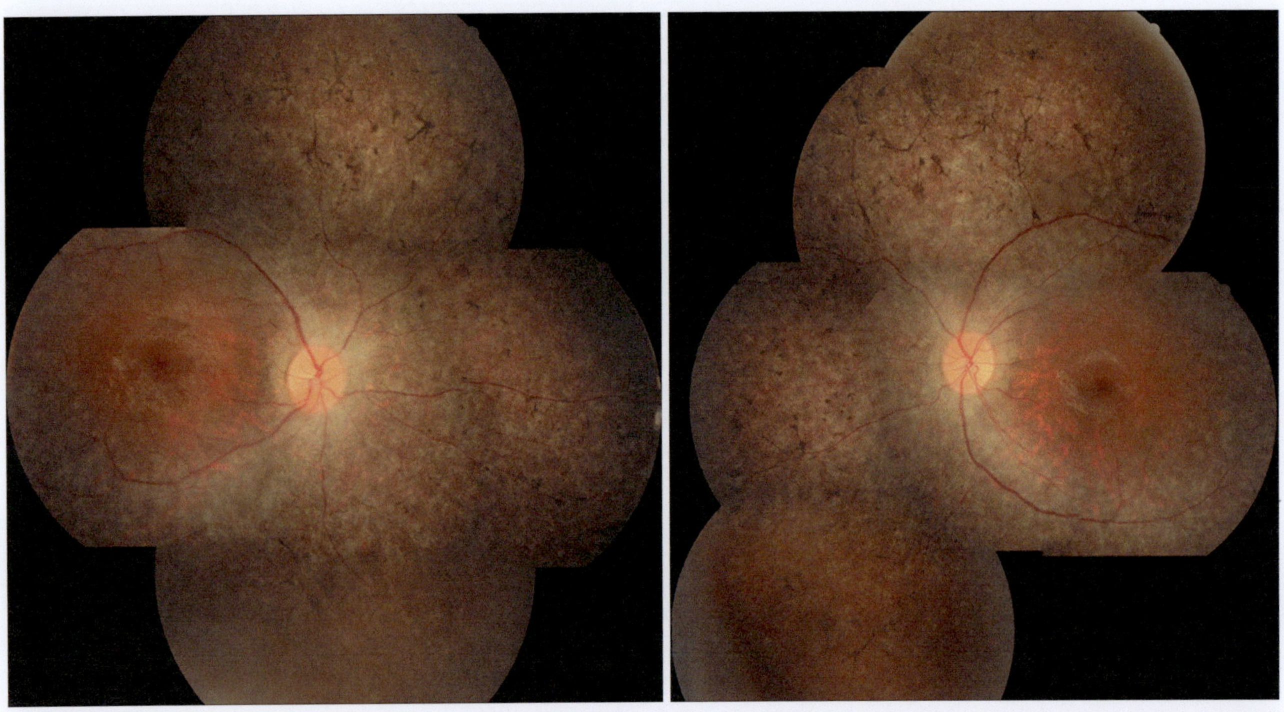

Fig. 1.49 A 23-year-old woman with night blindness since her early teens and hearing impairment since childhood. A fundus exam showed a typical retinitis pigmentosa appearance with preservation of the macula. Her parents and one brother have no ophthalmic or hearing-related problems. The clinical diagnosis was Usher Syndrome type II

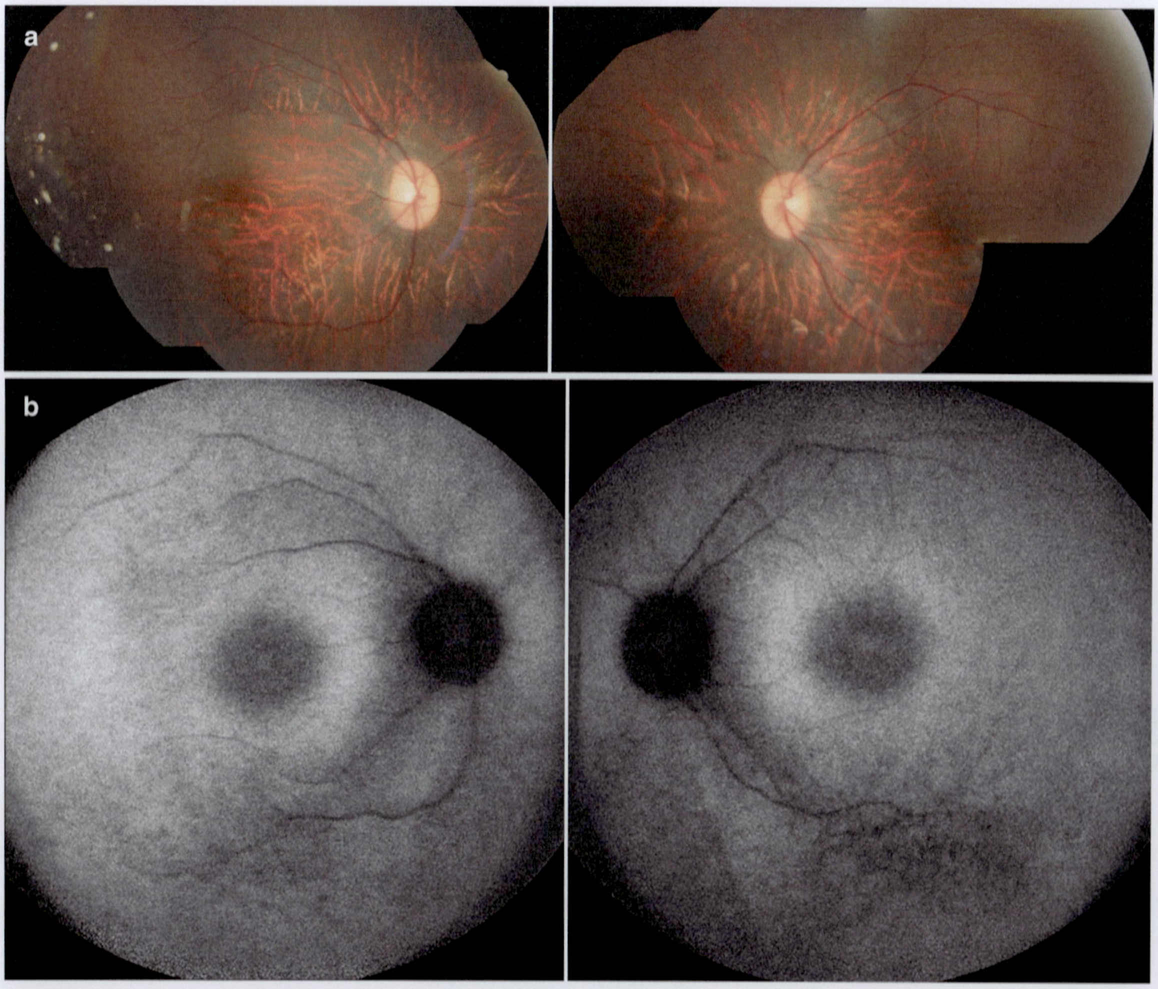

Fig. 1.50 A 17-year-old girl with Bardet–Biedl syndrome. She has diabetes mellitus, impaired renal function, vaginal atresia, and polydactyly in both feet. (**a**) Fundus photographs showing vessel attenuation, retinal hypopigmentation, and chorioretinal atrophy. The macula was preserved. (**b**) Fundus autofluorescence images display features of retinitis pigmentosa including mid-peripheral hypo-autofluorescence and perifoveal hyper-autofluorescent ring. The ERG study revealed severe rod and cone degeneration

Senior–Loken Syndrome

Senior–Loken syndrome is a rare autosomal recessive disorder affecting the eyes and the kidneys. The disease belongs to the spectrum of ciliopathy and causes RP- or LCA-like degenerative retinopathies and nephronophthisis, a cystic kidney disease which can lead to end-stage renal disease. The ocular findings consist of early onset night blindness or vision loss, nystagmus, and clinical features of RP (Ronquillo et al. 2012) (Fig. 1.51).

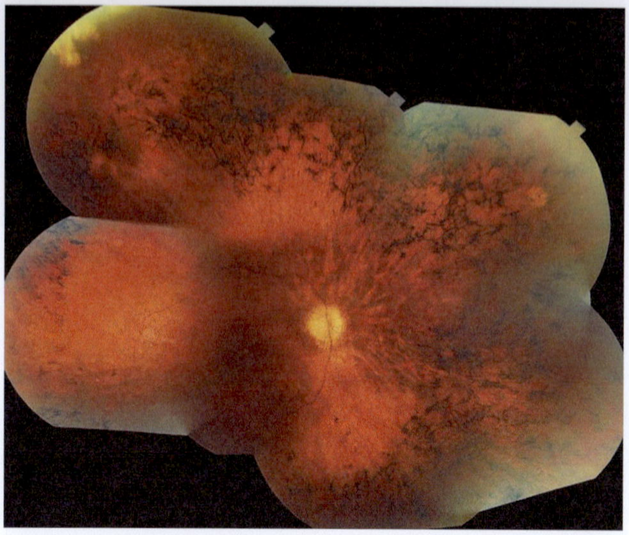

Fig. 1.51 The color fundus image of a patient with Senior–Loken syndrome demonstrates features of retinitis pigmentosa. (Reproduced from Ronquillo et al. 2012)

Kearns–Sayre Syndrome

Kearns–Sayre syndrome (KSS) is a group of rare mitochondrial diseases. Most patients initially present with ophthalmic abnormalities. The classic KSS triad includes progressive external ophthalmoplegia, pigmentary retinopathy, and onset age younger than 20 years. Additional

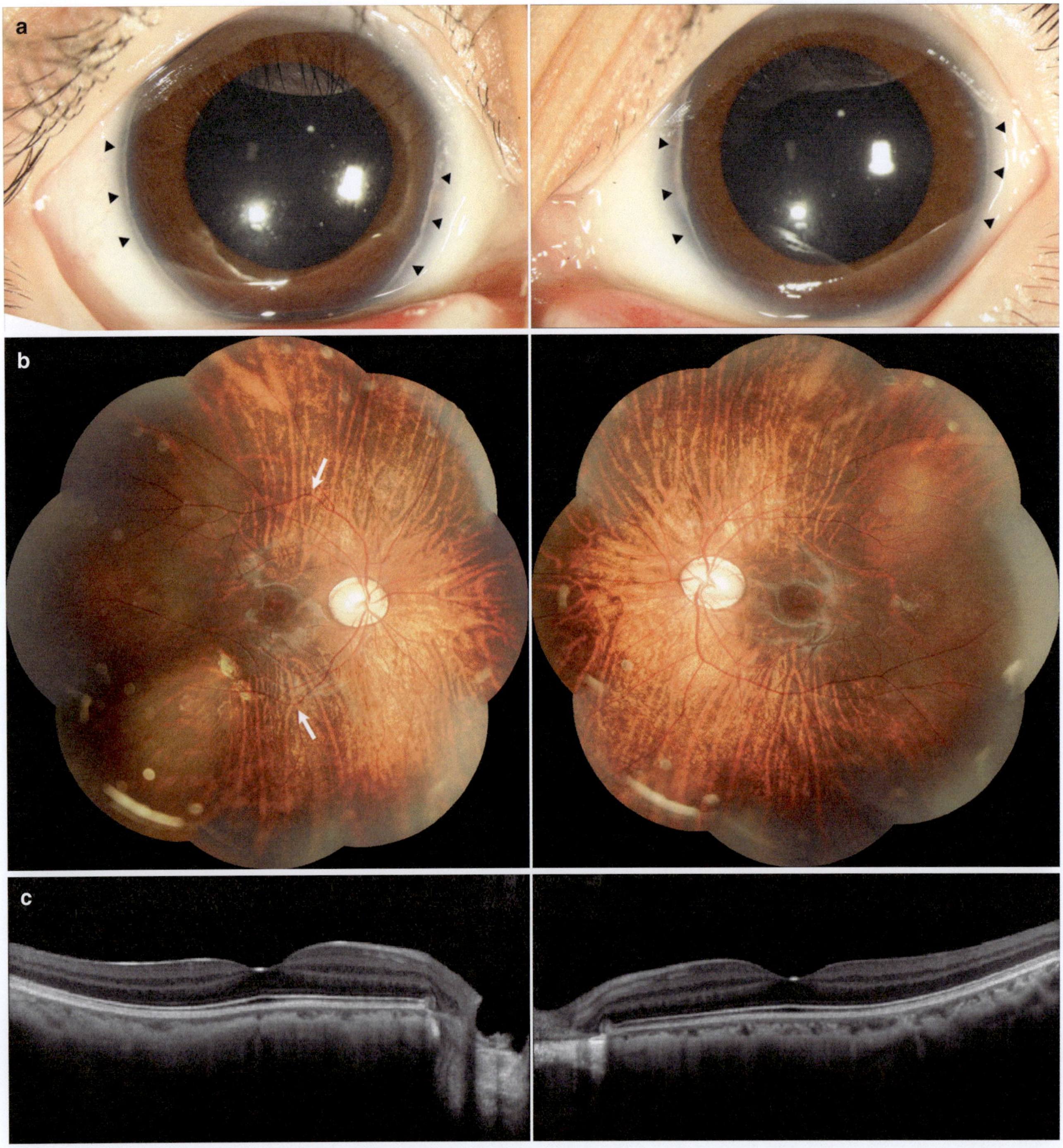

Fig. 1.52 A 9-year-old boy with Alagille syndrome and confirmed *human Jagged 1* (*JAG1*) gene mutation. His vision was 20/20 in both eyes. (**a**) Posterior embryotoxon (black arrowhead) is a key ophthalmic feature in Alagille syndrome. (**b**) Fundus photographs showing diffused hypopigmentation, retinal pigment epithelium alterations, oval-shaped optic nerve head anomaly with large cupping, and angulated retinal vessels (white arrow). (**c**) The optical coherence tomography images display decreased choroidal thickness for both eyes. (Reproduced from Shen et al. 2017)

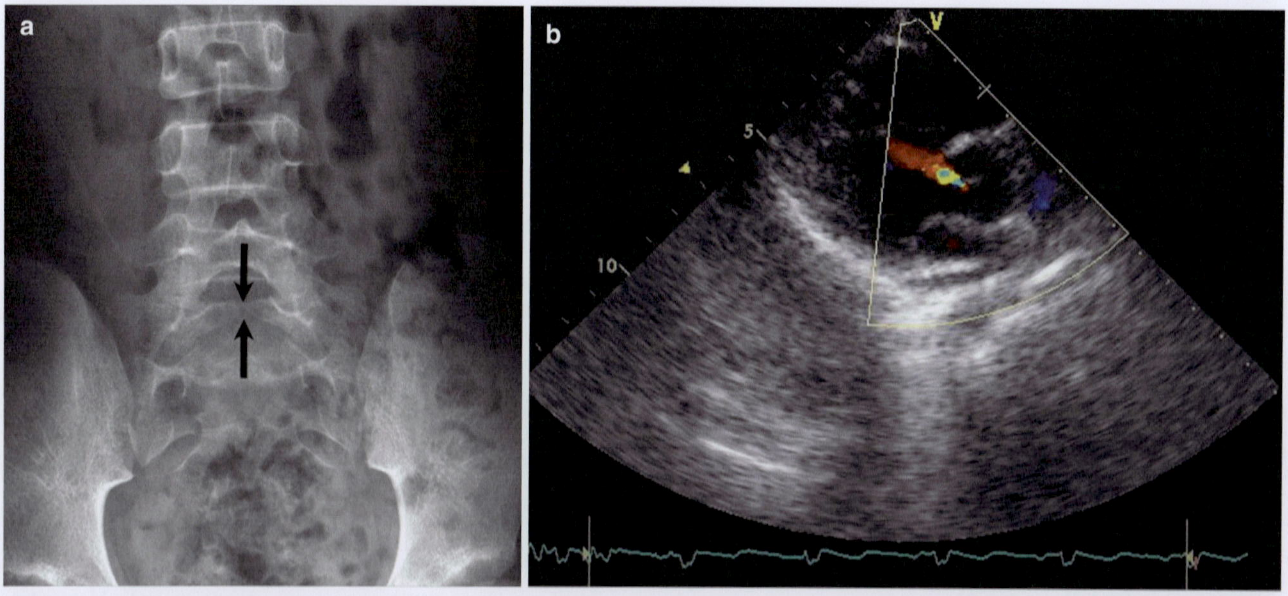

Fig. 1.53 The same Alagille syndrome patient in Fig. 1.52. (**a**) Lumbar X-ray showing inferior endplate depression and irregularity of the L5 body, and S1 spinal bifida (black arrows). No butterfly vertebrae were noted. (**b**) Cardiac echography showed mild aortic valve regurgitation, trivial tricuspid valve regurgitation, and equivocal mitral valve prolapse

diagnostic features include heart block, cerebellar ataxia, and increased cerebrospinal fluid protein level. The diagnosis is confirmed by muscle biopsy and genetic testing.

For ophthalmic disorders, 89% present with progressive external ophthalmoplegia, 86% with ptosis, and 71% with pigmentary retinopathy (Khambatta et al. 2014). The retinal pigments usually show a "salt and pepper" appearance instead of typical bone-spicules in RP.

Alagille Syndrome

Alagille syndrome (ALGS) is a rare multisystem disorder involving the eye. The primary manifestations are cholestasis, decreased bile duct numbers in a liver biopsy, congenital heart disease, butterfly vertebrae, characteristic facial features, and ocular abnormalities (Kim and Fulton 2007) (Figs. 1.52 and 1.53). The inheritance pattern is an autosomal dominant mutation that has been identified to be associated with the *human Jagged 1* (*JAG1*) gene.

Ophthalmologists can contribute to the early diagnosis of ALGS, especially in the circumstance of unexplained neonatal cholestasis. Over 90% of ALGS have been reported to have posterior embryotoxon (Hingorani et al. 1999) (Fig. 1.52). Other common ocular findings include microcornea, iris abnormalities, optic nerve head anomalies, retinal vessel changes, and retinopathies such as fundus hypopigmentation and RPE pigmentary changes (Fig. 1.52). Despite these ocular findings, ALGS patients usually have good visual acuity.

References

Aizawa S, Mitamura Y, Baba T, Hagiwara A, Ogata K, Yamamoto S. Correlation between visual function and photoreceptor inner/outer segment junction in patients with retinitis pigmentosa. Eye. 2009;23(2):304–8.

Alkharashi M, Fulton AB. Available evidence on Leber congenital amaurosis and gene therapy. Seminars in Ophthalmology. 2017;32(1):14–21.

Ammon FA. Klinische Darstellungen der Krankheiten und Bildungsfehler des menschlichen Auges. Berlin; 1838.

Audo I, Michaelides M, Robson AG, Hawlina M, Vaclavik V, Sandbach JM, Neveu MM, Hogg CR, Hunt DM, Moore AT, Bird AC, Webster AR, Holder GE. Phenotypic variation in enhanced S-cone syndrome. Investigative Ophthalmology & Visual Science. 2008;49(5):2082–93.

Auw-Haedrich C, Staubach F, Witschel H. Optic disk drusen. Surv Ophthalmol. 2002;47(6):515–32.

Ayala-Ramirez R, Graue-Wiechers F, Robredo V, Amato-Almanza M, Horta-Diez I, Zenteno JC. A new autosomal recessive syndrome consisting of posterior microphthalmos, retinitis pigmentosa, foveoschisis, and optic disc drusen is caused by a MFRP gene mutation. Mol Vis. 2006;12:1483–9.

Bainbridge JW, Smith AJ, Barker SS, Robbie S, Henderson R, Balaggan K, Viswanathan A, Holder GE, Stockman A, Tyler N, Petersen-Jones S, Bhattacharya SS, Thrasher AJ, Fitzke FW, Carter BJ, Rubin GS, Moore AT, Ali RR. Effect of gene therapy on visual function in Leber's congenital amaurosis. The New England Journal of Medicine. 2008;358(21):2231–9.

Bainbridge JW, Mehat MS, Sundaram V, Robbie SJ, Barker SE, Ripamonti C, Georgiadis A, Mowat FM, Beattie SG, Gardner PJ, Feathers KL, Luong VA, Yzer S, Balaggan K, Viswanathan A, de Ravel TJ, Casteels I, Holder GE, Tyler N, Fitzke FW, Weleber RG, Nardini M, Moore AT, Thompson DA, Petersen-Jones SM, Michaelides M, van den Born LI, Stockman A, Smith AJ, Rubin G,

Ali RR. Long-term effect of gene therapy on Leber's congenital amaurosis. The New England Journal of Medicine. 2015;372(20):1887–97.

Battu R, Khanna A, Hegde B, Berendschot TT, Grover S, Schouten JS. Correlation of structure and function of the macula in patients with retinitis pigmentosa. Eye. 2015;29(7):895–901.

Beales PL, Elcioglu N, Woolf AS, Parker D, Flinter FA. New criteria for improved diagnosis of Bardet-Biedl syndrome: results of a population survey. J Med Genet. 1999;36(6):437–46.

Ben-Arie-Weintrob Y, Berson EL, Dryja TP. Histopathologic-genotypic correlations in retinitis pigmentosa and allied diseases. Ophthalmic Genetics. 2005;26(2):91–100.

Benhamou N, Massin P, Haouchine B, Erginay A, Gaudric A. Macular retinoschisis in highly myopic eyes. Am J Ophthalmol. 2002;133(6):794–800.

Bernal S, Solans T, Gamundi MJ, Hernan I, de Jorge L, Carballo M, Navarro R, Tizzano E, Ayuso C, Baiget M. Analysis of the involvement of the NR2E3 gene in autosomal recessive retinal dystrophies. Clinical Genetics. 2008;73(4):360–6.

Berson EL, Rosner B, Sandberg MA, Hayes KC, Nicholson BW, Weigel-DiFranco C, Willett W. A randomized trial of vitamin A and vitamin E supplementation for retinitis pigmentosa. Arch Ophthalmol. 1993;111(6):761–72.

Berson EL, Rosner B, Sandberg MA, Weigel-DiFranco C, Moser A, Brockhurst RJ, Hayes KC, Johnson CA, Anderson EJ, Gaudio AR, Willett WC, Schaefer EJ. Clinical trial of docosahexaenoic acid in patients with retinitis pigmentosa receiving vitamin A treatment. Archives of Ophthalmology. 2004;122(9):1297–305.

Berson EL, Rosner B, Sandberg MA, Weigel-DiFranco C, Brockhurst RJ, Hayes KC, Johnson EJ, Anderson EJ, Johnson CA, Gaudio AR, Willett WC, Schaefer EJ. Clinical trial of lutein in patients with retinitis pigmentosa receiving vitamin A. Archives of Ophthalmology. 2010;128(4):403–11.

Bi A, Cui J, Ma YP, Olshevskaya E, Pu M, Dizhoor AM, Pan ZH. Ectopic expression of a microbial-type rhodopsin restores visual responses in mice with photoreceptor degeneration. Neuron. 2006;50(1):23–33.

Birch DG, Locke KG, Wen Y, Locke KI, Hoffman DR, Hood DC. Spectral-domain optical coherence tomography measures of outer segment layer progression in patients with X-linked retinitis pigmentosa. JAMA Ophthalmology. 2013;131(9):1143–50.

Boughman JA, Fishman GA. A genetic analysis of retinitis pigmentosa. Br J Ophthalmol. 1983;67(7):449–54.

Boughman JA, Conneally PM, Nance WE. Population genetic studies of retinitis pigmentosa. Am J Hum Genet. 1980;32(2):223–35.

Breuer DK, Yashar BM, Filippova E, Hiriyanna S, Lyons RH, Mears AJ, Asaye B, Acar C, Vervoort R, Wright AF, Musarella MA, Wheeler P, MacDonald I, Iannaccone A, Birch D, Hoffman DR, Fishman GA, Heckenlively JR, Jacobson SG, Sieving PA, Swaroop A. A comprehensive mutation analysis of RP2 and RPGR in a North American cohort of families with X-linked retinitis pigmentosa. American Journal of Human Genetics. 2002;70(6):1545–54.

Brito-Garcia N, Del Pino-Sedeno T, Trujillo-Martin MM, Coco RM, Rodriguez de la Rua E, Del Cura-Gonzalez I, Serrano-Aguilar P. Effectiveness and safety of nutritional supplements in the treatment of hereditary retinal dystrophies: A systematic review. Eye. 2017;31(2):273–85.

Bujakowska K, Audo I, Mohand-Said S, Lancelot ME, Antonio A, Germain A, Leveillard T, Letexier M, Saraiva JP, Lonjou C, Carpentier W, Sahel JA, Bhattacharya SS, Zeitz C. CRB1 mutations in inherited retinal dystrophies. Human Mutation. 2012;33(2):306–15.

Bulgakova NA, Knust E. The crumbs complex: From epithelial-cell polarity to retinal degeneration. Journal of Cell Science. 2009;122(Pt 15):2587–96.

Bumsted O'Brien KM, Cheng H, Jiang Y, Schulte D, Swaroop A, Hendrickson AE. Expression of photoreceptor-specific nuclear receptor NR2E3 in rod photoreceptors of fetal human retina. Investigative Ophthalmology & Visual Science. 2004;45(8):2807–12.

Busskamp V, Duebel J, Balya D, Fradot M, Viney TJ, Siegert S, Groner AC, Cabuy E, Forster V, Seeliger M, Biel M, Humphries P, Paques M, Mohand-Said S, Trono D, Deisseroth K, Sahel JA, Picaud S, Roska B. Genetic reactivation of cone photoreceptors restores visual responses in retinitis pigmentosa. Science. 2010;329(5990):413–7.

Chacon-Camacho OF, Zenteno JC. Review and update on the molecular basis of Leber congenital amaurosis. World Journal of Clinical Cases. 2015;3(2):112–24.

Chang MY, Pineles SL. Optic disk drusen in children. Survey of Ophthalmology. 2016;61(6):745–58.

Chen J, Rattner A, Nathans J. The rod photoreceptor-specific nuclear receptor Nr2e3 represses transcription of multiple cone-specific genes. The Journal of Neuroscience. 2005;25(1):118–29.

Chuang AT, Margo CE, Greenberg PB. Retinal implants: a systematic review. Br J Ophthalmol. 2014;98(7):852–6. https://doi.org/10.1136/bjophthalmol-2013-303708.

Coussa RG, Lopez Solache I, Koenekoop RK. Leber congenital amaurosis, from darkness to light: an ode to Irene Maumenee. Ophthalmic Genet. 2017;38(1):7–15. https://doi.org/10.1080/13816810.2016.1275021.

Crespi J, Buil JA, Bassaganyas F, Vela-Segarra JI, Diaz-Cascajosa J, Ayala-Ramirez R, Zenteno JC. A novel mutation confirms MFRP as the gene causing the syndrome of nanophthalmos-renititis pigmentosa-foveoschisis-optic disk drusen. Am J Ophthalmol. 2008;146(2):323–8. https://doi.org/10.1016/j.ajo.2008.04.029.

de Hollander AI, Heckenlively JR, van den Born LI, de Kok YJ, van der Velde-Visser SD, Kellner U, Jurklies B, van Schooneveld MJ, Blankenagel A, Rohrschneider K, Wissinger B, Cruysberg JR, Deutman AF, Brunner HG, Apfelstedt-Sylla E, Hoyng CB, Cremers FP. Leber congenital amaurosis and retinitis pigmentosa with coats-like exudative vasculopathy are associated with mutations in the crumbs homologue 1 (CRB1) gene. Am J Hum Genet. 2001;69(1):198–203. https://doi.org/10.1086/321263.

De Laey JJ. Leber's congenital amaurosis. Bull Soc Belge Ophtalmol. 1991;241:41–50.

den Hollander AI, Roepman R, Koenekoop RK, Cremers FP. Leber congenital amaurosis: genes, proteins and disease mechanisms. Prog Retin Eye Res. 2008;27(4):391–419. https://doi.org/10.1016/j.preteyeres.2008.05.003.

Dharmaraj S, Leroy BP, Sohocki MM, Koenekoop RK, Perrault I, Anwar K, Khaliq S, Devi RS, Birch DG, De Pool E, Izquierdo N, Van Maldergem L, Ismail M, Payne AM, Holder GE, Bhattacharya SS, Bird AC, Kaplan J, Maumenee IH. The phenotype of Leber congenital amaurosis in patients with AIPL1 mutations. Arch Ophthalmol. 2004;122(7):1029–37. https://doi.org/10.1001/archopht.122.7.1029.

Domanico D, Carnevale C, Fragiotta S, Verboschi F, Altimari S, Vingolo EM. Cystoid macular edema induced by low doses of nicotinic acid. Case Rep Ophthalmol Med. 2013;2013:713061. https://doi.org/10.1155/2013/713061.

Donders FC. Beitrage zur pathologischen Anatomie des Auges. II Pigmentbildung in der Netzhaut. Albrecht Von Graefes Arch Ophthalmol. 1857;3(1):139–50.

Dorenboim Y, Rehany U, Rumelt S. Central serous chorioretinopathy associated with retinitis pigmentosa. Graefes Arch Clin Exp Ophthalmol. 2004;242(4):346–9. https://doi.org/10.1007/s00417-003-0819-1.

Duncan JL, Pierce EA, Laster AM, Daiger SP, Birch DG, Ash JD, Iannaccone A, Flannery JG, Sahel JA, Zack DJ, Zarbin MA, the Foundation Fight Blindness Scientific Advisory Board. Inherited

retinal degenerations: Current landscape and knowledge gaps. Translational Vision Science & Technology. 2018;7(4):6.
Edwards A, Grover S, Fishman GA. Frequency of photographically apparent optic disc and parapapillary nerve fiber layer drusen in Usher syndrome. Retina. 1996;16(5):388–92.
Fazzi E, Signorini SG, Scelsa B, Bova SM, Lanzi G. Leber's congenital amaurosis: an update. Eur J Paediatr Neurol. 2003;7(1):13–22.
Ferrucci S, Anderson SF, Townsend JC. Retinitis pigmentosa inversa. Optom Vis Sci. 1998;75(8):560–70.
Fishman GA. Retinitis pigmentosa. Genetic percentages. Arch Ophthalmol. 1978;96(5):822–6.
Fishman GA, Farber MD, Derlacki DJ. X-linked retinitis pigmentosa. Profile of clinical findings. Arch Ophthalmol. 1988;106(3):369–75.
Flynn MF, Fishman GA, Anderson RJ, Roberts DK. Retrospective longitudinal study of visual acuity change in patients with retinitis pigmentosa. Retina. 2001;21(6):639–46.
Forsythe E, Beales PL. Bardet-Biedl syndrome. Eur J Hum Genet. 2013;21(1):8–13. https://doi.org/10.1038/ejhg.2012.115.
Franceschetti D. Importance diagnostique et prognostique de l'é lectroré tinogramme (ERG). dans les dé gé né rescences ré tré cissement du champ. Confin Neurol. 1954;14:184–6.
Grant CA, Berson EL. Treatable forms of retinitis pigmentosa associated with systemic neurological disorders. Int Ophthalmol Clin. 2001;41(1):103–10.
Greenstein VC, Duncker T, Holopigian K, Carr RE, Greenberg JP, Tsang SH, Hood DC. Structural and functional changes associated with normal and abnormal fundus autofluorescence in patients with retinitis pigmentosa. Retina. 2012;32(2):349–57. https://doi.org/10.1097/IAE.0b013e31821dfc17.
Grover S, Fishman GA, Brown J Jr. Frequency of optic disc or parapapillary nerve fiber layer drusen in retinitis pigmentosa. Ophthalmology. 1997;104(2):295–8.
Grover S, Fishman GA, Brown J Jr. Patterns of visual field progression in patients with retinitis pigmentosa. Ophthalmology. 1998;105(6):1069–75. https://doi.org/10.1016/s0161-6420(98)96009-2.
Hagiwara A, Yamamoto S, Ogata K, Sugawara T, Hiramatsu A, Shibata M, Mitamura Y. Macular abnormalities in patients with retinitis pigmentosa: prevalence on OCT examination and outcomes of vitreoretinal surgery. Acta Ophthalmol. 2011;89(2):e122–5. https://doi.org/10.1111/j.1755-3768.2010.01866.x.
Haim M. Retinitis pigmentosa: problems associated with genetic classification. Clin Genet. 1993;44(2):62–70.
Hartong DT, Berson EL, Dryja TP. Retinitis pigmentosa. Lancet. 2006;368(9549):1795–809. https://doi.org/10.1016/s0140-6736(06)69740-7.
Hashimoto Y, Kase S, Saito W, Ishida S. Abnormalities of fundus autofluorescence in pigmented paravenous chorioretinal atrophy. Open Ophthalmol J. 2012;6:125–8. https://doi.org/10.2174/1874364101206010125.
Hauswirth WW, Aleman TS, Kaushal S, Cideciyan AV, Schwartz SB, Wang L, Conlon TJ, Boye SL, Flotte TR, Byrne BJ, Jacobson SG. Treatment of leber congenital amaurosis due to RPE65 mutations by ocular subretinal injection of adeno-associated virus gene vector: short-term results of a phase I trial. Hum Gene Ther. 2008;19(10):979–90. https://doi.org/10.1089/hum.2008.107.
Heckenlively JR, Rodriguez JA, Daiger SP. Autosomal dominant sectoral retinitis pigmentosa. Two families with transversion mutation in codon 23 of rhodopsin. Arch Ophthalmol. 1991;109(1):84–91.
Hingorani M, Nischal KK, Davies A, Bentley C, Vivian A, Baker AJ, Mieli-Vergani G, Bird AC, Aclimandos WA. Ocular abnormalities in Alagille syndrome. Ophthalmology. 1999;106(2):330–7. https://doi.org/10.1016/s0161-6420(99)90072-6.
Hood DC, Lazow MA, Locke KG, Greenstein VC, Birch DG. The transition zone between healthy and diseased retina in patients with retinitis pigmentosa. Invest Ophthalmol Vis Sci. 2011;52(1):101–8. https://doi.org/10.1167/iovs.10-5799.
Huckfeldt RM, Comander J. Management of cystoid macular edema in retinitis pigmentosa. Semin Ophthalmol. 2017;32(1):43–51. https://doi.org/10.1080/08820538.2016.1228404.
Iannaccone A, Rispoli E, Vingolo EM, Onori P, Steindl K, Rispoli D, Pannarale MR. Correlation between Goldmann perimetry and maximal electroretinogram response in retinitis pigmentosa. Doc Ophthalmol. 1995;90(2):129–42.
Ikeda Y, Yoshida N, Murakami Y, Nakatake S, Notomi S, Hisatomi T, Enaida H, Ishibashi T. Long-term surgical outcomes of epiretinal membrane in patients with retinitis pigmentosa. Sci Rep. 2015;5:13078. https://doi.org/10.1038/srep13078.
Jacobson SG. Crumbs homolog 1 (CRB1) mutations result in a thick human retina with abnormal lamination. Hum Mol Genet. 2003;12(9):1073–8. https://doi.org/10.1093/hmg/ddg117.
Jacobson SG, Cideciyan AV. Treatment possibilities for retinitis pigmentosa. N Engl J Med. 2010;363(17):1669–71. https://doi.org/10.1056/NEJMcibr1007685.
Jacobson SG, Aleman TS, Sumaroka A, Cideciyan AV, Roman AJ, Windsor EA, Schwartz SB, Rehm HL, Kimberling WJ. Disease boundaries in the retina of patients with Usher syndrome caused by MYO7A gene mutations. Invest Ophthalmol Vis Sci. 2009;50(4):1886–94. https://doi.org/10.1167/iovs.08-3122.
Jacobson SG, Roman AJ, Aleman TS, Sumaroka A, Herrera W, Windsor EA, Atkinson LA, Schwartz SB, Steinberg JD, Cideciyan AV. Normal central retinal function and structure preserved in retinitis pigmentosa. Invest Ophthalmol Vis Sci. 2010;51(2):1079–85. https://doi.org/10.1167/iovs.09-4372.
Jacobson SG, Cideciyan AV, Roman AJ, Sumaroka A, Schwartz SB, Heon E, Hauswirth WW. Improvement and decline in vision with gene therapy in childhood blindness. N Engl J Med. 2015;372(20):1920–6. https://doi.org/10.1056/NEJMoa1412965.
Katz ML, Drea CM, Eldred GE, Hess HH, Robison WG Jr. Influence of early photoreceptor degeneration on lipofuscin in the retinal pigment epithelium. Exp Eye Res. 1986;43(4):561–73.
Khambatta S, Nguyen DL, Beckman TJ, Wittich CM. Kearns-Sayre syndrome: a case series of 35 adults and children. Int J Gen Med. 2014;7:325–32. https://doi.org/10.2147/ijgm.s65560.
Khan JA, Ide CH, Strickland MP. Coats'-type retinitis pigmentosa. Surv Ophthalmol. 1988;32(5):317–32.
Kim BJ, Fulton AB. The genetics and ocular findings of Alagille syndrome. Semin Ophthalmol. 2007;22(4):205–10. https://doi.org/10.1080/08820530701745108.
Kiratli H, Ozturkmen C. Coats-like lesions in Usher syndrome type II. Graefes Arch Clin Exp Ophthalmol. 2004;242(3):265–7. https://doi.org/10.1007/s00417-003-0818-2.
Klein D, Ammann F. The syndrome of Laurence-Moon-Bardet-Biedl and allied diseases in Switzerland. Clinical, genetic and epidemiological studies. J Neurol Sci. 1969;9(3):479–513.
Koenekoop RK. An overview of Leber congenital amaurosis: a model to understand human retinal development. Surv Ophthalmol. 2004;49(4):379–98. https://doi.org/10.1016/j.survophthal.2004.04.003.
Koenekoop RK, Wang H, Majewski J, Wang X, Lopez I, Ren H, Chen Y, Li Y, Fishman GA, Genead M, Schwartzentruber J, Solanki N, Traboulsi EI, Cheng J, Logan CV, McKibbin M, Hayward BE, Parry DA, Johnson CA, Nageeb M, Poulter JA, Mohamed MD, Jafri H, Rashid Y, Taylor GR, Keser V, Mardon G, Xu H, Inglehearn CF, Fu Q, Toomes C, Chen R. Mutations in NMNAT1 cause Leber congenital amaurosis and identify a new disease pathway for retinal degeneration. Nat Genet. 2012;44(9):1035–9. https://doi.org/10.1038/ng.2356.
Krill AE, Archer D, Martin D. Sector retinitis pigmentosa. Am J Ophthalmol. 1970;69(6):977–87.

Lagali PS, Balya D, Awatramani GB, Munch TA, Kim DS, Busskamp V, Cepko CL, Roska B. Light-activated channels targeted to ON bipolar çells restore visual function in retinal degeneration. Nat Neurosci. 2008;11(6):667–75. https://doi.org/10.1038/nn.2117.

Lambert SR, Kriss A, Taylor D, Coffey R, Pembrey M. Follow-up and diagnostic reappraisal of 75 patients with Leber's congenital amaurosis. Am J Ophthalmol. 1989;107(6):624–31.

Langenbeck BCR. De retina. Observations anatomico-pathologica. Göttingen: Sumptibus; 1836.

Leber TV. Uber retinitis pigmentosa und angeborene amaurose. Graefes Arch Clin Exp Ophthalmol. 1869;15(3):1–25.

Lenassi E, Troeger E, Wilke R, Hawlina M. Correlation between macular morphology and sensitivity in patients with retinitis pigmentosa and hyperautofluorescent ring. Invest Ophthalmol Vis Sci. 2012;53(1):47–52. https://doi.org/10.1167/iovs.11-8048.

Lima LH, Cella W, Greenstein VC, Wang NK, Busuioc M, Smith RT, Yannuzzi LA, Tsang SH. Structural assessment of hyperautofluorescent ring in patients with retinitis pigmentosa. Retina. 2009;29(7):1025–31. https://doi.org/10.1097/IAE.0b013e3181ac2418.

Lima LH, Burke T, Greenstein VC, Chou CL, Cella W, Yannuzzi LA, Tsang SH. Progressive constriction of the hyperautofluorescent ring in retinitis pigmentosa. Am J Ophthalmol. 2012;153(4):718–27, 727.e711–712. https://doi.org/10.1016/j.ajo.2011.08.043.

Lorenz B, Wabbels B, Wegscheider E, Hamel CP, Drexler W, Preising MN. Lack of fundus autofluorescence to 488 nanometers from childhood on in patients with early-onset severe retinal dystrophy associated with mutations in RPE65. Ophthalmology. 2004;111(8):1585–94. https://doi.org/10.1016/j.ophtha.2004.01.033.

Luo YH, da Cruz L. The Argus((R)) II retinal prosthesis system. Prog Retin Eye Res. 2016;50:89–107. https://doi.org/10.1016/j.preteyeres.2015.09.003.

Lupo S, Grenga PL, Vingolo EM. Fourier-domain optical coherence tomography and microperimetry findings in retinitis pigmentosa. Am J Ophthalmol. 2011;151(1):106–11. https://doi.org/10.1016/j.ajo.2010.07.026.

Maguire AM, Simonelli F, Pierce EA, Pugh EN Jr, Mingozzi F, Bennicelli J, Banfi S, Marshall KA, Testa F, Surace EM, Rossi S, Lyubarsky A, Arruda VR, Konkle B, Stone E, Sun J, Jacobs J, Dell'Osso L, Hertle R, Ma JX, Redmond TM, Zhu X, Hauck B, Zelenaia O, Shindler KS, Maguire MG, Wright JF, Volpe NJ, McDonnell JW, Auricchio A, High KA, Bennett J. Safety and efficacy of gene transfer for Leber's congenital amaurosis. N Engl J Med. 2008;358(21):2240–8. https://doi.org/10.1056/NEJMoa0802315.

Mathur P, Yang J. Usher syndrome: hearing loss, retinal degeneration and associated abnormalities. Biochim Biophys Acta. 2015;1852(3):406–20. https://doi.org/10.1016/j.bbadis.2014.11.020.

Matsuo T, Morimoto N. Visual acuity and perimacular retinal layers detected by optical coherence tomography in patients with retinitis pigmentosa. Br J Ophthalmol. 2007;91(7):888–90. https://doi.org/10.1136/bjo.2007.114538.

Marmor MF, Jacobson SG, Foerster MH, Kellner U, Weleber RG. Diagnostic clinical findings of a new syndrome with night blindness, maculopathy, and enhanced S cone sensitivity. American Journal of Ophthalmology. 1990;110(2):124–34.

McBain VA, Forrester JV, Lois N. Fundus autofluorescence in the diagnosis of cystoid macular oedema. Br J Ophthalmol. 2008;92(7):946–9. https://doi.org/10.1136/bjo.2007.129957.

McKay GJ, Clarke S, Davis JA, Simpson DA, Silvestri G. Pigmented paravenous chorioretinal atrophy is associated with a mutation within the crumbs homolog 1 (CRB1) gene. Invest Ophthalmol Vis Sci. 2005;46(1):322–8. https://doi.org/10.1167/iovs.04-0734.

Meunier I, Ben Salah S, Arndt C, Hamel C. [Retinitis pigmentosa and central serous choroiditis. Retinal imaging and optical coherence tomography views]. J Fr Ophtalmol. 2008;31(7):735.

Mohamed MD, Topping NC, Jafri H, Raashed Y, McKibbin MA, Inglehearn CF. Progression of phenotype in Leber's congenital amaurosis with a mutation at the LCA5 locus. Br J Ophthalmol. 2003;87(4):473–5.

Moisseiev E, Moisseiev J, Loewenstein A. Optic disc pit maculopathy: when and how to treat? A review of the pathogenesis and treatment options. Int J Retina Vitreous. 2015;1:13. https://doi.org/10.1186/s40942-015-0013-8.

Murakami T, Akimoto M, Ooto S, Suzuki T, Ikeda H, Kawagoe N, Takahashi M, Yoshimura N. Association between abnormal autofluorescence and photoreceptor disorganization in retinitis pigmentosa. Am J Ophthalmol. 2008;145(4):687–94. https://doi.org/10.1016/j.ajo.2007.11.018.

Murthy R, Honavar SG. Secondary vasoproliferative retinal tumor associated with Usher syndrome type 1. J AAPOS. 2009;13(1):97–8. https://doi.org/10.1016/j.jaapos.2008.07.012.

Ogura S, Yasukawa T, Kato A, Usui H, Hirano Y, Yoshida M, Ogura Y. Wide-field fundus autofluorescence imaging to evaluate retinal function in patients with retinitis pigmentosa. Am J Ophthalmol. 2014;158(5):1093–8. https://doi.org/10.1016/j.ajo.2014.07.021.

Oishi A, Ogino K, Makiyama Y, Nakagawa S, Kurimoto M, Yoshimura N. Wide-field fundus autofluorescence imaging of retinitis pigmentosa. Ophthalmology. 2013;120(9):1827–34. https://doi.org/10.1016/j.ophtha.2013.01.050.

Omphroy CA. Sector retinitis pigmentosa and chronic angle-closure glaucoma: a new association. Ophthalmologica. 1984;189(1–2):12–20.

Osman SA, Aylin Y, Arikan G, Celikel H. Photodynamic treatment of a secondary vasoproliferative tumour associated with sector retinitis pigmentosa and Usher syndrome type I. Clin Exp Ophthalmol. 2007;35(2):191–3. https://doi.org/10.1111/j.1442-9071.2007.01440.x.

Pasadhika S, Fishman GA, Stone EM, Lindeman M, Zelkha R, Lopez I, Koenekoop RK, Shahidi M. Differential macular morphology in patients with RPE65-, CEP290-, GUCY2D-, and AIPL1-related Leber congenital amaurosis. Invest Ophthalmol Vis Sci. 2010;51(5):2608–14. https://doi.org/10.1167/iovs.09-3734.

Paun CC, Pijl BJ, Siemiatkowska AM, Collin RW, Cremers FP, Hoyng CB, den Hollander AI. A novel crumbs homolog 1 mutation in a family with retinitis pigmentosa, nanophthalmos, and optic disc drusen. Mol Vis. 2012;18:2447–53.

Pelletier V, Jambou M, Delphin N, Zinovieva E, Stum M, Gigarel N, Dollfus H, Hamel C, Toutain A, Dufier JL, Roche O, Munnich A, Bonnefont JP, Kaplan J, Rozet JM. Comprehensive survey of mutations in RP2 and RPGR in patients affected with distinct retinal dystrophies: genotype-phenotype correlations and impact on genetic counseling. Hum Mutat. 2007;28(1):81–91. https://doi.org/10.1002/humu.20417.

Pocha SM, Knust E. Complexities of crumbs function and regulation in tissue morphogenesis. Curr Biol. 2013;23(7):R289–93. https://doi.org/10.1016/j.cub.2013.03.001.

Pruett R. Retinitis pigmentosa: clinical observations and correlations. Trans Am Ophthalmol Soc. 1983;81:693–735.

Pyo Park S, Hwan Hong I, Tsang SH, Chang S. Cellular imaging demonstrates genetic mosaicism in heterozygous carriers of an X-linked ciliopathy gene. Eur J Hum Genet. 2013;21(11):1240–8. https://doi.org/10.1038/ejhg.2013.21.

Rayapudi S, Schwartz SG, Wang X, Chavis P. Vitamin A and fish oils for retinitis pigmentosa. Cochrane Database Syst Rev. 2013;(12):CD008428. https://doi.org/10.1002/14651858.CD008428.pub2.

RetNet. https://sph.uth.edu/retnet/. Accessed 4 Nov 2019.

Robson AG, El-Amir A, Bailey C, Egan CA, Fitzke FW, Webster AR, Bird AC, Holder GE. Pattern ERG correlates of abnormal fundus autofluorescence in patients with retinitis pigmentosa and normal visual acuity. Invest Ophthalmol Vis Sci. 2003;44(8):3544–50.

Robson AG, Saihan Z, Jenkins SA, Fitzke FW, Bird AC, Webster AR, Holder GE. Functional characterisation and serial imaging of abnormal fundus autofluorescence in patients with retinitis pigmentosa and normal visual acuity. Br J Ophthalmol. 2006;90(4):472–9. https://doi.org/10.1136/bjo.2005.082487.

Ronquillo CC, Bernstein PS, Baehr W. Senior-Loken syndrome: a syndromic form of retinal dystrophy associated with nephronophthisis. Vis Res. 2012;75:88–97. https://doi.org/10.1016/j.visres.2012.07.003.

Ruete C. Bildliche Darstellung der Krankheiten des Menschlichen Auges. Teubner, Leipzig: Druck und Verlag von B.G; 1855.

Sandberg MA, Weigel-DiFranco C, Rosner B, Berson EL. The relationship between visual field size and electroretinogram amplitude in retinitis pigmentosa. Invest Ophthalmol Vis Sci. 1996;37(8):1693–8.

Sandberg MA, Brockhurst RJ, Gaudio AR, Berson EL. The association between visual acuity and central retinal thickness in retinitis pigmentosa. Invest Ophthalmol Vis Sci. 2005;46(9):3349–54. https://doi.org/10.1167/iovs.04-1383.

Sayman Muslubas I, Karacorlu M, Arf S, Hocaoglu M, Ersoz MG. Features of the macula and central visual field and fixation pattern in patients with retinitis pigmentosa. Retina. 2017;38:424–31. https://doi.org/10.1097/iae.0000000000001532.

Scholl HP, Chong NH, Robson AG, Holder GE, Moore AT, Bird AC. Fundus autofluorescence in patients with Leber congenital amaurosis. Invest Ophthalmol Vis Sci. 2004;45(8):2747–52. https://doi.org/10.1167/iovs.03-1208.

Sharon D, Sandberg MA, Rabe VW, Stillberger M, Dryja TP, Berson EL. RP2 and RPGR mutations and clinical correlations in patients with X-linked retinitis pigmentosa. Am J Hum Genet. 2003;73(5):1131–46. https://doi.org/10.1086/379379.

Shen JH, Chen KJ, Wang NK. Leptochoroid in a case of alagille syndrome (arteriohepatic dysplasia). Ophthalmology. 2017;124(8):1135.

Sheth S, Rush R, Narayanan R. Retinitis pigmentosa inversa with unilateral high myopia with fellow eye optic disc pitting. Eur J Ophthalmol. 2011;21(4):509–12. https://doi.org/10.5301/ejo.2011.6264.

Slavotinek AM. The family of crumbs genes and human disease. Mol Syndromol. 2016;7(5):274–81. https://doi.org/10.1159/000448109.

Steidl SM, Pruett RC. Macular complications associated with posterior staphyloma. Am J Ophthalmol. 1997;123(2):181–7.

Strong S, Liew G, Michaelides M. Retinitis pigmentosa-associated cystoid macular oedema: pathogenesis and avenues of intervention. Br J Ophthalmol. 2017;101(1):31–7. https://doi.org/10.1136/bjophthalmol-2016-309376.

Sujirakul T, Lin MK, Duong J, Wei Y, Lopez-Pintado S, Tsang SH. Multimodal imaging of central retinal disease progression in a 2-year mean follow-up of retinitis pigmentosa. Am J Ophthalmol. 2015;160(4):786–798.e784. https://doi.org/10.1016/j.ajo.2015.06.032.

Swaroop A, Wang QL, Wu W, Cook J, Coats C, Xu S, Chen S, Zack DJ, Sieving PA. Leber congenital amaurosis caused by a homozygous mutation (R90W) in the homeodomain of the retinal transcription factor CRX: direct evidence for the involvement of CRX in the development of photoreceptor function. Hum Mol Genet. 1999;8(2):299–305.

Takahashi Y, Moiseyev G, Chen Y, Nikolaeva O, Ma JX. An alternative isomerohydrolase in the retinal Muller cells of a cone-dominant species. FEBS J. 2011;278(16):2913–26. https://doi.org/10.1111/j.1742-4658.2011.08216.x.

Talib M, van Schooneveld MJ, van Genderen MM, Wijnholds J, Florijn RJ, Ten Brink JB, Schalij-Delfos NE, Dagnelie G, Cremers FPM, Wolterbeek R, Fiocco M, Thiadens AA, Hoyng CB, Klaver CC, Bergen AA, Boon CJF. Genotypic and phenotypic characteristics of CRB1-associated retinal dystrophies: A long-term follow-up study. Ophthalmology. 2017;124(6):884–95.

Testa F, Rossi S, Colucci R, Gallo B, Di Iorio V, della Corte M, Azzolini C, Melillo P, Simonelli F. Macular abnormalities in Italian patients with retinitis pigmentosa. Br J Ophthalmol. 2014;98(7):946–50. https://doi.org/10.1136/bjophthalmol-2013-304082.

Thobani A, Fishman GA, Genead M, Anastasakis A. Visual acuity loss in recessive retinitis pigmentosa and its correlation with macular lesions. Retina. 2011;31(5):967–72. https://doi.org/10.1097/IAE.0b013e3181f441e1.

Tosi J, Tsui I, Lima LH, Wang NK, Tsang SH. Case report: Autofluorescence imaging and phenotypic variance in a sibling pair with early-onset retinal dystrophy due to defective CRB1 function. Current Eye Research. 2009;34(5):395–400.

Usher C. On a few hereditary eye affections. Trans Ophthal Soc U K. 1935;55:164–245.

van den Born LI, van Soest S, van Schooneveld MJ, Riemslag FC, de Jong PT, Bleeker-Wagemakers EM. Autosomal recessive retinitis pigmentosa with preserved para-arteriolar retinal pigment epithelium. Am J Ophthalmol. 1994;118(4):430–9.

Trigt ACV. Dissertatio ophthalmologica inauguralis de speculo oculi. Utrecht: Utrecht University Library; 1853.

Wakabayashi T, Sawa M, Gomi F, Tsujikawa M. Correlation of fundus autofluorescence with photoreceptor morphology and functional changes in eyes with retinitis pigmentosa. Acta Ophthalmologica. 2010;88(5):e177–83.

Wang NK, Fine HF, Chang S, Chou CL, Cella W, Tosi J, Lin CS, Nagasaki T, Tsang SH. Cellular origin of fundus autofluorescence in patients and mice with a defective NR2E3 gene. The British Journal of Ophthalmology. 2009;93(9):1234–40.

Wang NK, Lai CC, Liu CH, Yeh LK, Chou CL, Kong J, Nagasaki T, Tsang SH, Chien CL. Origin of fundus hyperautofluorescent spots and their role in retinal degeneration in a mouse model of Goldmann-Favre syndrome. Disease Models & Mechanisms. 2013;6(5):1113–22.

Wegscheider E, Preising MN, Lorenz B. Fundus autofluorescence in carriers of X-linked recessive retinitis pigmentosa associated with mutations in RPGR, and correlation with electrophysiological and psychophysical data. Graefes Archive for Clinical and Experimental Ophthalmology. 2004;242(6):501–11.

Witkin AJ, Ko TH, Fujimoto JG, Chan A, Drexler W, Schuman JS, Reichel E, Duker JS. Ultra-high resolution optical coherence tomography assessment of photoreceptors in retinitis pigmentosa and related diseases. American Journal of Ophthalmology. 2006;142(6):945–52.

Wolsley CJ, Silvestri G, O'Neill J, Saunders KJ, Anderson RS. The association between multifocal electroretinograms and OCT retinal thickness in retinitis pigmentosa patients with good visual acuity. Eye. 2009;23(7):1524–31.

Wright AF. Long-term effects of retinal gene therapy in childhood blindness. The New England Journal of Medicine. 2015;372(20):1954–5.

Wu AL, Wang JP, Tseng YJ, Liu L, Kang YC, Chen KJ, Chao AN, Yeh LK, Chen TL, Hwang YS, Wu WC, Lai CC, Wang NK. Multimodal imaging of mosaic retinopathy in carriers of hereditary X-linked recessive diseases. Retina. 2018;38(5):1047–57.

Wuthisiri W, Lingao MD, Capasso JE, Levin AV. Lyonization in ophthalmology. Current Opinion in Ophthalmology. 2013;24(5):389–97.

Yzer S, Hollander AI, Lopez I, Pott JW, de Faber JT, Cremers FP, Koenekoop RK, van den Born LI. Ocular and extra-ocular features of patients with Leber congenital amaurosis and mutations in CEP290. Mol Vis. 2012;18:412–25.

Yzer S, Barbazetto I, Allikmets R, van Schooneveld MJ, Bergen A, Tsang SH, Jacobson SG, Yannuzzi LA. Expanded clinical spectrum of enhanced S-cone syndrome. JAMA Ophthalmology. 2013;131(10):1324–30.

Best Disease

2

Christine Anggun Putri, Edward Pritchard, and Fahd Quhill

Introduction

Best disease or Best vitelliform macular dystrophy was named after Dr. Franz Best, a German Ophthalmologist who first described the pedigree in 1905 (Best 1905). It is typically an autosomal dominant disorder which presents in childhood with characteristic 'egg-yolk' macular lesion (Deutman 1971). This yellow lesion gradually gets reabsorbed, resulting in retinal pigment epithelium (RPE) atrophy and subretinal fibrosis (Budiene et al. 2014). Usual onset of Best disease is from 3 to 15 years of age (Wabbels et al. 2006). At the onset of disease, patients usually have normal visual function. As the disease progresses, patients experience decline in the central visual acuity and metamorphopsia. This eventually leads to visual impairment at a later age. Patients usually retain reading vision until the fifth decade of life (Booij et al. 2010).

Best disease is the second most common juvenile macular degeneration; however, it only attributes to 1% of all cases of macular degeneration (Yanoff and Fine 2002). This is a rare disorder and its prevalence is unknown. Best disease is most commonly described in Caucasians, although it has also been reported in individuals of African, Asian and Hispanic ancestry (Shibuya and Hayasaka 1993).

Important differential diagnoses of Best disease to consider include other dystrophies of the central part of retina and choroid, central chorioretinitis, serous RPE detachment, colobomas of the central retina, age-related macular degeneration and foveal changes in angioid streaks (Michaelides et al. 2003).

Etiopathogenesis

Best disease is a hereditary disease with autosomal dominant pattern of inheritance, even though sporadic cases have been reported (Budiene et al. 2014). Mutations in the *BEST1* gene (formerly *VMD2*) located on chromosome 11q13 are responsible for Best disease (Petrukhin et al. 1998). This gene codes for a 585-amino acid transmembrane protein with size of 68 kDa named bestrophin-1. This $Ca2^{+}$-sensitive chloride channel is located in the basolateral plasma membrane of RPE cells and is essential for normal ocular development (Marano et al. 2000; Marmorstein et al. 2000; Rosenthal et al. 2006). Abnormal $Ca2^{+}$-sensitive chloride channel results in abnormal chloride conductance across the basolateral membrane of RPE. Mutations in *BEST1* lead to altered function of bestrophin and ion transport by the RPE, resulting in the accumulation of fluid and/or debris between RPE and photoreceptors and also between RPE and Bruch's membrane. These changes eventually lead to detachment and secondary photoreceptor degeneration (Michaelides et al. 2003; Weingeist et al. 1982; Marmorstein et al. 2009).

There are at least 253 reported *BEST1* gene mutations and majority of these are missense mutations. In addition to Best disease, mutations in *BEST1* have been reported in adult-onset vitelliform macular dystrophy, autosomal dominant vitreoretinochoroidopathy and autosomal recessive bestrophinopathy (Budiene et al. 2014). Mutation in *BEST1* gene has also been linked to retinitis pigmentosa (RP) (Davidson et al. 2009).

A histopathological study confirmed that in Best disease, the RPE cells were flattened with deposition of abnormal lipofuscin and pleomorphic melanolipofuscin granules. A PAS-positive, acid-mucopolysaccharide-negative, electron-dense, finely granular material was deposited in the inner segments of the degenerating photoreceptors and the Muller cells. An abnormal fibrillar material was present underneath and in close association with the RPE cells, just beneath the area of photoreceptor cell loss (Frangieh et al. 1982).

C. A. Putri · E. Pritchard · F. Quhill (✉)
Sheffield Teaching Hospitals NHS Foundation Trust, Sheffield, UK
e-mail: C.putri@nhs.net; Edward.Pritchard@nhs.net; F.quhill@nhs.net

G. Cheung (ed.), *Hereditary Chorioretinal Disorders*, Retina Atlas, https://doi.org/10.1007/978-981-15-0414-3_2

Choroidal neovascularization may develop as a late complication due to the breakdown of RPE and Bruch's membrane (Miller et al. 1976).

Clinical Features

The onset of disease typically starts in childhood between 3 and 15 years of age, with the mean age of 6 years (Wabbels et al. 2006). At the early stage of the disease, patients may be asymptomatic as the visual function remains sufficient for many years. Progressive visual decline usually happens after the fourth decade especially in patients with longstanding atrophic changes. Patients may experience symptoms such as metamorphopsia, blurred vision and decrease of central vision (Budiene et al. 2014).

There are several classifications proposed for Best disease, based on the aspect of lesion on ophthalmoscopy. There are several stages that define the progression of Best disease.

In stage 1, fundus appears normal but eletro-oculogram (EOG) is abnormal. The Arden ratio (the ratio of the light peak divided by the dark trough) is reduced in Best disease with ratio of <1.5, most often between 1.0 and 1.3 (normal ratio is 1.8) (Francois et al. 1967). This signifies that the disease process is more widespread and not only confined to the macula (Skoog and Nilsson 1981). EOG in asymptomatic carrier of Best disease is also abnormal; therefore, EOG plays a role in screening these individuals. Occasionally, individuals who display clinical features of stage 1 Best disease and a variant of *BEST1* may have normal EOG findings (Testa et al. 2008). Full-field electroretinogram (ERG) result is normal in stage 1 Best disease. A focal ERG or multifocal ERG, concentrating on macular function, reveals abnormal function consistent with the anatomical location of disease (Glybina and Frank 2006).

In stage 2 (previtelliform stage), patients may have normal fundus or subtle RPE changes with abnormal EOG. Fluorescein angiogram (FA) shows window defects. In 75% of sufferers, visual acuity remains 20/20 at this stage of disease.

Stage 3 (vitelliform stage) consists of circular, well-circumscribed, elevated, orange or yellow-opaque, 0.5–5 mm 'yolk-like' macular lesions (Fig. 2.1a). The rest of the fundus typically has a normal appearance. Rarely, these lesions may be multifocal. FA shows hypofluorescence due to blockage of choroidal fluorescence by the vitelliform lesion (Fig. 2.1b). VA at this stage is typically 20/20 to 20/50.

In stage 4 (vitelliruptive or 'scrambled egg' stage), yellow vitelline substance breaks through RPE and accumulates in the subretinal space forming a cyst. The cyst is granular and lumpy in appearance, thus resembling a 'scrambled egg'. FA reveals area of hypofluorescence due to FA partially blocked by vitelline material with superior hyperfluorescence. VA is usually 20/50 or better.

In stage 5 (pseudohypopyon stage), a horizontal level of yellow vitelline substance is observed in the inferior part of the lesion. Above the level of this vitelline substance, the lesion contains relatively transparent fluid. The vitelliruptive stage and pseudohypopyon stage may revert back and forth for many years (Fig. 2.2a). FA typically shows inferior hypofluorescence secondary to the blockage by the vitelline substance and superior hyperfluorescent area. At this stage, VA markedly reduces to 20/100.

Stage 6 (atropic/neovascular stage) is a result of progressive chorioretinal atrophy, and this is characterized by hypertrophic scar and atrophic maculopathy (Fig. 2.3a). FA shows hyperfluorescence due to window defect without leakage. VA significantly reduces to 20/200. This stage may be associated with the development of choroidal neovascularization where FA shows hyperfluorescence secondary to leakage (Fig. 2.3d).

Apart from the above investigative modalities, optical coherence tomography (OCT) and fundus autofluorescence (FAF) also show changes related to Best disease. OCT shows normal retinal architecture or subtle changes in the outer retina in previtelliform clinical stages. In intermediate clinical stages, splitting and elevation at the outer retina-RPE letvel is apparent (Fig. 2.1c and 2.2c) . Thinning of the retina and RPE is the hallmark of the atrophic clinical stage (Fig. 2.3b) (Pianta et al. 2003; Querques et al. 2008). FAF detects metabolic changes in the RPE and photoreceptor layers, and lesion seen in fundus corresponds to increase in autofluorescence in several retinal dystrophies including Best disease (Fig. 2.2b) (Boon et al. 2008).

Management

Supportive Management

Individuals with Best disease should be monitored regularly and referred for visual rehabilitation. Social and psychological support should be offered to individuals affected, adapted to their age and individual needs. Visual aids such as magnifiers, special eye wear, enhanced-vision TV systems and computers and various aids for mobility should be considered (Budiene et al. 2014). Smoking cessation has been shown to prevent neovascularization of retina, thus this should be encouraged (Clemons et al. 2005). Genetic counselling with information on nature, inheritance and implication as well as prenatal testing of Best disease should be offered to individuals affected to provide them with reproductive options (Macdonald and Lee 1993–2017).

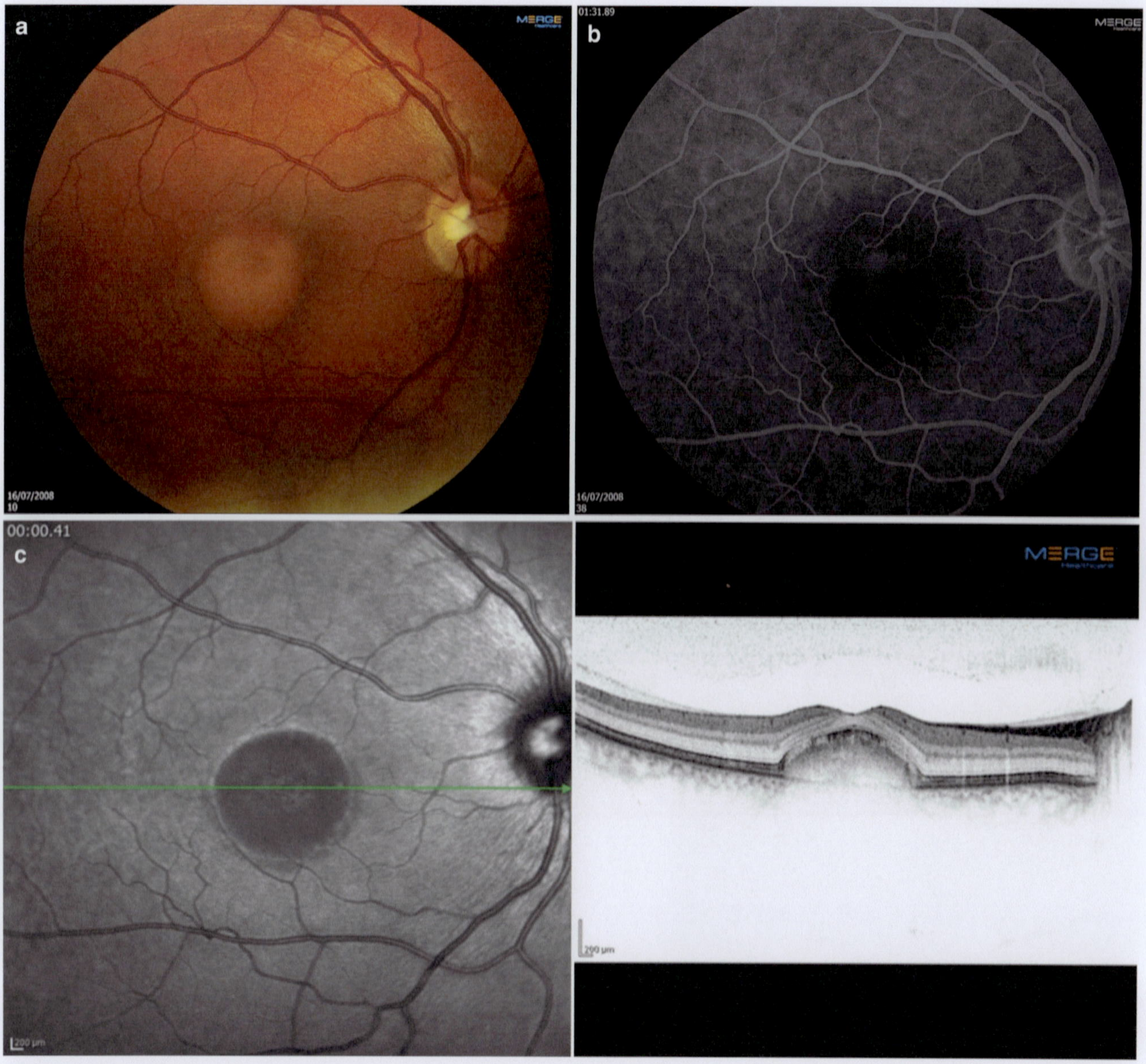

Fig. 2.1 Vitelliform stage (stage 3). (**a**) Fundus photograph showing a well-circumscribed circular elevated orange lesion at the macula. (**b**) Fluorescein angiogram showing typically hypofluorescence at the macula. (**c**) Macular OCT shows buildup of vitelline substance below the RPE

Anti-VEGF

Best disease can be complicated by choroidal neovascularization (Miller et al. 1976). Anti-VEGFs such as ranibizumab and bevacizumab have been reported to be beneficial for the preservation of vision in eyes complicated by choroidal neovascular membrane (Leu et al. 2007; Rishi et al. 2010; Heidary et al. 2011). Further study is necessary to determine the long-term visual outcome, recurrence rate and optimum number of intravitreal injections required. Anti-VEGF affects normal retinal vasculogenesis, revascularization and organogenesis, and its pharmacokinetics in pediatric population is not yet fully understood. Therefore, it is important to consider both risks and benefits before commencing treatment with anti-VEGF in children (Chaudhary et al. 2013).

Photodynamic Therapy (PDT)

Treatment of subfoveal neovascularization with hemorrhage in Best disease with PDT has been reported with significant improvement in vision within 1 year of treatment, and this remained stable throughout 7 years of follow-up. Treatment with PDT resulted in resolution of subretinal fluid and regression of choroidal neovascularization (Frennesson et al. 2014).

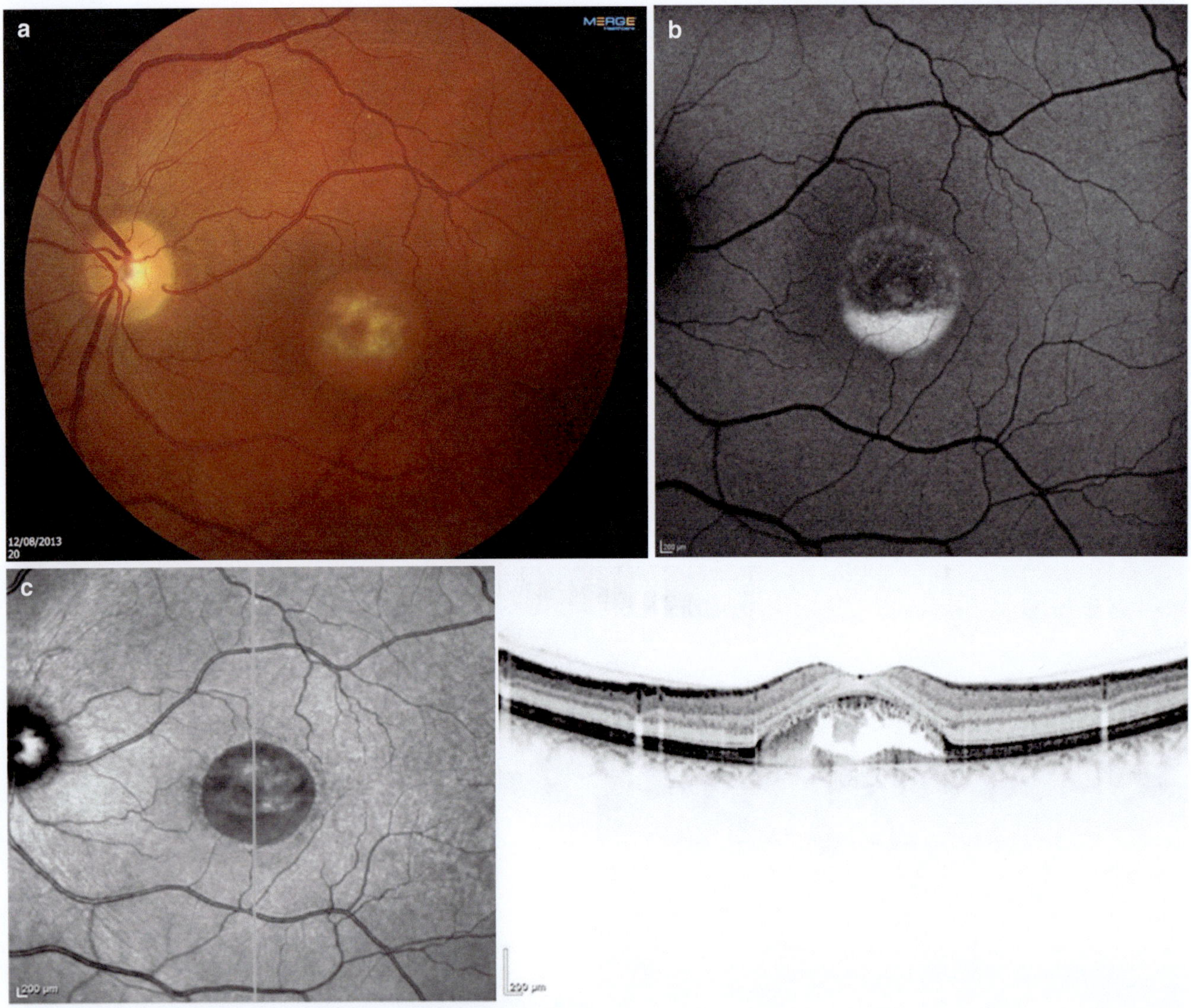

Fig. 2.2 Pseudohypopyon (stage 5). (**a**) Fundus photograph. (**b**) Fundus autofluorescence showing inferior hyperfluorescence. (**c**) Macular OCT demonstrating cross-section through pseudohypopyon

Future Treatment

Gene therapy is a promising treatment for inherited retinal dystrophy and other genetic diseases. Canine multifocal retinopathy (CMR) displays the full spectrum of clinical and molecular features observed in human bestrophinopathies and serves a valuable disease model for the development and testing of therapeutic strategies. Using this disease model, Guziewicz et al reported transfer of recombinant AAV (deno-associated virus) - mediated BEST1 to RPE was safe, specific and stable, thus should be considered for further development of gene augmentation therapies in bestrophinopathies (Guziewicz et al. 2013).

Autosomal Recessive Bestrophinopathy

Autosomal recessive bestrophinopathy (ARB), a phenotypic spectrum associated with *BEST1* mutation, is characterized by progressive reduction in central vision, marked FAF changes, absence of EOG light rise and reduced full-field ERGs. Vitelliform lesions are not typical of ARB. A spectrum of fundus abnormalities is observed in ARB including multifocal yellowish subretinal deposits, subretinal fibrous scars and cystoid intraretinal fluid collections in the macula (Burgess et al. 2008; Boon et al. 2013). ARB is caused by either compound heterozygous or homozygous *BEST1* mutations (Burgess et al. 2008; Boon et al. 2009).

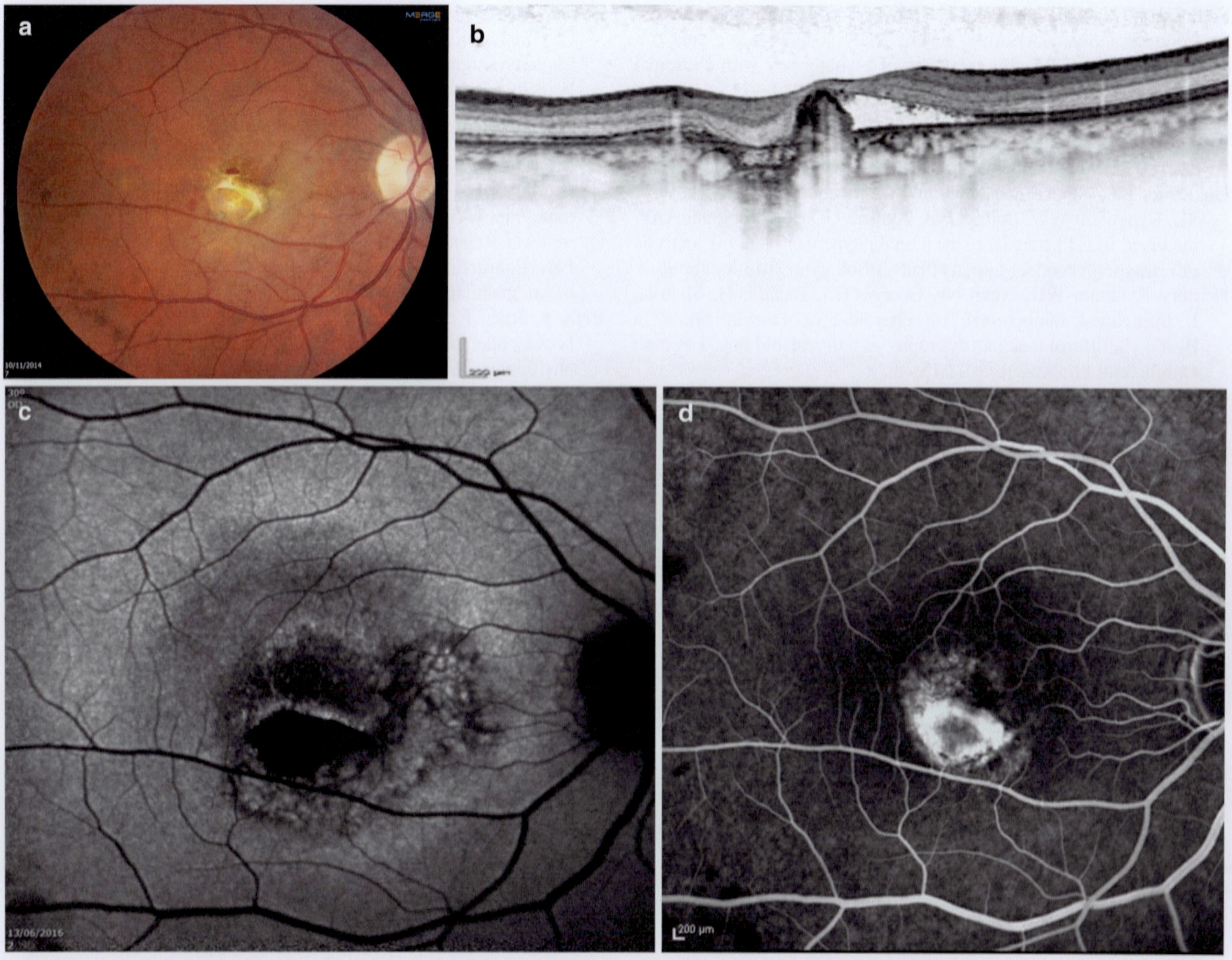

Fig. 2.3 Atrophic/neovascular (stage 6). (**a**) Fundus photograph showing RPE changes, retinal scarring and macular hemorrhage. (**b**) Macular OCT showing disruption of the RPE, atrophic changes and associated subretinal fluid (c) Fundus autofluorescence showing macular hypofluorescence. (d) Fluorescein angiogram showing macular leakage in the late venous phase due to choroidal neovascularization

References

Best F. Ubereine hereditare Maculaaffektion. Beitrage zur Vererbungslehre. Z Augenheilkd. 1905;13:199–212.

Booij JC, Boon CJ, Van Schooneveld MJ, Ten Brink JB, Bakker A, De Jong PT, Hoyng CB, Bergen AA, Klaver CC. Course of visual decline in relation to the Best1 genotype in vitelliform macular dystrophy. Ophthalmology. 2010;117:1415–22.

Boon CJ, Jeroen Klevering B, Keunen JE, Hoyng CB, Theelen T. Fundus autofluorescence imaging of retinal dystrophies. Vis Res. 2008;48:2569–77.

Boon CJ, Klevering BJ, Leroy BP, Hoyng CB, Keunen JE, Den Hollander AI. The spectrum of ocular phenotypes caused by mutations in the BEST1 gene. Prog Retin Eye Res. 2009;28:187–205.

Boon CJ, Van Den Born LI, Visser L, Keunen JE, Bergen AA, Booij JC, Riemslag FC, Florijn RJ, Van Schooneveld MJ. Autosomal recessive bestrophinopathy: differential diagnosis and treatment options. Ophthalmology. 2013;120:809–20.

Budiene B, Liutkeviciene R, Zaliuniene D. Best vitelliform macular dystrophy: literature review. Cent Eur J Med. 2014;9:784–95.

Burgess R, Millar ID, Leroy BP, Urquhart JE, Fearon IM, De Baere E, Brown PD, Robson AG, Wright GA, Kestelyn P, Holder GE, Webster AR, Manson FD, Black GC. Biallelic mutation of BEST1 causes a distinct retinopathy in humans. Am J Hum Genet. 2008;82:19–31.

Chaudhary KM, Mititelu M, Lieberman RM. An evidence-based review of vascular endothelial growth factor inhibition in pediatric retinal diseases: part 2. Coats' disease, best disease, and uveitis with childhood neovascularization. J Pediatr Ophthalmol Strabismus. 2013;50:11–9.

Clemons TE, Milton RC, Klein R, Seddon JM, Ferris FL 3rd. Risk factors for the incidence of advanced age-related macular degeneration in the age-related eye disease study (AREDS) AREDS report no. 19. Ophthalmology. 2005;112:533–9.

Davidson AE, Millar ID, Urquhart JE, Burgess-Mullan R, Shweikh Y, Parry N, O'Sullivan J, Maher GJ, Mckibbin M, Downes SM, Lotery AJ, Jacobson SG, Brown PD, Black GC, Manson FD. Missense mutations in a retinal pigment epithelium protein, bestrophin-1, cause retinitis pigmentosa. Am J Hum Genet. 2009;85:581–92.

Deutman A. The hereditary dystrophies of the posterior pole of the eye. Assen: Van Gorcum & Co.; 1971.

Francois J, De Rouck A, Fernandez-Sasso D. Electro-oculography in vitelliform degeneration of the macula. Arch Ophthalmol. 1967;77:726–33.

Frangieh G, Green WR, Fine SL. A histopathologic study of Best's macular dystrophy. Arch Ophthalmol. 1982;100:1115–21.

Frennesson CI, Wadelius C, Nilsson SE. Best vitelliform macular dystrophy in a Swedish family: genetic analysis and a seven-year follow-up of photodynamic treatment of a young boy with choroidal neovascularization. Acta Ophthalmol. 2014;92:238–42.

Glybina IV, Frank RN. Localization of multifocal electroretinogram abnormalities to the lesion site: findings in a family with Best disease. Arch Ophthalmol. 2006;124:1593–600.

Guziewicz KE, Zangerl B, Komaromy AM, Iwabe S, Chiodo VA, Boye SL, Hauswirth WW, Beltran WA, Aguirre GD. Recombinant AAV-mediated BEST1 transfer to the retinal pigment epithelium: analysis of serotype-dependent retinal effects. PLoS One. 2013;8:e75666.

Heidary F, Hitam WH, Ngah NF, George TM, Hashim H, Shatriah I. Intravitreal ranibizumab for choroidal neovascularization in Best's vitelliform macular dystrophy in a 6-year-old boy. J Pediatr Ophthalmol Strabismus. 2011;15:48.

Leu J, Schrage NF, Degenring RF. Choroidal neovascularisation secondary to Best's disease in a 13-year-old boy treated by intravitreal bevacizumab. Graefes Arch Clin Exp Ophthalmol. 2007;245:1723–5.

Macdonald I, Lee T. Best vitelliform macular dystrophy [Online]. Seattle: University of Washington; 1993–2017. https://www.ncbi.nlm.nih.gov/books/NBK1167/. Accessed 16 Aug 2017.

Marano F, Deutman AF, Leys A, Aandekerk AL. Hereditary retinal dystrophies and choroidal neovascularization. Graefes Arch Clin Exp Ophthalmol. 2000;238:760–4.

Marmorstein AD, Marmorstein LY, Rayborn M, Wang X, Hollyfield JG, Petrukhin K. Bestrophin, the product of the Best vitelliform macular dystrophy gene (VMD2), localizes to the basolateral plasma membrane of the retinal pigment epithelium. Proc Natl Acad Sci U S A. 2000;97:12758–63.

Marmorstein AD, Cross HE, Peachey NS. Functional roles of bestrophins in ocular epithelia. Prog Retin Eye Res. 2009;28:206–26.

Michaelides M, Hunt DM, Moore AT. The genetics of inherited macular dystrophies. J Med Genet. 2003;40:641–50.

Miller SA, Bresnick GH, Chandra SR. Choroidal neovascular membrane in Best's vitelliform macular dystrophy. Am J Ophthalmol. 1976;82:252–5.

Petrukhin K, Koisti MJ, Bakall B, Li W, Xie G, Marknell T, Sandgren O, Forsman K, Holmgren G, Andreasson S, Vujic M, Bergen AA, Mcgarty-Dugan V, Figueroa D, Austin CP, Metzker ML, Caskey CT, Wadelius C. Identification of the gene responsible for Best macular dystrophy. Nat Genet. 1998;19:241–7.

Pianta MJ, Aleman TS, Cideciyan AV, Sunness JS, Li Y, Campochiaro BA, Campochiaro PA, Zack DJ, Stone EM, Jacobson SG. In vivo micropathology of Best macular dystrophy with optical coherence tomography. Exp Eye Res. 2003;76:203–11.

Querques G, Regenbogen M, Quijano C, Delphin N, Soubrane G, Souied EH. High-definition optical coherence tomography features in vitelliform macular dystrophy. Am J Ophthalmol. 2008;146:501–7.

Rishi E, Rishi P, Mahajan S. Intravitreal bevacizumab for choroidal neovascular membrane associated with Best's vitelliform dystrophy. Indian J Ophthalmol. 2010;58:160–2.

Rosenthal R, Bakall B, Kinnick T, Peachey N, Wimmers S, Wadelius C, Marmorstein A, Strauss O. Expression of bestrophin-1, the product of the VMD2 gene, modulates voltage-dependent Ca2+ channels in retinal pigment epithelial cells. FASEB J. 2006;20:178–80.

Shibuya Y, Hayasaka S. Various fundus manifestations in a Japanese family with Best's vitelliform macular dystrophy. Jpn J Ophthalmol. 1993;37:478–84.

Skoog KO, Nilsson SE. The c-wave of the electroretinogram in vitelliruptive macular degeneration (alvdalssjukan). Acta Ophthalmol. 1981;59:756–8.

Testa F, Rossi S, Passerini I, Sodi A, Di Iorio V, Interlandi E, Della Corte M, Menchini U, Rinaldi E, Torricelli F, Simonelli F. A normal electro-oculography in a family affected by best disease with a novel spontaneous mutation of the BEST1 gene. Br J Ophthalmol. 2008;92:1467–70.

Wabbels B, Preising MN, Kretschmann U, Demmler A, Lorenz B. Genotype-phenotype correlation and longitudinal course in ten families with Best vitelliform macular dystrophy. Graefes Arch Clin Exp Ophthalmol. 2006;244:1453–66.

Weingeist TA, Kobrin JL, Watzke RC. Histopathology of Best's macular dystrophy. Arch Ophthalmol. 1982;100:1108–14.

Yanoff M, Fine BS. Ocular pathology. St. Louis: Mosby; 2002.

X-Linked Retinoschisis

3

Eugene Yu-Chuan Kang and Nan-Kai Wang

Introduction

X-linked retinoschisis (XLRS, MIM 312700, also called X-linked juvenile retinoschisis) is an inherited vitreoretinal dystrophy that affects the macula of young men with the prevalence of 1:5000 to 1:25,000 (George et al. 1995; Retinoschisis Consortium 1998). Functional implications of the spectrum of mutations were found in 234 cases with XLRS (Retinoschisis Consortium 1998). XLRS was first described by Austrian ophthalmologist Josef Haas in 1898 (Haas 1898). He diagnosed two brothers with "Veränderungen der Retina und Choroidea," that is, radiating cystic maculopathy and peripheral choroidal atrophy (Fig. 3.1). Since then, this disease has been diagnosed using ophthalmoscopy and has been mentioned in the literature under a variety of names according to different clinical manifestations and etiologies. Thomson reported it as a "familial neuroretinal disease" for four males in 1932 (Thomson 1932), and Anderson helped diagnose a 2-year-old boy with an "anterior dialysis of the young" in the same year (Anderson 1932). In 1938, Mann and Macrae reported "congenital vascular veils in the vitreous" in three male patients and stated that this was different from the congenital retinal fold (Mann and Macrae 1938). In 1951, Magnus discovered an unusual detachment; the membrane was very thin and could have been part of the retina of a 14-year-old boy, which Magnus termed "congenital cystic retinal detachment" (Magnus 1951). Pagenstecher described the first family

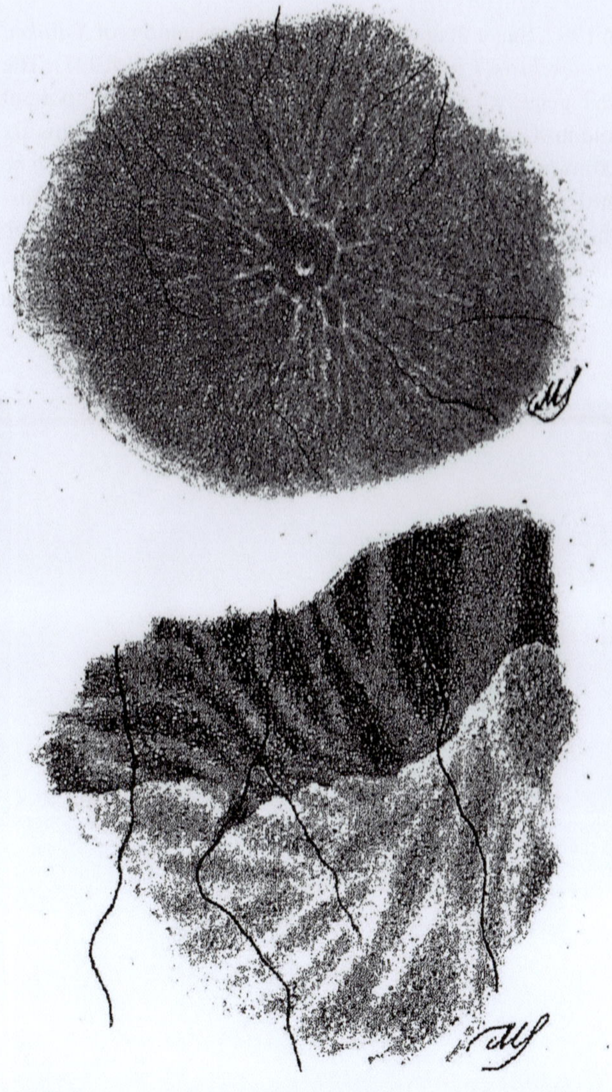

Fig. 3.1 The image shows the first XLRS feature described by Haas in 1898. It shows a cartwheel pattern around the fovea and peripheral retinal splitting

E. Y.-C. Kang
Department of Ophthalmology, Chang Gung Memorial Hospital, Linkou Medical Center, Taoyuan, Taiwan

College of Medicine, Chang Gung University, Taoyuan, Taiwan

N.-K. Wang (✉)
Department of Ophthalmology, Chang Gung Memorial Hospital, Linkou Medical Center, Taoyuan, Taiwan

College of Medicine, Chang Gung University, Taoyuan, Taiwan

Department of Ophthalmology, Edward S. Harkness Eye Institute, Columbia University, New York, USA

G. Cheung (ed.), *Hereditary Chorioretinal Disorders*, Retina Atlas, https://doi.org/10.1007/978-981-15-0414-3_3

with an X-chromosomal transmission pattern in 1913 (Pagenstecher 1913), and Wilczek first coined the term "retinoschisis" (schisis: cleavage) in 1935 (Wilczek 1935). In 1953, Jager coined the term "X-linked retinoschisis" for this disease (Jager 1953). In the 1960s, abnormal electroretinograms (ERGs) (Forsius et al. 1963) and b/a ratio (Hirose et al. 1977; Krill 1977) were found in almost all cases with XLRS. Since then, ERGs have played an important role in the diagnosis of XLRS, which shows electronegative ERGs. Recently, family members with XLRS were reported to have more phenotypic variability due to the availability of genetic abnormality.

Pathogenesis

In 1997, Sauer diagnosed a patient with mutations of *X-linked retinoschisis-1 gene*, or the *RS1* gene (Sauer et al. 1997). The *RS1* gene, which is located on Xp22.2, plays an important role in XLRS (Sauer et al. 1997). The *RS1* gene contains six exons and produces a 700-base transcript, which can then be further translated to a 224-amino acid protein, called retinoschisin (Sauer et al. 1997; Hu et al. 2017; Grayson et al. 2000). The protein was thought to have cell adhesion and to be able to maintain the structural integrity of the retina (Retinoschisis Consortium 1998; Grayson et al. 2000; Wu and Molday 2003; Wu et al. 2005). Mutation of the *RS1* gene impairs cell–cell interaction and results in the degeneration of photoreceptors and schisis formation (Kirsch et al. 1996; Sauer et al. 1997). Examples of mutations related to XLRS include missense, nonsense, deletion, and frame shifting (Weber and Kellner 2007). The missense mutation was the leading cause of the disease and caused several ocular complications (Hu et al. 2017; Retinoschisis Consortium 1998). Although the mutations and the pathogenesis of XLRS have been thoroughly investigated, the correlation between the genotype and the phenotype remains unclear (Eksandh et al. 2000; Renner et al. 2008; Riveiro-Alvarez et al. 2009; Hewitt et al. 2005; Vincent et al. 2013), and their variability is wide (Hu et al. 2017; Wang et al. 2015).

Clinical Features

Patients with XLRS usually present with decreased visual acuity, with other symptoms such as amblyopia, leukocoria (Fig. 3.2), strabismus, vitreous hemorrhage (Fig. 3.3), and neovascular glaucoma. Even though it mostly affects young men (George et al. 1996), some studies have discovered

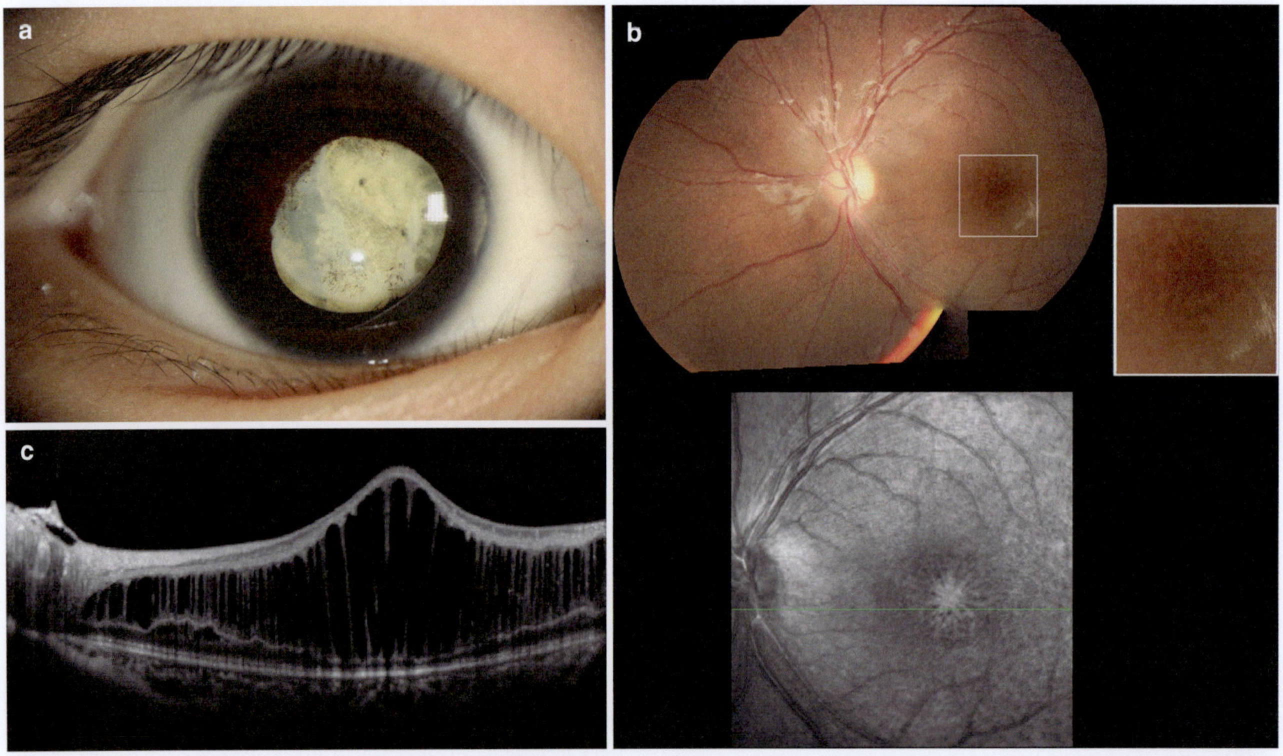

Fig. 3.2 A 4-year-old boy with an initial impression of Coats' disease at birth was diagnosed ultimately with XLRS. (**a**) Image of the patient's right eye showed his lens completely opacified. (**b**) A typical cartwheel pattern around the fovea was found in a color fundus image, and the cartwheel pattern was more prominent in the near-infrared (NIR) image. (**c**) A foveolamellar schisis was seen in the OCT of the left eye. (Images reprinted with permission from NK Wang, 2015, *Clinical presentations of X-linked retinoschisis in Taiwanese patients confirmed with genetic sequencing*, © 2015 Molecular Vision)

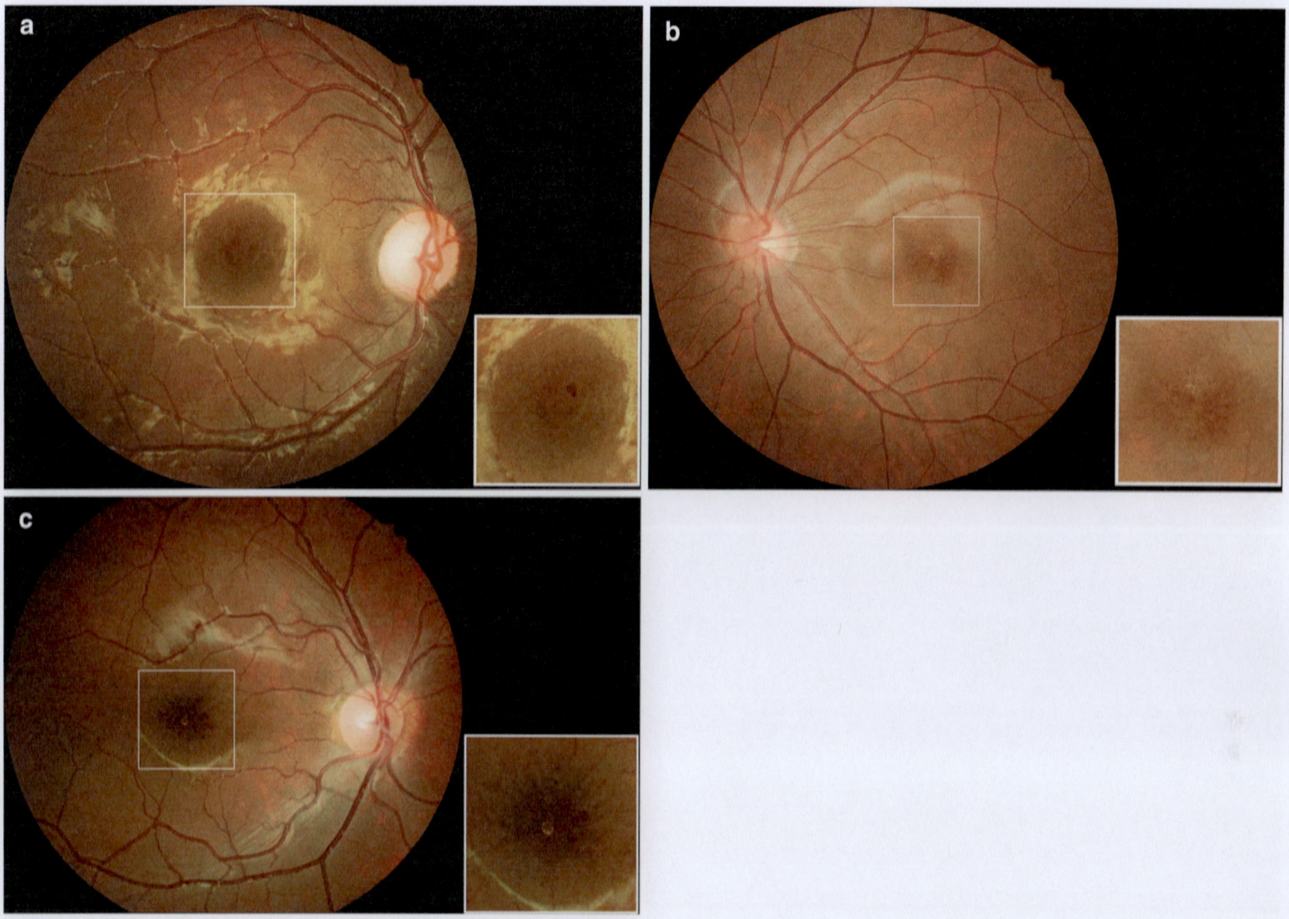

Fig. 3.3 The typical cartwheel-like appearance in the fundus images in (**a**) a 4-year-old, (**b**) a 12-year-old, and (**c**) an 8-year-old

retinal lesion could be present even at birth (Lee et al. 2009; Prasad et al. 2006; Renner et al. 2008). In the advanced stage of the disease, choroidal sclerosis, retinal detachment, and retinal atrophy are present (Tantri et al. 2004; Grayson et al. 2000). Female carriers are mostly asymptomatic, but minor retinal abnormality may be present (Kim et al. 2007). Foveal schisis is most commonly found in young individuals with XLRS (Kellner et al. 1990) with macular atrophy or retinal pigment epithelium (RPE) irregularities in later years (Forsius et al. 1973; George et al. 1996). However, its fundus appearance varies widely, especially in older patients, who are more challenging to identify if XLRS is present. Young patients may also present with lens opacity that mimics other congenital ophthalmic disorders (Wang et al. 2015) (Fig. 3.2). Hence, XLRS should be suspected as one of the differential diagnoses in patients with unsatisfactory best-corrected vision from childhood. For accurate diagnosis, combined examinations of fundus autofluorescence, optical coherence tomography, ERG, and molecular genetic testing have been suggested (Renner et al. 2008). Visual acuity in XLRS patients has a wide variability, although the vision is usually less than 20/100 (Forsius et al. 1973; Roesch et al. 1998).

Color Fundus Imaging

Hass first discovered the typical fundus presentation of XLRS in 1898, which includes radiating cystic maculopathy and peripheral retinal splitting (Fig. 3.1) (Haas 1898). This typical spoke- or cartwheel-like pattern in the macula area is a feature of XLRS fundus (Figs. 3.2, 3.3, 3.4, and 3.5) and near-infrared (NIR) images (Fig. 3.2). Retinal splitting with and without retinal pigmentation can be seen using montage or ultrawide fundus imaging (Figs. 3.6 and 3.7). Some patients have vitreous hemorrhage, subretinal fibrosis, a golden yellow reflection, or white dots in the posterior fundus mimicking fundus albipunctatus (Figs. 3.4, 3.5, 3.7, 3.8, and 3.9). The macular pigment changes (Fig. 3.8) that mimic maculopathy and diffused pigments (Fig. 3.8) can be seen in older patients with XLRS.

Fundus Autofluorescence (FAF)

FAF is a useful tool in retinal degeneration and dystrophy. Typical FAF feature of XLRS is a spoke-like pattern (Fig. 3.4) of hyper- and hypo-AF in the macula area due to

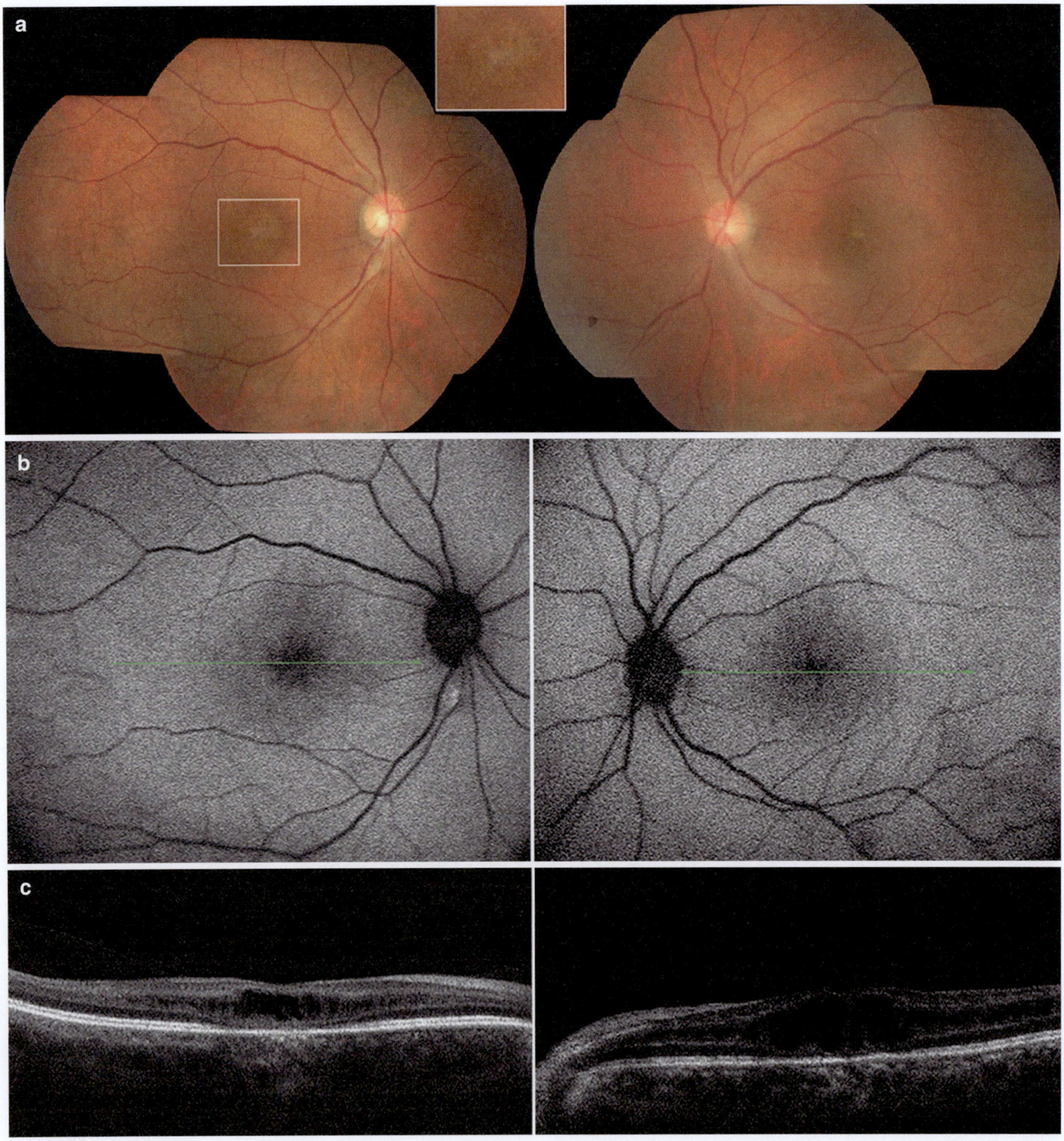

Fig. 3.4 Images of a 56-year-old male with poor night vision since childhood. He underwent cataract surgery but vision did not improve much. (**a**) Color fundus images showed cartwheel-like patterns around the fovea and a reduced foveal reflex in both eyes. (**b**) FAF revealed a spoke-like pattern around the macula. (**c**) OCT revealed foveal atrophy in the right eye and cystoid macula edema in the left eye (central retina thickness: OD: 183 μm, and OS: 359 μm)

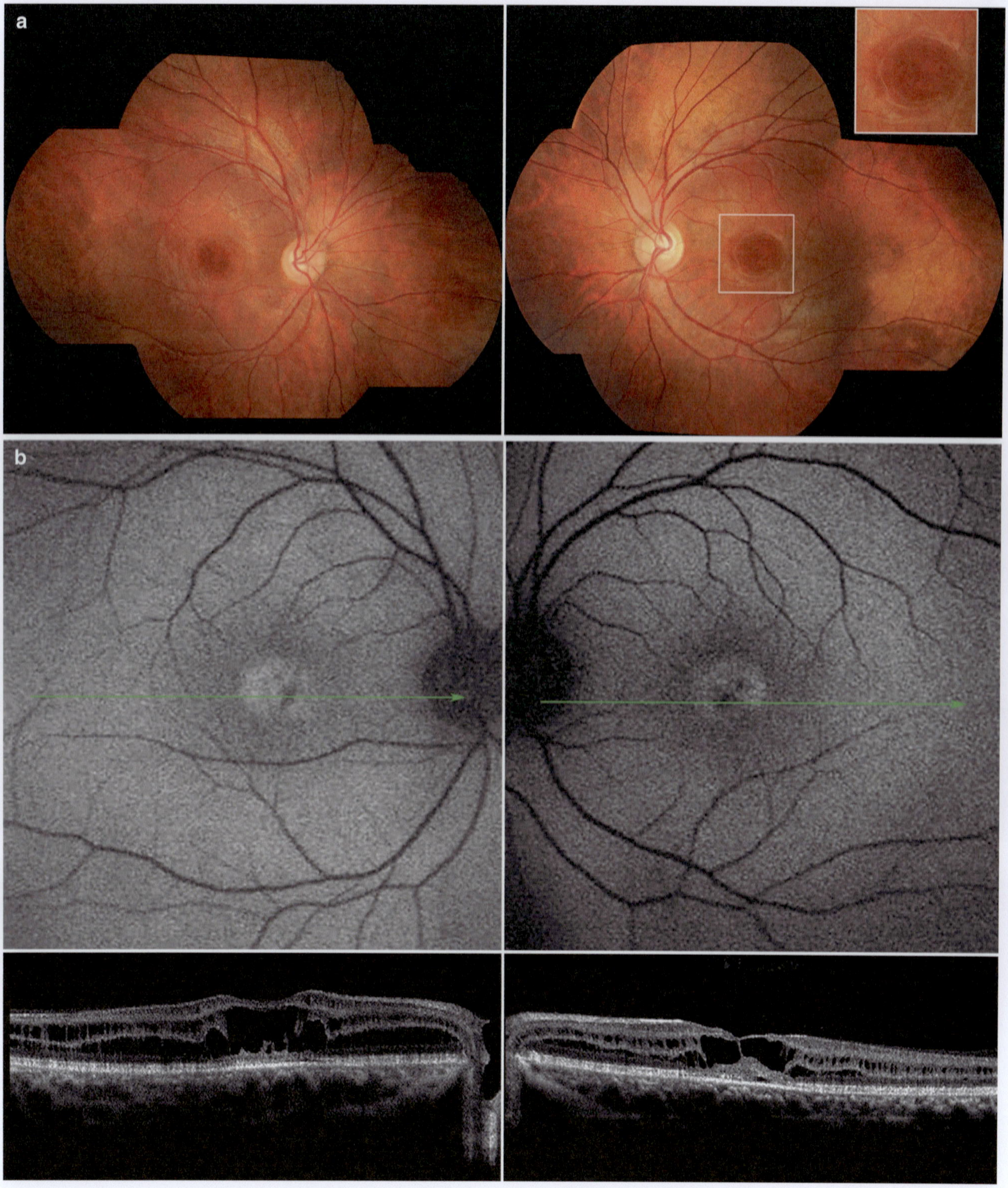

Fig. 3.5 Images of a 22-year-old male with amblyopia. His best-corrected vision was OD: 20/200 and OS: 20/200. (**a**) Color fundus images showed cartwheel-like patterns around the fovea and a golden yellow reflection at the temporal retina. (Images reprinted with permission from NK Wang, 2015, *Clinical presentations of X-linked retinoschisis in Taiwanese patients confirmed with genetic sequencing*, © 2015 Molecular Vision.) (**b**) OCT revealed foveolamellar schisis in both eyes, a lamellar hole in the left eye, and an increase in thickness of the fovea in the right eye. FAF showed concentric areas of hyper-AF

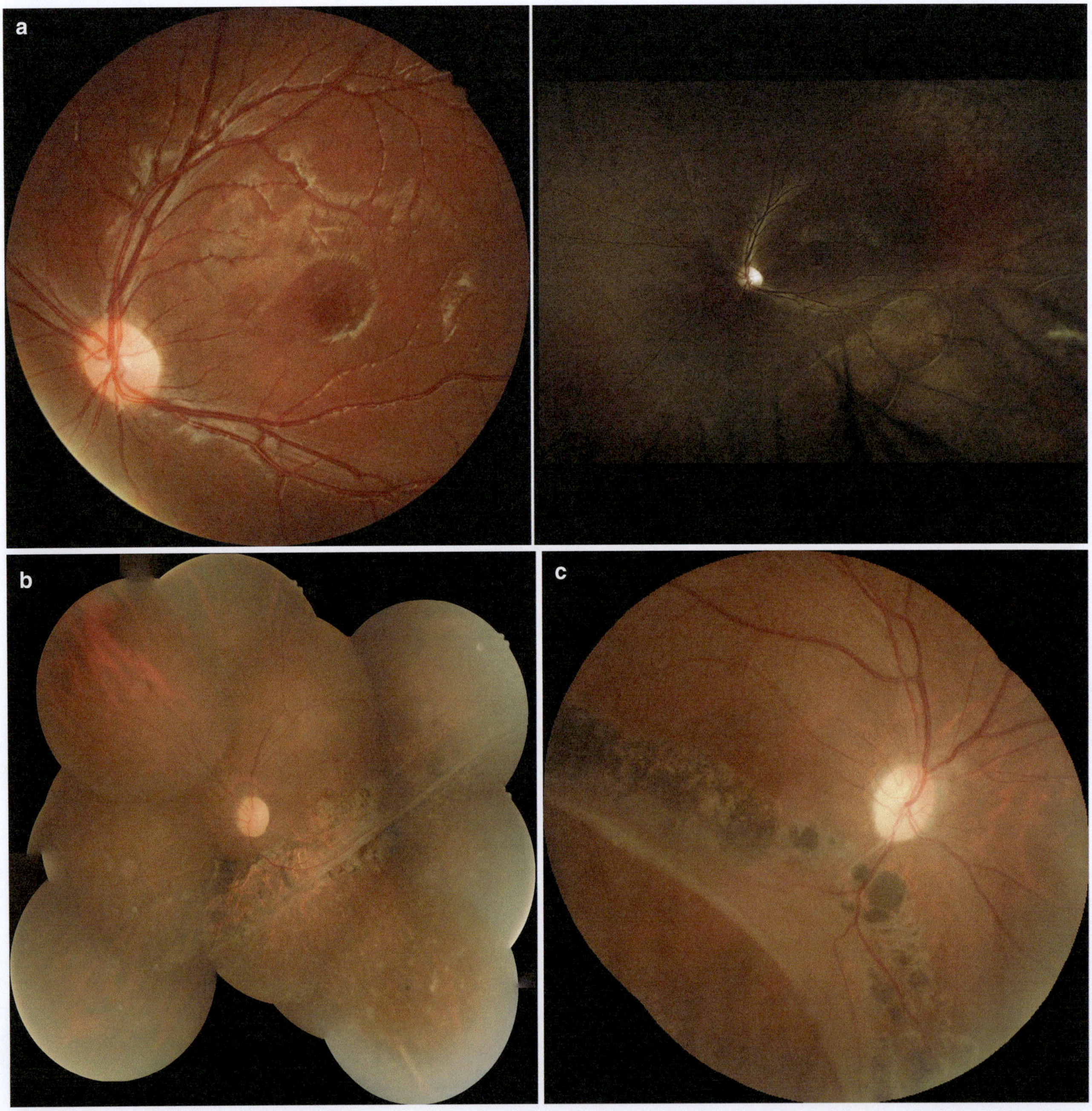

Fig. 3.6 (**a**) Color fundus and Optos images of a 7-year-old boy with XLRS. An inferior retinal schisis can be easily seen in the Optos image. (**b**) Image of a 41-year-old male shows retinal splitting across the macula and white dots at the inferior temporal retina. (Images reprinted with permission from NK Wang, 2015, *Clinical presentations of X-linked retinoschisis in Taiwanese patients confirmed with genetic sequencing*, © 2015 Molecular Vision.) (**c**) Retinal splitting in a 38-year-old male. (**d**) Bullous retinoschisis approaching the arcade with a laser scar in a 5-year-old boy

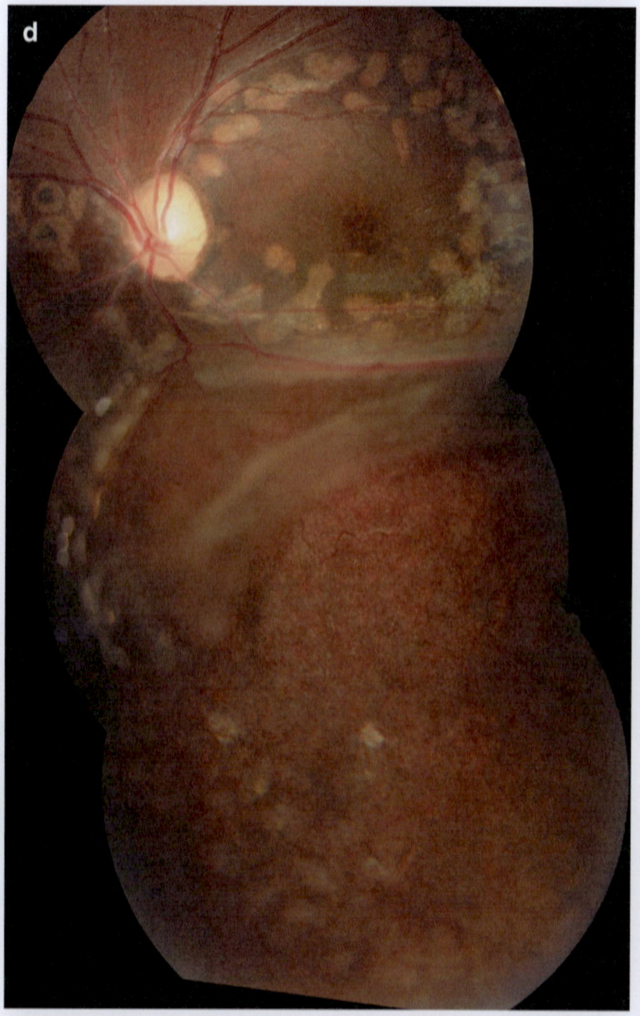

Fig. 3.6 (continued)

altered light transmission in the area of retinoschisis (Molday et al. 2012). Some patients may have irregular hyper-AF (Fig. 3.7), irregular hypo-AF (Fig. 3.9), and concentric hyper-AF (Figs. 3.5 and 3.10). These FAF findings are not specific features of XLRS and need to be differentiated from other maculopathies or retinal dystrophies.

Optical Coherence Tomography (OCT)

Stanga et al. first demonstrated a cleavage plane in the neural retina using OCT (Stanga et al. 2001). Prenner et al. proposed a classification system based on clinical examination and OCT (Prenner et al. 2006). Lesch et al. further modified that system and divided XLRS into six cystic subtypes and one atrophic type (Table 3.1) (Lesch et al. 2008). Typical OCT findings of XLRS include foveal cystic schisis (Figs. 3.2, 3.5, and 3.10), as well as intraretinal cysts without the increased thickness of the macula (Figs. 3.10 and 3.11), a lamellar macular hole (Fig. 3.11), and foveal atrophy (Figs. 3.4 and 3.7). Spectral-domain or swept-source OCT is a simple and quick examination to evaluate the macula status in young patients when dilated ophthalmoscopy, FAF, whereas ERG may not be easy to perform.

Previous reports have shown that cystic macular lesions in XLRS may spontaneously resolve and further form an atrophic macular lesion which can be detected on OCT scans (George et al. 1995, 1996). Carbonic anhydrase inhibitors have been reported to be effective in improving cystoid macular edema in patients with XLRS (Thobani and Fishman 2011; Khandhadia et al. 2011; Genead et al. 2010; Walia et al. 2009; Wang et al. 2015). However, even though some patients had positive responses to topical dorzolamide, their vision did not improve significantly (Fig. 3.12).

Fluorescein Angiography (FA)

FA in XLRS is characterized as non-FA leakage cystoid macula edema (Fig. 3.10). Other diseases share this feature, including enhanced S-cone syndrome (Goldmann–Favre syndrome), nicotinic acid maculopathy, and optic pit. Even though FA is not a necessary examination for diagnosing XLRS, physicians should be aware of the possibility of XLRS in patients with non-FA leakage cystoid macula edema.

Electroretinography (ERG)

A typical feature of ERGs in XLRS is a "negative ERG" (Fig. 3.13) due to a marked reduction in the b-wave's amplitude, which results in an abnormal b/a ratio (Vincent et al. 2013; Hirose et al. 1977). A wider range of ERG abnormalities is associated with the missense mutation of the *RS1* gene (Vincent et al. 2013). Several studies have reported that negative ERG was only found in 50–60% of XLRS patients (Renner et al. 2008; Wang et al. 2015). Therefore, a normal b/a ratio cannot exclude the diagnosis of XLRS (Fig. 3.14). In addition, a multifocal ERG may show a widespread cone dysfunction (Piao et al. 2003).

Differential Diagnosis

XLRS is a heterogeneous disease, characterized by its X-linked inheritance, non-FA leakage cystoid macular edema, foveal schisis, and electronegative ERG.

The cystoid change and/or retinal schisis in the macula can also be found in some disorders such as diabetic macula edema, retinal vascular occlusion, nicotinic acid maculopathy (Gass 1973), high myopia with long axial length, enhanced

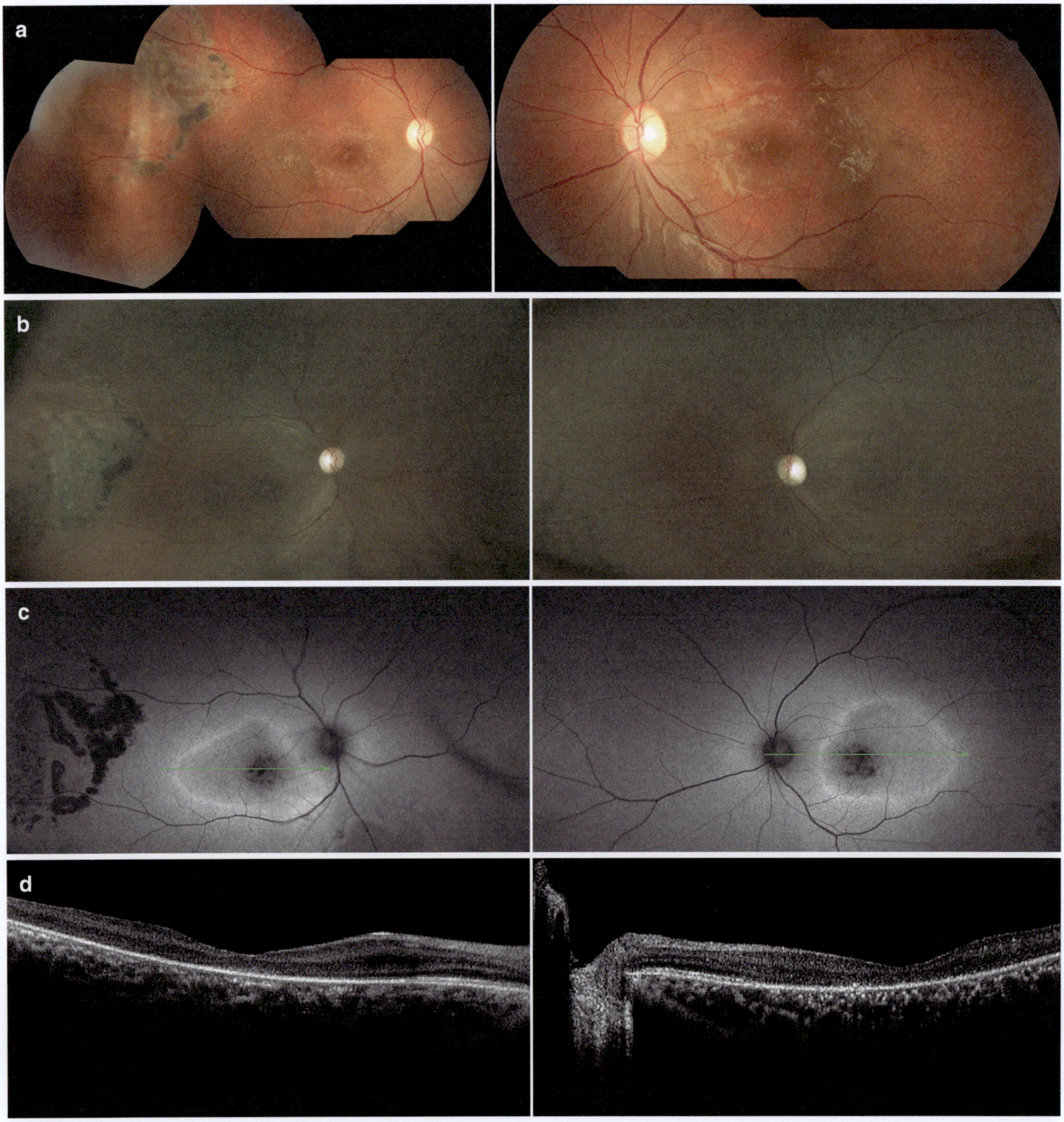

Fig. 3.7 A 26-year-old male patient with XLRS. His best-corrected vision was OD: 20/200 and OS: 20/200. (**a**) The color fundus montage shows peripheral retinal splitting in the right eye and scattered white pigments in both eyes. (**b**) The Optos image shows the change in the peripheral retinal splitting in one shot. (**c**) FAF revealed irregularly shaped areas of hyper- and hypo-AF. (**d**) OCT shows decreased retinal thickness in both eyes (central retina thickness: OD: 193 μm, OS: 190 μm)

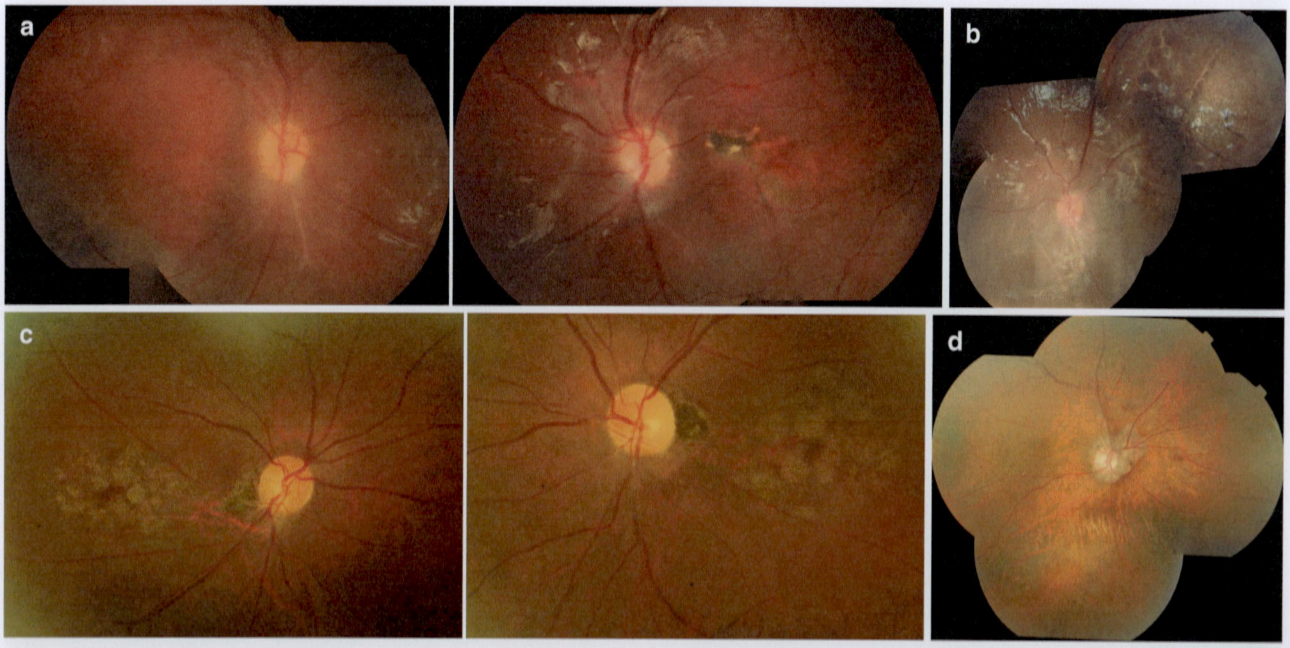

Fig. 3.8 (**a**) Vitreous hemorrhage was found in the right eye of an 18-year-old patient with XLRS. An atrophic lesion around the fovea was also found in his left eye. (**b**) Image of a 6-year-old boy with subretinal fibrosis and peripheral retinal splitting. (Images reprinted with permission from NK Wang, 2015, *Clinical presentations of X-linked retinoschisis in Taiwanese patients confirmed with genetic sequencing*, © 2015 Molecular Vision.) (**c**) Image of a 48-year-old male with macular RPE and photoreceptor atrophy in both eyes. (**d**) Image of a 72-year-old male with peripheral retinal pigmentation

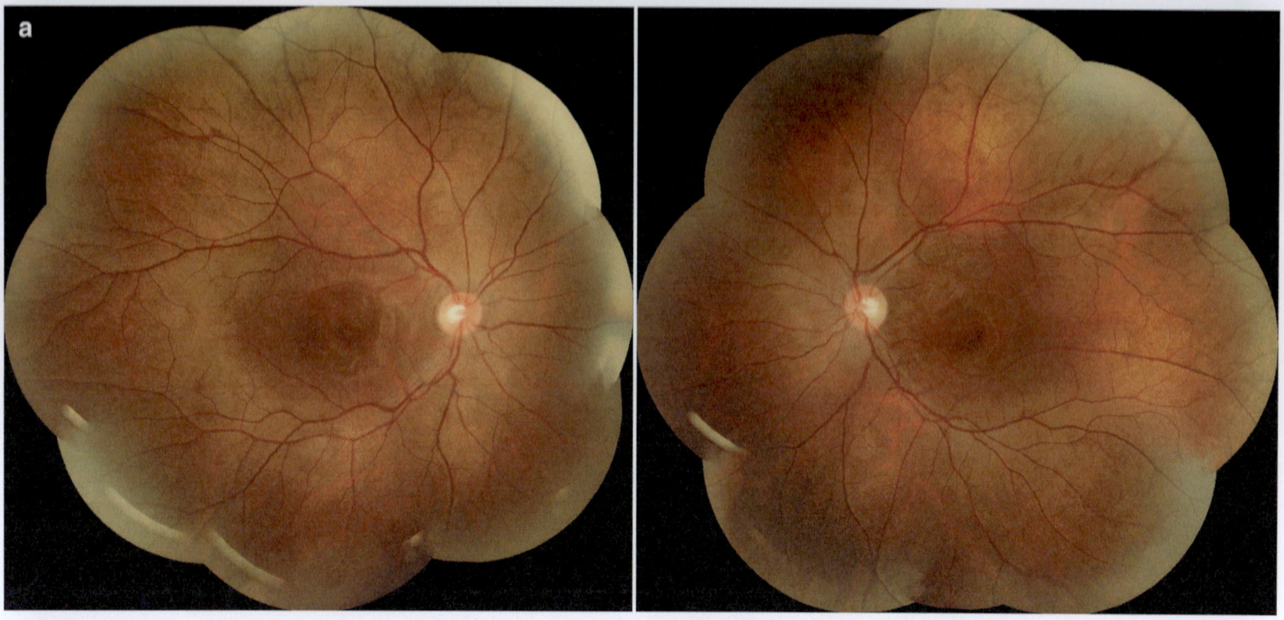

Fig. 3.9 (**a**) Fundus image of a 35-year-old male with a golden yellow reflection over the temporal retina. (**b**) FAF shows an irregular hypo-AF (right) and hyper-AF (left) area in the macula

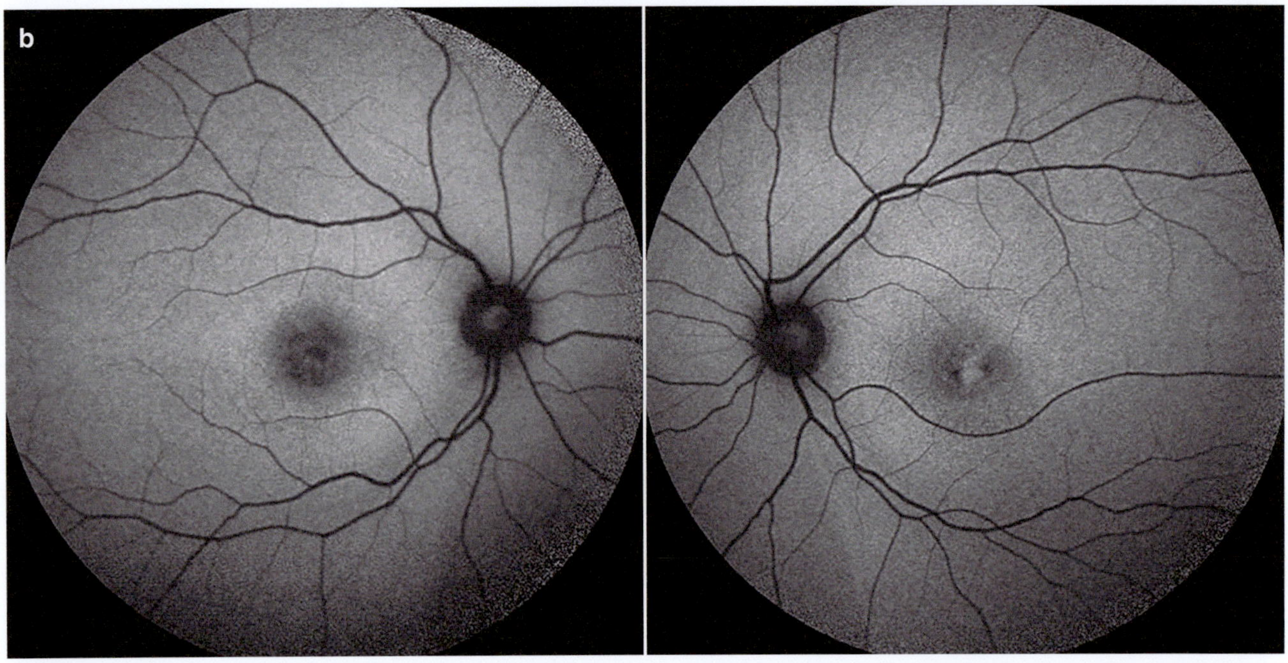

Fig. 3.9 (continued)

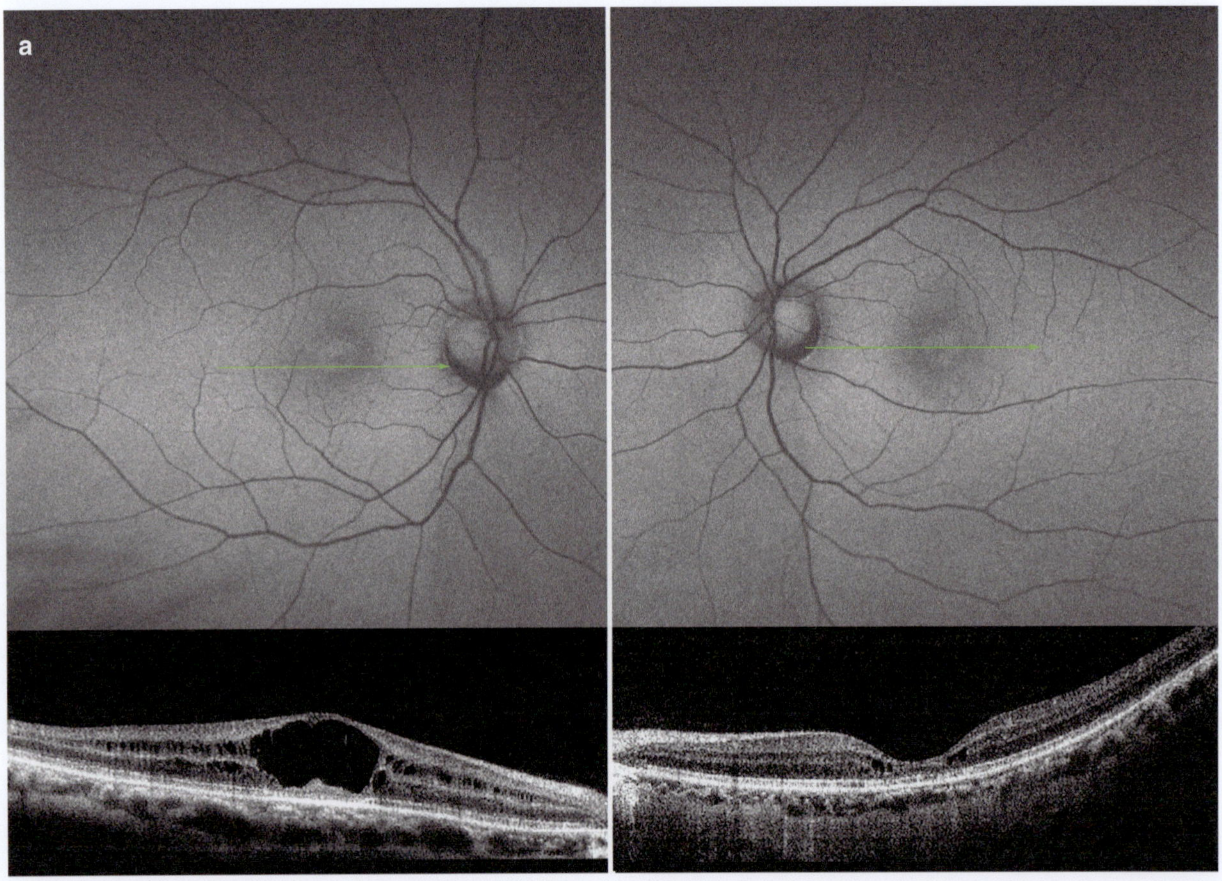

Fig. 3.10 Images of a 51-year-old male with XLRS. His initial best-corrected visual acuity was OD: 20/200 and OS: 20/70. (**a**) FAF showed concentric areas of hyper-AF in the right eye; OCT revealed intraretinal cysts in both eyes and lamellar retinal schisis in his right eye (central retina thickness: OD: 455 μm, OS: 173 μm). (**b**) Fluorescence angiography revealed no leakage in the central macula even though OCT showed intraretinal cysts

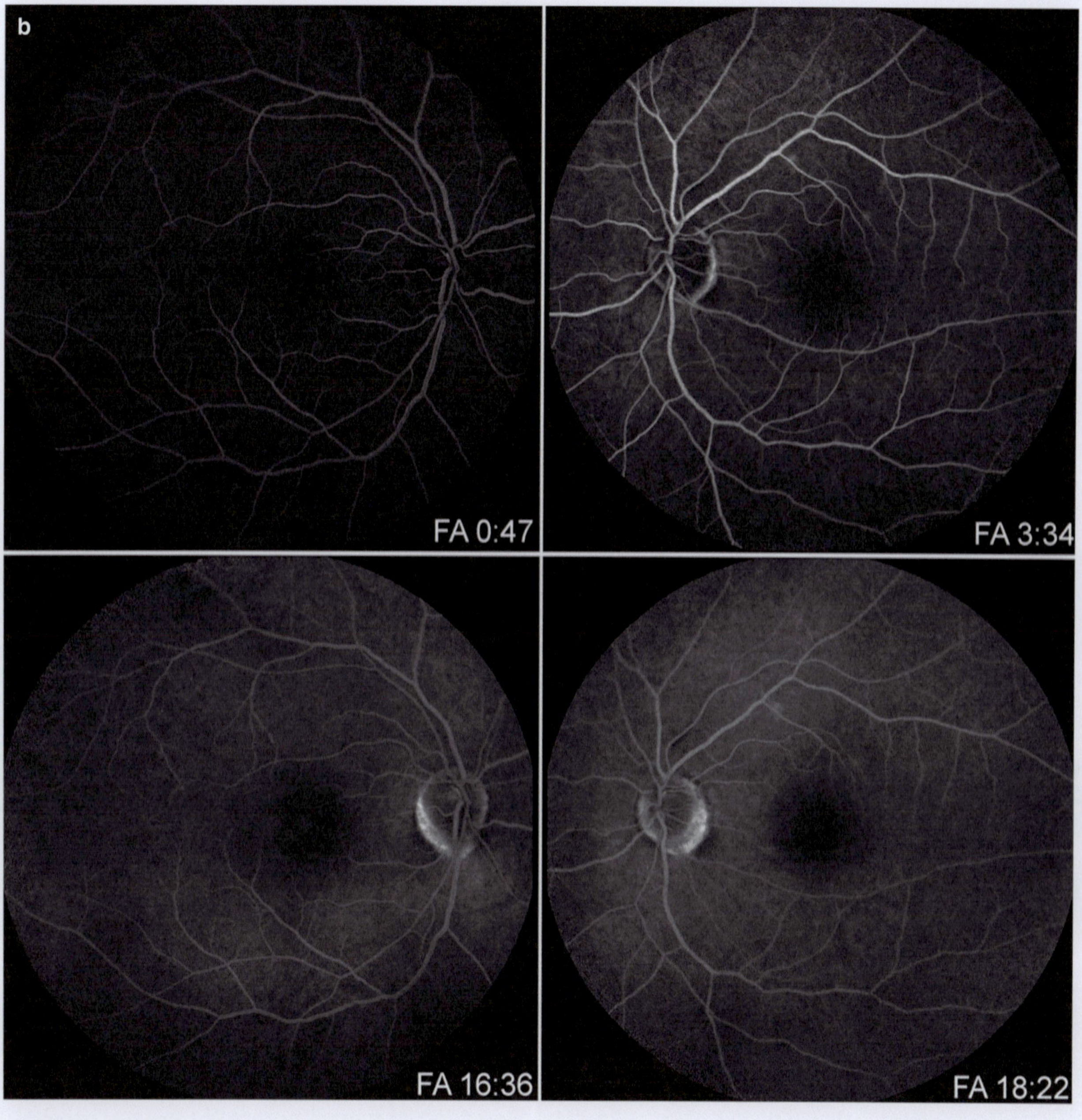

Fig. 3.10 (continued)

Table 3.1 Classification scheme of XLRS

XLRS form	Type	Foveal cystic schisis	Macular lamellar schisis	Peripheral schisis
Cystic	Type 1: fovea	+	–	–
	Type 2: lamellar	–	+	–
	Type 3: foveolamellar	+	+	–
	Type 4: complex	+	+	+
	Type 5: foveoperipheral	+	–	+
	Type 6: peripheral	–	–	+
Atrophic	Type 7: nonspecific	–	–	–

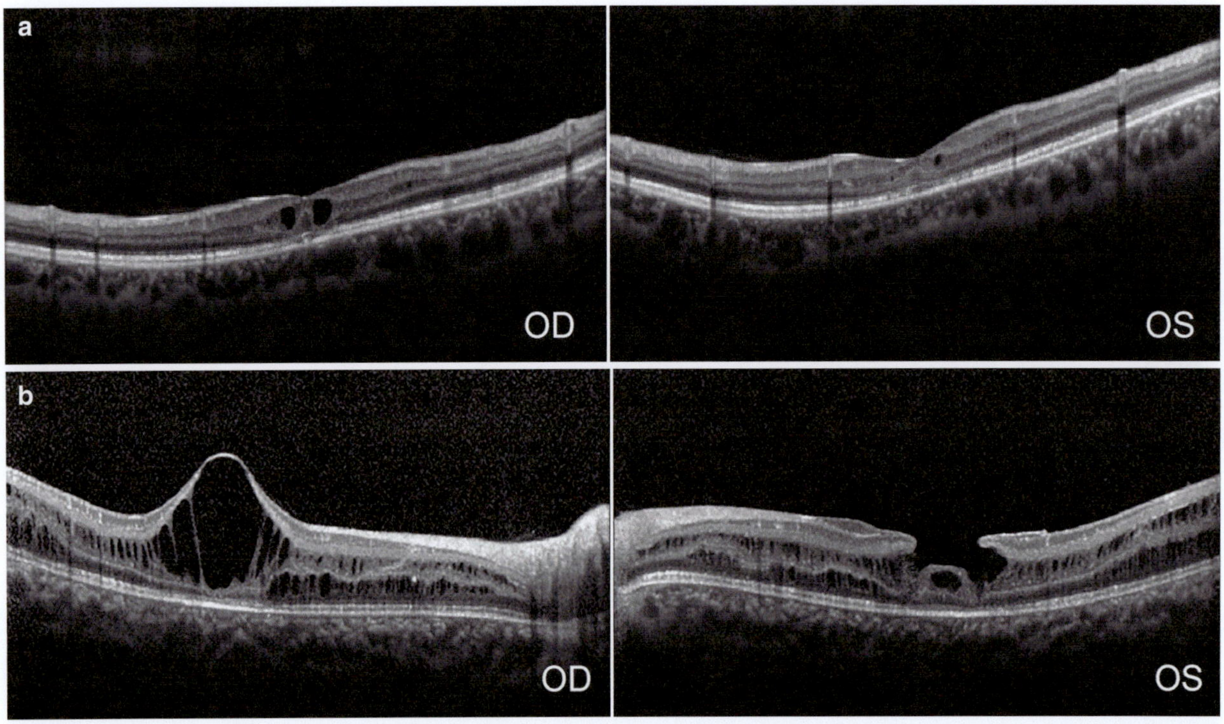

Fig. 3.11 (**a**) Images of a 30-year-old male with intraretinal cysts without increased thickness of the macula in both eyes. Central retina thickness was OD: 230 μm and OS: 220 μm. (**b**) Image of a 6-year-old boy with a lamellar macular hole in the left eye and foveal schisis in the right eye

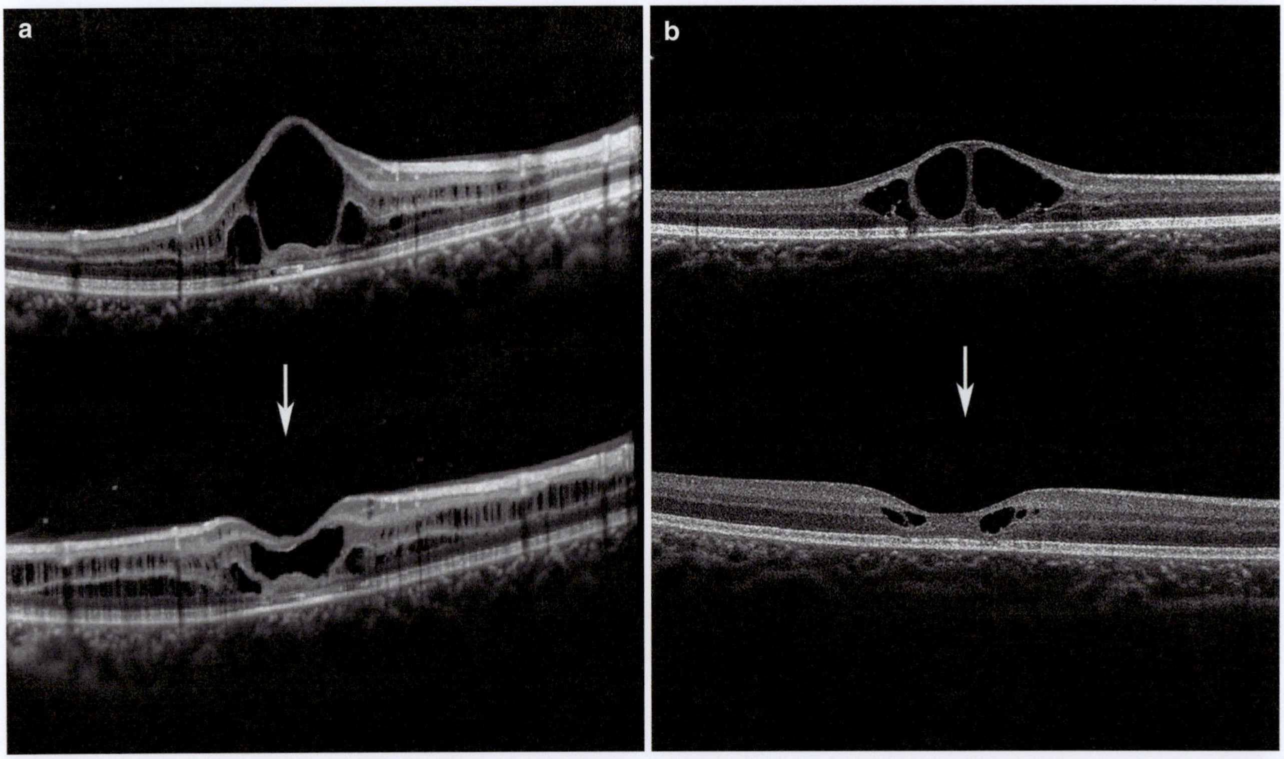

Fig. 3.12 Two eyes with XLRS received topical dorzolamide solution. Partial resolution of the foveal cysts and a decrease in the central foveal thickness were observed after the treatment, but with no significant improvement in vision. (**a**) Images of a 23-year-old male who received dorzolamide treatment for 5 months. After treatment, OCT of his right eye showed improvement of intraretinal cysts, and the central retinal thickness decreased from 609 to 388 μm. The vision was 20/200 before and after the treatment. (**b**) Images of an 8-year-old boy who received dorzolamide treatment for 7 months. OCT of his right eye showed a decrease of intraretinal cysts, and the central retinal thickness decreased from 471 to 214 μm. The initial visual acuity was 20/40, and this remained the same after the treatment

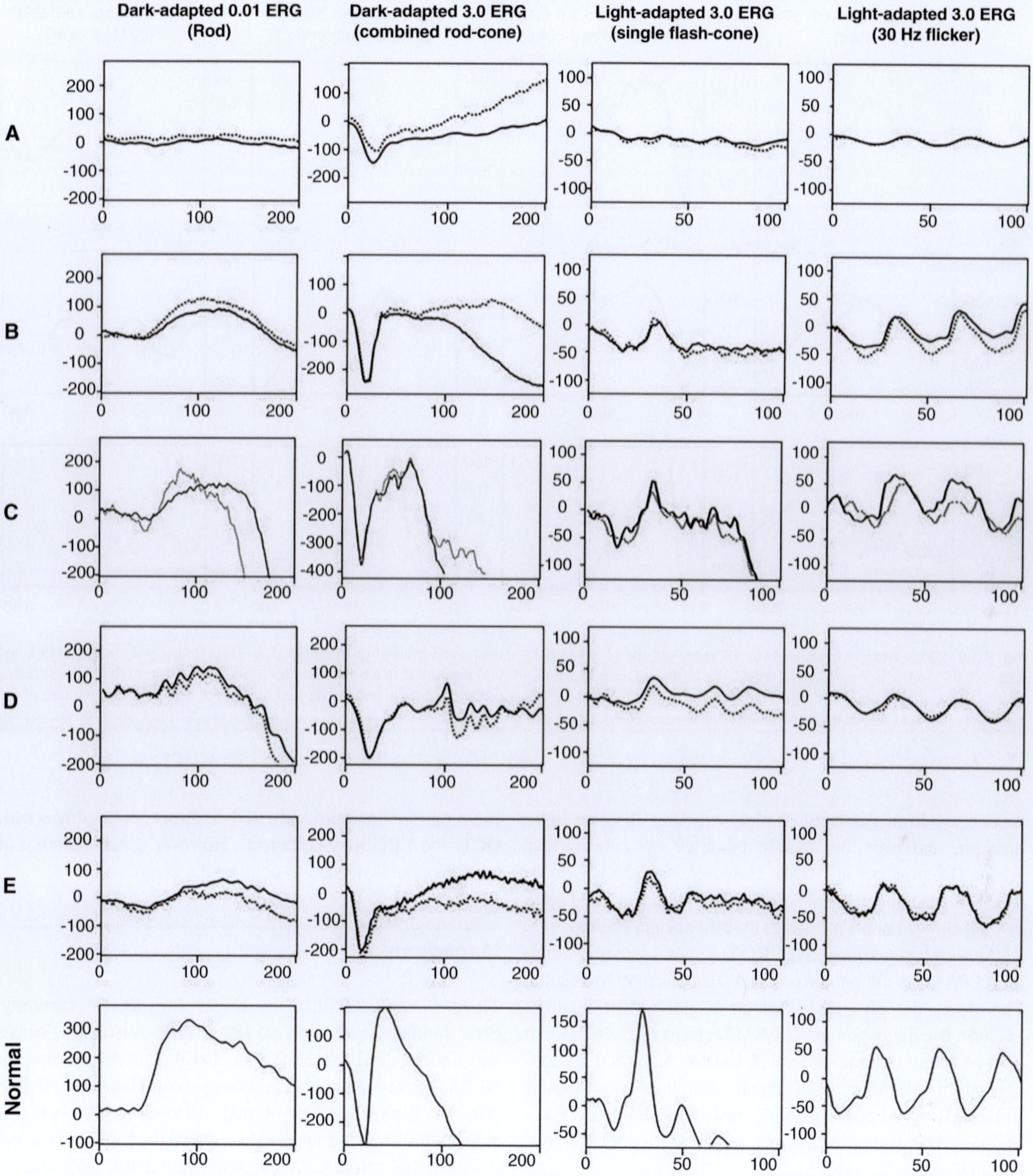

Fig. 3.13 ERGs from five patients (**a**: 23 years old, **b**: 51 years old, **c**: 22 years old, **d**: 42 years old, **e**: 30 years old) with XLRS and a normal control ERG. In the patients tested, the dark-adapted (DA) 0.01 ERG was reduced, the DA 3.0 ERG showed a reduced b/a ratio, the light-adapted (LA) 3.0 ERG b-waves were delayed and decreased in amplitude, and the LA 30 Hz flicker peak time was delayed and decreased in amplitude. The solid lines represent the average traces of the right eyes, and the dashed lines represent the average traces of the left eyes

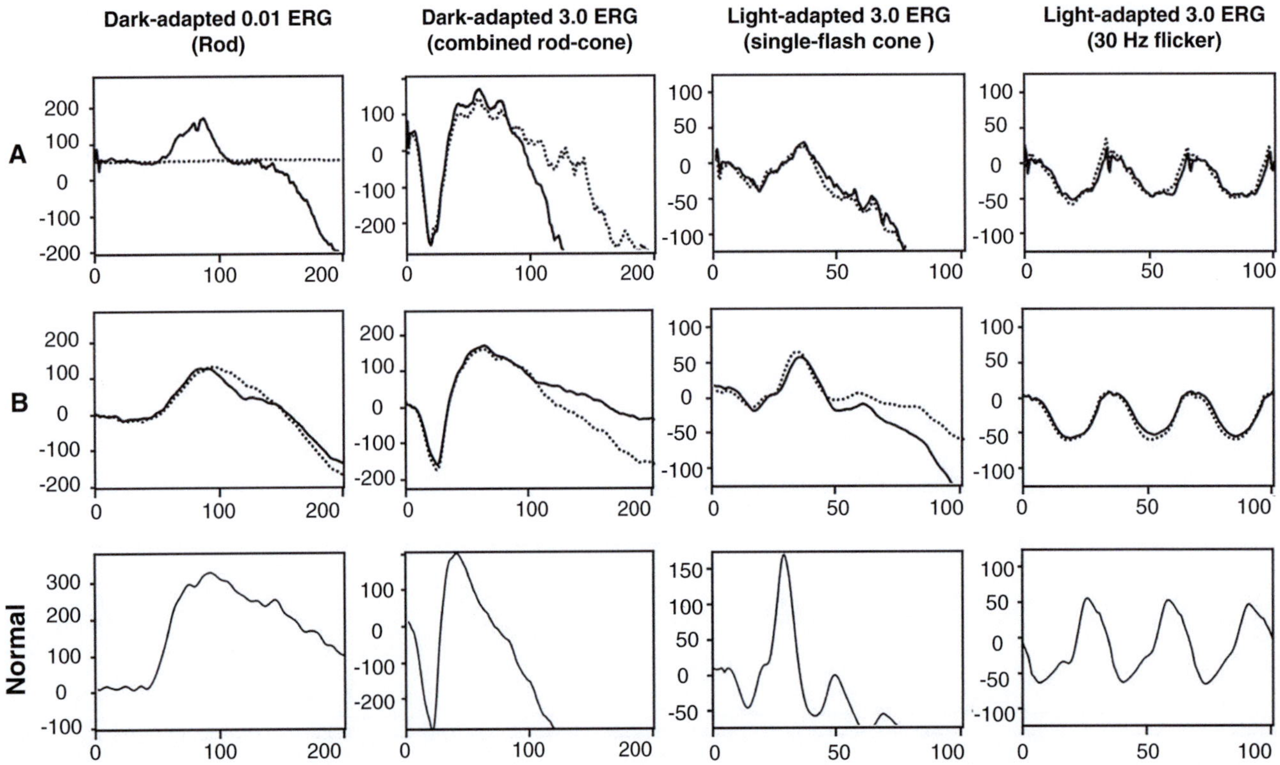

Fig. 3.14 ERGs from two patients (**a**: 18 years old, **b**: 11 years old) with XLRS and a normal control ERG. In both patients, the dark-adapted (DA) 0.01 ERG was reduced, the DA 3.0 ERG showed a b/a ratio > 1, the light-adapted (LA) 3.0 ERG b-waves were delayed and decreased in amplitude, and the LA 30 Hz flicker peak time was delayed and decreased in amplitude. The solid lines represent the average traces of the right eyes, and the dashed lines represent the average traces of the left eyes

S-cone syndrome, autosomal recessive Best disease, optic disc pit, and even dominantly inherited cystoid macular edema (Deutman et al. 1976). However, only XLRS, nicotinic acid maculopathy, enhanced S-cone syndrome, and optic disc pit showed non-FA leakage cystoid macula edema.

Although electronegative ERG is a characteristic finding in XLRS, not all patients reveal electronegative results. Therefore, the absence of electronegative ERG cannot exclude the diagnosis of XLRS. Electronegative ERG can also be found in patients with X-linked congenital stationary night blindness, autosomal dominant neovascular inflammatory vitreoretinopathy, birdshot retinopathy, ischemic retinal vascular occlusion, melanoma-associated retinopathy, and siderosis.

In the advanced stage of XLRS and macular atrophy, the diffusion of retinal pigmentary change without retinal schisis in the OCT may develop, which makes the diagnosis more challenging.

Patients with XLRS could be diagnosed as having amblyopia, strabismus, traumatic vitreous hemorrhage and/or retinal detachment, retinitis pigmentosa or exudative retinal detachment, with or without neovascular glaucoma, which mimics Coats' disease. A thorough family history, retinal examination including dilated indirect ophthalmoscopy, OCT, and ERG may be crucial. However, genetic testing of the *RS1* gene is needed to confirm the diagnosis.

Management

There is no definitive treatment for XLRS currently. Prescription of low-vision aid was given in most cases (Weber and Kellner 2007; Molday et al. 2012). Current practice for XLRS focuses on the interventions for complications, such as vitreous hemorrhage or retinal detachment (Weber and Kellner 2007). Some studies have shown the benefit of topical dorzolamide solution, a carbonic anhydrase inhibitor, to reduce the severity of the disease (Fig. 3.12) (Khandhadia et al. 2011; Molday et al. 2012; Wang et al. 2015), which can help to decrease the thickness of the fovea and enhance retinal adhesiveness (Wolfensberger 1999); however, vision does not improve to a great extent (Khandhadia et al. 2011; Wang et al. 2015). Gene therapy with delivery of an adeno-associated virus (AAV) containing the normal human *RS1* gene has been used in animal models and has proven to be successful and safe (Molday et al. 2012; Min et al. 2005;

Janssen et al. 2008; Kjellstrom et al. 2007; Park et al. 2009; Marangoni et al. 2016; Bush et al. 2016). These studies suggest a possible long-term solution for impaired retinal function in XLRS using gene therapy. Currently, many gene therapies for hereditary retinal diseases including XLRS have already been advanced to clinical trials. To date, two clinical trials of an intravitreal injection with AAV vectors for treating XLRS have been performed (Lam 2017).

Acknowledgments N. K. Wang is supported by the Taiwan Ministry of Science and Technology MOST 106-2314-B-182A-041 and the Chang Gung Memorial Hospital CMRPG3F1241-3F1242.

References

Anderson JR. Anterior dialysis of the retina: disinsertion or avulsion at ora serrata. Br J Ophthalmol. 1932;16(12):641–70.

Bush RA, Zeng Y, Colosi P, Kjellstrom S, Hiriyanna S, Vijayasarathy C, Santos M, Li J, Wu Z, Sieving PA. Preclinical dose-escalation study of intravitreal AAV-RS1 gene therapy in a mouse model of X-linked retinoschisis: dose-dependent expression and improved retinal structure and function. Hum Gene Ther. 2016;27(5):376–89.

Deutman AF, Pinckers AJ, Aan de Kerk AL. Dominantly inherited cystoid macular edema. Am J Ophthalmol. 1976;82(4):540–8.

Eksandh LC, Ponjavic V, Ayyagari R, Bingham EL, Hiriyanna KT, Andreasson S, Ehinger B, Sieving PA. Phenotypic expression of juvenile X-linked retinoschisis in Swedish families with different mutations in the XLRS1 gene. Arch Ophthalmol. 2000;118(8):1098–104.

Forsius H, Eriksson A, Vainio-Mattila B. [Sex-related hereditary retinoschisis in 2 families in Finland]. Klinische Monatsblatter fur Augenheilkunde. 1963;143:806–816.

Forsius H, Krause U, Helve J, Vuopala V, Mustonen E, Vainio-Mattila B, Fellman J, Eriksson AW. Visual acuity in 183 cases of X-chromosomal retinoschisis. Can J Ophthalmol. 1973;8(3):385–93.

Gass JD. Nicotinic acid maculopathy. Am J Ophthalmol. 1973;76(4):500–10.

Genead MA, Fishman GA, Walia S. Efficacy of sustained topical dorzolamide therapy for cystic macular lesions in patients with X-linked retinoschisis. Arch Ophthalmol. 2010;128(2):190–7.

George ND, Yates JR, Moore AT. X linked retinoschisis. Br J Ophthalmol. 1995;79(7):697–702.

George ND, Yates JR, Moore AT. Clinical features in affected males with X-linked retinoschisis. Arch Ophthalmol. 1996;114(3):274–80.

Grayson C, Reid SN, Ellis JA, Rutherford A, Sowden JC, Yates JR, Farber DB, Trump D. Retinoschisin, the X-linked retinoschisis protein, is a secreted photoreceptor protein, and is expressed and released by Weri-Rb1 cells. Hum Mol Genet. 2000;9(12):1873–9.

Haas J. Über das Zusammenvorkommen von Veränderungen der Retina und Choroidea. Arch Augenheilkd. 1898;37:343–8.

Hewitt AW, FitzGerald LM, Scotter LW, Mulhall LE, McKay JD, Mackey DA. Genotypic and phenotypic spectrum of X-linked retinoschisis in Australia. Clin Exp Ophthalmol. 2005;33(3):233–9.

Hirose T, Wolf E, Hara A. Electrophysiological and psychophysical studies in congenital retinoschisis of X-linked recessive inheritance. In: Lawwill T, editor. ERG, VER and psychophysics, vol. 13. Netherlands: Springer; 1977. p. 173–84.

Hu QR, Huang LZ, Chen XL, Xia HK, Li TQ, Li XX. Genetic analysis and clinical features of X-linked retinoschisis in Chinese patients. Sci Rep. 2017;7:44060.

Jager GM. A hereditary retinal disease. Trans Ophthalmol Soc U K. 1953;73:617–9.

Janssen A, Min SH, Molday LL, Tanimoto N, Seeliger MW, Hauswirth WW, Molday RS, Weber BH. Effect of late-stage therapy on disease progression in AAV-mediated rescue of photoreceptor cells in the retinoschisin-deficient mouse. Mol Ther. 2008;16(6):1010–7.

Kellner U, Brummer S, Foerster MH, Wessing A. X-linked congenital retinoschisis. Graefes Arch Clin Exp Ophthalmol. 1990;228(5):432–7.

Khandhadia S, Trump D, Menon G, Lotery AJ. X-linked retinoschisis maculopathy treated with topical dorzolamide, and relationship to genotype. Eye. 2011;25(7):922–8.

Kim LS, Seiple W, Fishman GA, Szlyk JP. Multifocal ERG findings in carriers of X-linked retinoschisis. Doc Ophthalmol. 2007;114(1):21–6.

Kirsch LS, Brownstein S, de Wolff-Rouendaal D. A histopathological, ultrastructural and immunohistochemical study of congenital hereditary retinoschisis. Can J Ophthalmol. 1996;31(6):301–10.

Kjellstrom S, Bush RA, Zeng Y, Takada Y, Sieving PA. Retinoschisin gene therapy and natural history in the Rs1h-KO mouse: long-term rescue from retinal degeneration. Invest Ophthalmol Vis Sci. 2007;48(8):3837–45.

Krill AE. Krill's hereditary retinal and choroidal diseases, vol. 1. Hagerstown, Cambridge, London, New York: Harper & Row; 1977.

Lam BL. Update on gene therapy for the treatment of hereditary retinal diseases: retinal gene therapy is on the brink of clinical reality. Retina Today; 2017.

Lee JJ, Kim JH, Kim SY, Park SS, Yu YS. Infantile vitreous hemorrhage as the initial presentation of X-linked juvenile retinoschisis. Korean J Ophthalmol. 2009;23(2):118–20.

Lesch B, Szabo V, Kanya M, Somfai GM, Vamos R, Varsanyi B, Pamer Z, Knezy K, Salacz G, Janaky M, Ferencz M, Hargitai J, Papp A, Farkas A. Clinical and genetic findings in Hungarian patients with X-linked juvenile retinoschisis. Mol Vis. 2008;14:2321–32.

Magnus JA. Case of retinal detachment in a child (?cystic ?congenital). Trans Ophthalmol Soc U K. 1951;71:728–30.

Mann I, Macrae A. Congenital vascular veils in the vitreous. Br J Ophthalmol. 1938;22(1):1–10.

Marangoni D, Bush RA, Zeng Y, Wei LL, Ziccardi L, Vijayasarathy C, Bartoe JT, Palyada K, Santos M, Hiriyanna S, Wu Z, Colosi P, Sieving PA. Ocular and systemic safety of a recombinant AAV8 vector for X-linked retinoschisis gene therapy: GLP studies in rabbits and Rs1-KO mice. Mol Ther Methods Clin Dev. 2016;5:16011.

Min SH, Molday LL, Seeliger MW, Dinculescu A, Timmers AM, Janssen A, Tonagel F, Tanimoto N, Weber BH, Molday RS, Hauswirth WW. Prolonged recovery of retinal structure/function after gene therapy in an Rs1h-deficient mouse model of x-linked juvenile retinoschisis. Mol Ther. 2005;12(4):644–51.

Molday RS, Kellner U, Weber BH. X-linked juvenile retinoschisis: clinical diagnosis, genetic analysis, and molecular mechanisms. Prog Retin Eye Res. 2012;31(3):195–212.

Pagenstecher HE. Über eine unter dem Bilde der Netzhautablösung verlaufende, erbliche Erkrankung der Retina. Graefes Arch Ophthalmol. 1913;86(3):457–62.

Park TK, Wu Z, Kjellstrom S, Zeng Y, Bush RA, Sieving PA, Colosi P. Intravitreal delivery of AAV8 retinoschisin results in cell type-specific gene expression and retinal rescue in the Rs1-KO mouse. Gene Ther. 2009;16(7):916–26.

Piao CH, Kondo M, Nakamura M, Terasaki H, Miyake Y. Multifocal electroretinograms in X-linked retinoschisis. Invest Ophthalmol Vis Sci. 2003;44(11):4920–30.

Prasad A, Wagner R, Bhagat N. Vitreous hemorrhage as the initial manifestation of X-linked retinoschisis in a 9-month-old infant. J Pediatr Ophthalmol Strabismus. 2006;43(1):56–8.

Prenner JL, Capone A Jr, Ciaccia S, Takada Y, Sieving PA, Trese MT. Congenital X-linked retinoschisis classification system. Retina. 2006;26(7 Suppl):S61–4.

Renner AB, Kellner U, Fiebig B, Cropp E, Foerster MH, Weber BH. ERG variability in X-linked congenital retinoschisis patients with mutations in the RS1 gene and the diagnostic importance of fundus autofluorescence and OCT. Doc Ophthalmol. 2008;116(2):97–109.

Retinoschisis Consortium. Functional implications of the spectrum of mutations found in 234 cases with X-linked juvenile retinoschisis. The Retinoschisis Consortium. Hum Mol Genet. 1998;7(7):1185–92.

Riveiro-Alvarez R, Trujillo-Tiebas MJ, Gimenez-Pardo A, Garcia-Hoyos M, Lopez-Martinez MA, Aguirre-Lamban J, Garcia-Sandoval B, Vazquez-Fernandez del Pozo S, Cantalapiedra D, Avila-Fernandez A, Baiget M, Ramos C, Ayuso C. Correlation of genetic and clinical findings in Spanish patients with X-linked juvenile retinoschisis. Invest Ophthalmol Vis Sci. 2009;50(9):4342–50.

Roesch MT, Ewing CC, Gibson AE, Weber BH. The natural history of X-linked retinoschisis. Can J Ophthalmol. 1998;33(3):149–58.

Sauer CG, Gehrig A, Warneke-Wittstock R, Marquardt A, Ewing CC, Gibson A, Lorenz B, Jurklies B, Weber BH. Positional cloning of the gene associated with X-linked juvenile retinoschisis. Nat Genet. 1997;17(2):164–70.

Stanga PE, Chong NH, Reck AC, Hardcastle AJ, Holder GE. Optical coherence tomography and electrophysiology in X-linked juvenile retinoschisis associated with a novel mutation in the XLRS1 gene. Retina. 2001;21(1):78–80.

Tantri A, Vrabec TR, Cu-Unjieng A, Frost A, Annesley WH Jr, Donoso LA. X-linked retinoschisis: a clinical and molecular genetic review. Surv Ophthalmol. 2004;49(2):214–30.

Thobani A, Fishman GA. The use of carbonic anhydrase inhibitors in the retreatment of cystic macular lesions in retinitis pigmentosa and X-linked retinoschisis. Retina. 2011;31(2):312–5.

Thomson E. Memorandum regarding a family in which neuroretinal disease of an unusual kind occurred only in males. Br J Ophthalmol. 1932;16(12):681–6.

Vincent A, Robson AG, Neveu MM, Wright GA, Moore AT, Webster AR, Holder GE. A phenotype-genotype correlation study of X-linked retinoschisis. Ophthalmology. 2013;120(7):1454–64.

Walia S, Fishman GA, Molday RS, Dyka FM, Kumar NM, Ehlinger MA, Stone EM. Relation of response to treatment with dorzolamide in X-linked retinoschisis to the mechanism of functional loss in retinoschisin. Am J Ophthalmol. 2009;147(1):111–5.e111.

Wang NK, Liu L, Chen HM, Tsai S, Chang TC, Tsai TH, Yang CM, Chao AN, Chen KJ, Kao LY, Yeung L, Yeh LK, Hwang YS, Wu WC, Lai CC. Clinical presentations of X-linked retinoschisis in Taiwanese patients confirmed with genetic sequencing. Mol Vis. 2015;21:487–501.

Weber BHF, Kellner U. X-linked juvenile retinoschisis. In: Tombran-Tink J, Barnstable CJ, editors. Ophthalmology research: retinal degenerations: biology, diagnostics, and therapeutics. Totowa: Humana Press Inc.; 2007.

Wilczek M. Ein Fall der Netzhautspaltung (Retinoschisis) mit einer Öffnung. Zeit Augenhlkd. 1935;85:108–16.

Wolfensberger TJ. The role of carbonic anhydrase inhibitors in the management of macular edema. Doc Ophthalmol. 1999;97(3–4):387–97.

Wu WW, Molday RS. Defective discoidin domain structure, subunit assembly, and endoplasmic reticulum processing of retinoschisin are primary mechanisms responsible for X-linked retinoschisis. J Biol Chem. 2003;278(30):28139–46.

Wu WW, Wong JP, Kast J, Molday RS. RS1, a discoidin domain-containing retinal cell adhesion protein associated with X-linked retinoschisis, exists as a novel disulfide-linked octamer. J Biol Chem. 2005;280(11):10721–30.

Progressive Cone/Cone-Rod Dystrophy

4

Andrew Tsai, Adrian Koh, Ranjana Mathur, and Gemmy C. M. Cheung

Abbreviations

CRD	Cone-rod dystrophy
ELM	External limiting membrane
ERG	Electroretinogram
EZ	Ellipsoid zone
FAF	Fundus autofluorescence
IZ	Interdigitation zone
mfERG	Multifocal electroretinogram
OCT	Optical coherence tomography
RP	Retinitis pigmentosa
RPE	Retinal pigment epithelium
SD-OCT	Spectral domain optical coherence tomography

Introduction

Progressive cone/cone-rod dystrophies (CRD) are a heterogeneous group of disorders characterized by early deterioration of visual acuity and color vision, and in some cases nystagmus. The prevalence is estimated to be 1/40,000. Patients usually present in childhood or early adult life. In later life, patients with cone dystrophies can progress to have rod dysfunction. Hence CRD may be a more appropriate terminology, to reflect widespread retinal dysfunction, with cones usually more affected than rods. When there is involvement of both cone and rod systems, it may be difficult clinically to differentiate CRD from retinitis pigmentosa (RP). Therefore, electrophysiology can be helpful, as reduction or absence of cone ERG responses, with less reduction in rod responses would indicate CRD. However, in advanced disease, both cone and rod ERG responses may become undetectable. Compared to rod-cone dystrophies, CRD are less often associated with syndromes, but CRD may be part of Bardet–Biedl syndrome and spinocerebellar ataxia type 7.

A. Tsai · R. Mathur · G. C. M. Cheung (✉)
Singapore National Eye Centre, Singapore Eye Research Institute, Singapore, Singapore

Duke NUS Graduate Medical School, Singapore, Singapore
e-mail: gemmy.cheung.c.m@snec.com.sg

A. Koh
Singapore National Eye Centre, Singapore Eye Research Institute, Singapore, Singapore

Etiopathogenesis

Autosomal dominant, recessive, and X-linked inheritance patterns have been described in CRD (Moore 1992). Many different genetic mutations have been described to cause CRD, with more being identified as technology for genetic sequencing improves (Roosing et al. 2014). Major genes include *ABCA4*, *CRX*, *GUCY2D*, and *RPGR* (Hamel 2007). CRD has been found to be associated with mutations in the gene *GUCY2D*, and cone dystrophy-3 (COD3) has been associated with mutations in GUCA1A (Payne et al. 1998; Wilkie et al. 2001). *GUCY2D* and *GUCA1A* encode the retina-specific guanylate cyclase (RETGC-1) (Kelsell et al. 1998) and its activating protein guanylate cyclase activating protein-1 (GCAP-1), respectively. GCAPs play an important role in regulating the function of RETGC-1 in a calcium-dependent manner. However, it is unclear how defects in these proteins result in degeneration which is limited to cones.

Clinical Features

Clinical features include photophobia, nystagmus, color vision defects, and visual field abnormalities. Various visual field defects have been reported, which include central scotoma, peripheral field loss, generalized loss of sensitivity, and ring scotoma (Simunovic and Moore 1998). In later stages of the disease when the rod photoreceptors are involved, night blindness may also become a prominent symptom.

G. Cheung (ed.), *Hereditary Chorioretinal Disorders*, Retina Atlas, https://doi.org/10.1007/978-981-15-0414-3_4

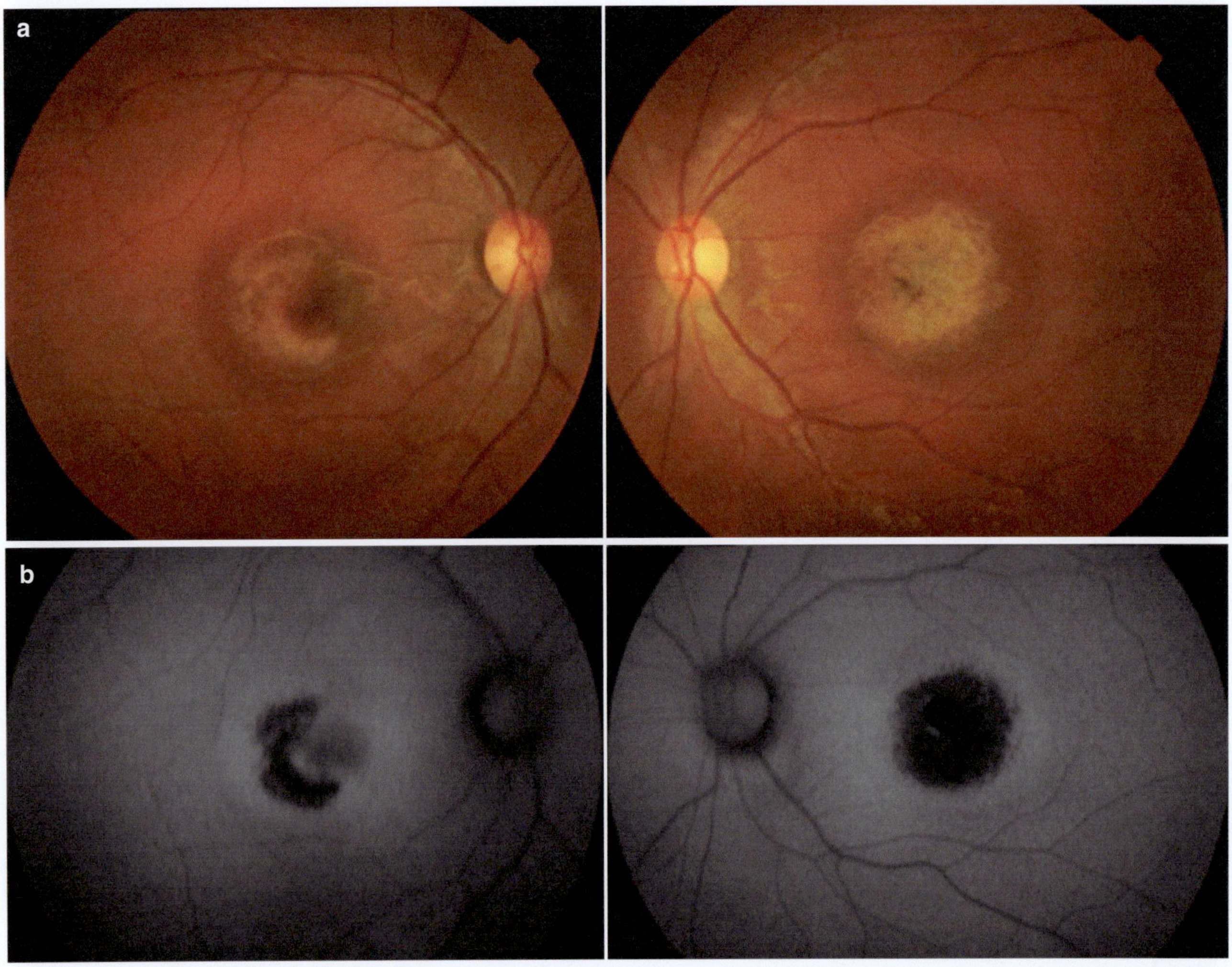

Fig. 4.1 A 23-year-old male with cone dystrophy with decreased vision in both eyes. Visual acuity (VA) 6/15 OD and 6/45 OS. (**a**) Color fundus photographs showing retinal pigment epithelium (RPE) atrophy at the macular (left worse than right). (**b**) Corresponding fundus autofluorescence (FAF) showing hypoautofluorescence at areas of RPE atrophy

Fundus examination findings can range from a normal macula to bull's eye configuration in late disease (Roosing et al. 2014). White flecks at the level of RPE, and tapetum-like sheen have also been described (Simunovic and Moore 1998). When there is widespread retinal involvement, there can be presence of bone spicules resembling RP. Late stages of CRD may be indistinguishable from RP.

Here we showcase various forms of cone and cone rod dystrophies (Figs. 4.1, 4.2, 4.3, 4.4, 4.5, and 4.6).

Investigations

Optical coherence tomography (OCT) characteristic of cone dystrophy in the early stages may be subtle, such as loss of interdigitation zone (IZ) with or without foveal cavitation. There is a less distinct border in the periphery between the EZ and the ELM with lower intensity and thinning of the EZ band. At the macula, the EZ band can show irregular foveal loss or segmental foveal loss. Another pattern of OCT abnormality that has been observed in cone dystrophy is central foveal thickening with irregular perifoveal loss of the EZ band. In the later stages, the ELM and EZ may be completely lost at the macular region but preserved in the peripheral regions of the fundus. There is also generalized thinning of the RPE layer. Overall, cone and cone-rod dystrophy show characteristic changes on OCT that affects predominantly the macula area in the early stages and correlates with the level of visual impairment.

Fundus autofluorescence (FAF) findings in cone/cone-rod dystrophy can be variable and may depend on the stage of disease. A ring of hyperautofluorescence surrounded by an area of macula RPE atrophy has been described (Robson et al. 2010) (Fig. 4.4b).

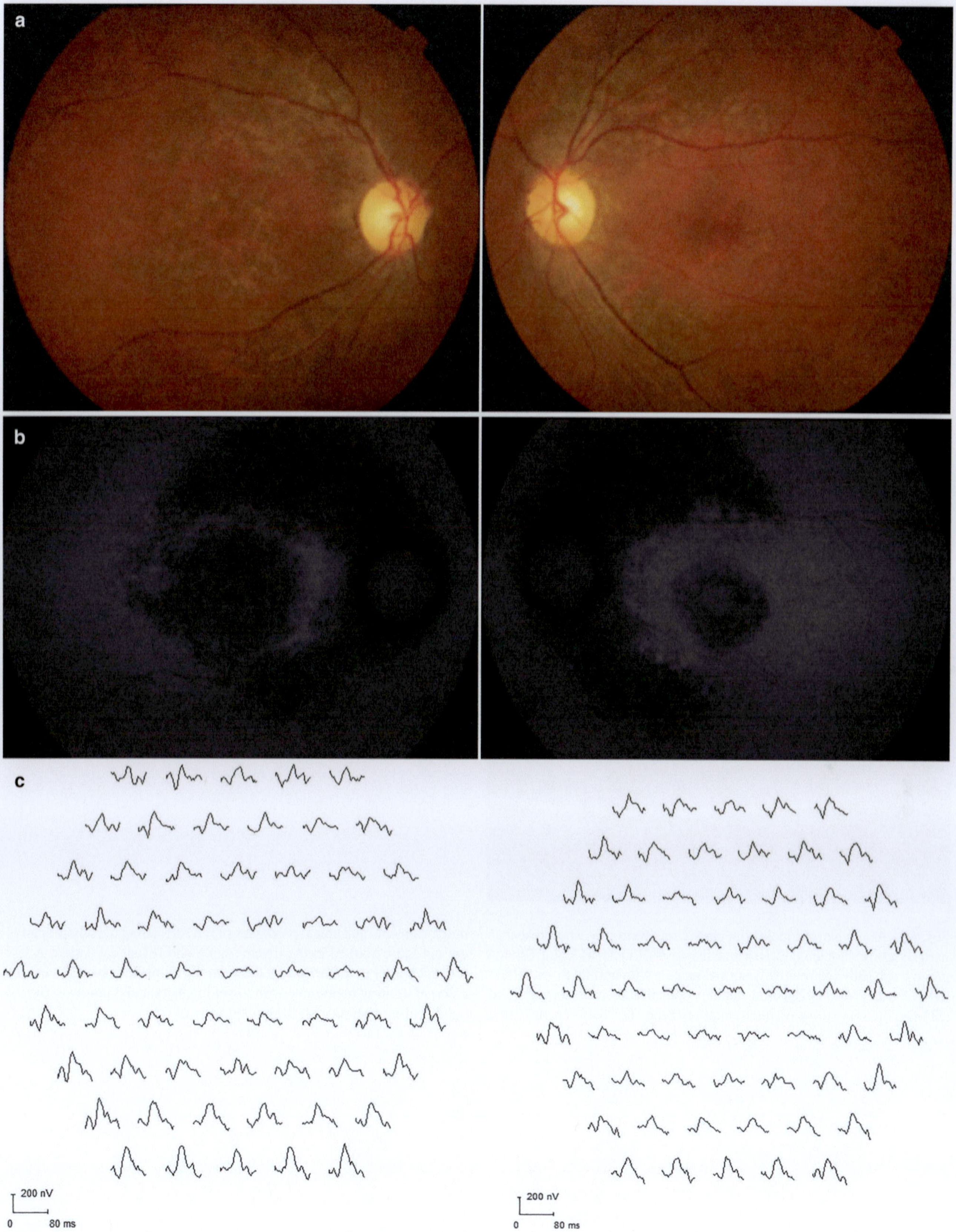

Fig. 4.2 A 68-year-old female with cone-rod dystrophy with right eye blur vision for 2 years. VA count fingers OD 6/12 OS. (**a**) Color fundus photographs showing RPE mottling at the macula, with associated RPE disturbance in the mid periphery. (**b**) FAF showing hypoautofluorescent areas in the macula and beyond the macula region, suggesting more widespread RPE dysfunction (right worse than left). (**c**) Multifocal electroretinogram (mfERG) showing reduced and delayed responses in the central 2–3 rings in both eyes. OD (picture on left), OS (picture of right)

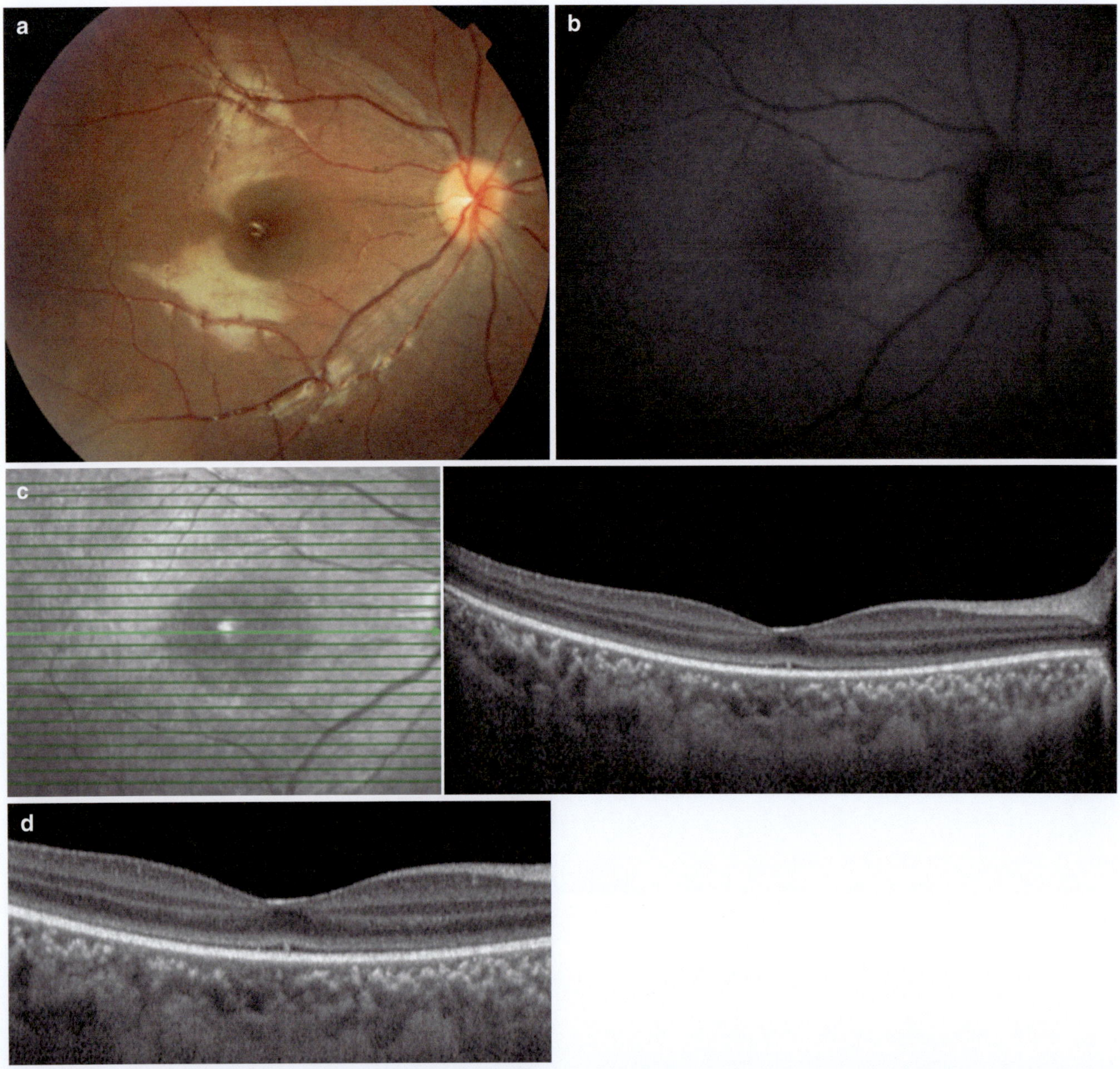

Fig. 4.3 A 12-year-old male with early cone dystrophy who presented with dyschromatopsia and visual acuity of 6/24 OU. (**a**) Color fundus photograph showing relatively normal macula with normal fovea reflex. (**b**) Normal FAF. (**c**) Spectral domain optical coherence tomography (SD-OCT) shows loss of interdigitation zone (IZ) between the cone outer segments and apical processes of the RPE along the whole span of cut but more marked in the foveal region and foveal cavitation. A less distinct border in the periphery between the ellipsoid zone (EZ) and the external limiting membrane with lower intensity and thinning of the EZ band is also observed. (**d**) Magnified view of (**c**)

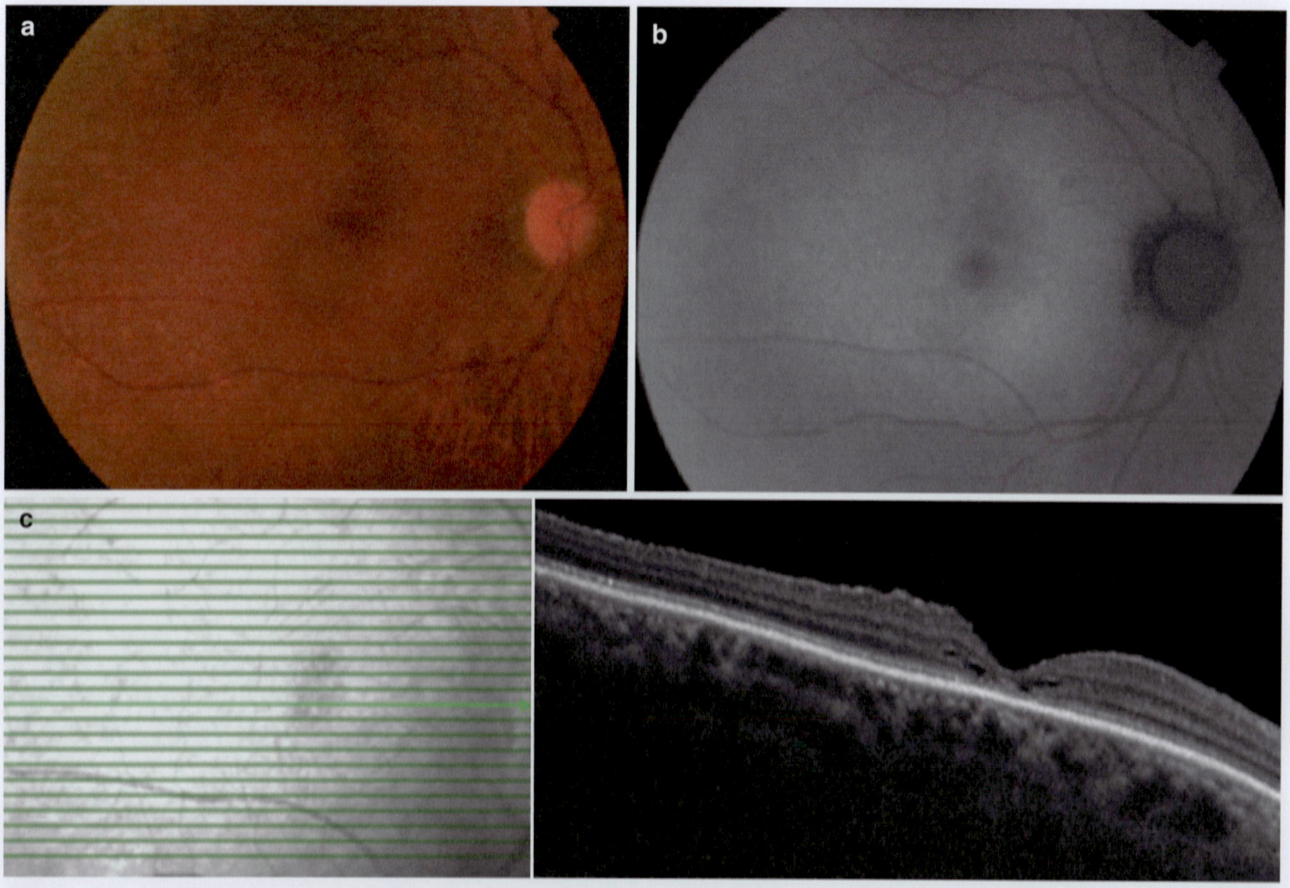

Fig. 4.4 A 67-year-old female with cone dystrophy with poor vision for many years. VA 6/120 OD, 6/90 OS. (**a**) Color fundus photograph showing subtle mottling at the macula. This patient also has age-related peripheral drusen. (**b**) FAF showing abnormal hyperautofluorescence in the parafoveal area, with a wider ring of hypoautofluorescence in the macula region. (**c**) SD-OCT of right macula showing RPE atrophy, loss of ellipsoid zone, and degenerative cysts

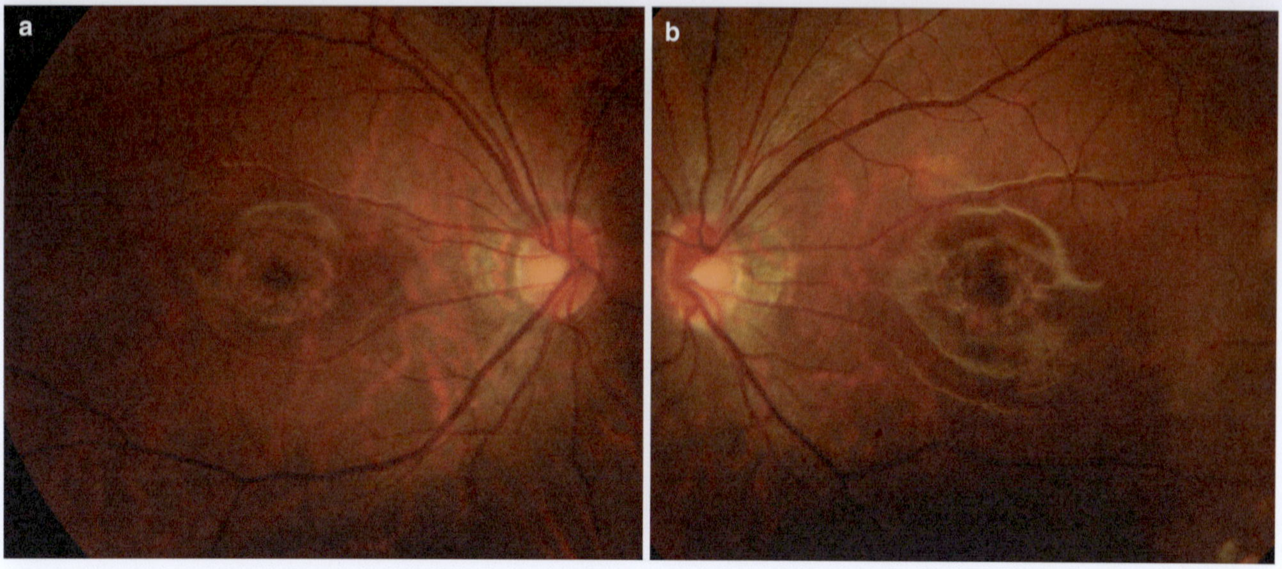

Fig. 4.5 A 20-year-old male with bilateral central blurring of vision. VA 6/21 OU. (**a**, **b**) Bull's eye maculopathy is seen in both eyes. Peripheral retina was unremarkable. However, ERG showed both rod and cone dysfunction, suggesting a *cone-rod dystrophy*. (**c**, **d**) FAF shows a central ring of iso-autofluorescence, surrounded by a ring of hypoautofluorescence, then a peripheral ring of hyperautofluorescence, typical of bull's eye lesion. (**e**, **f**) SD-OCT showing EZ disruption corresponding to area of hypoautofluorescence. There is hypertransmission of light into the choroid in areas of atrophy

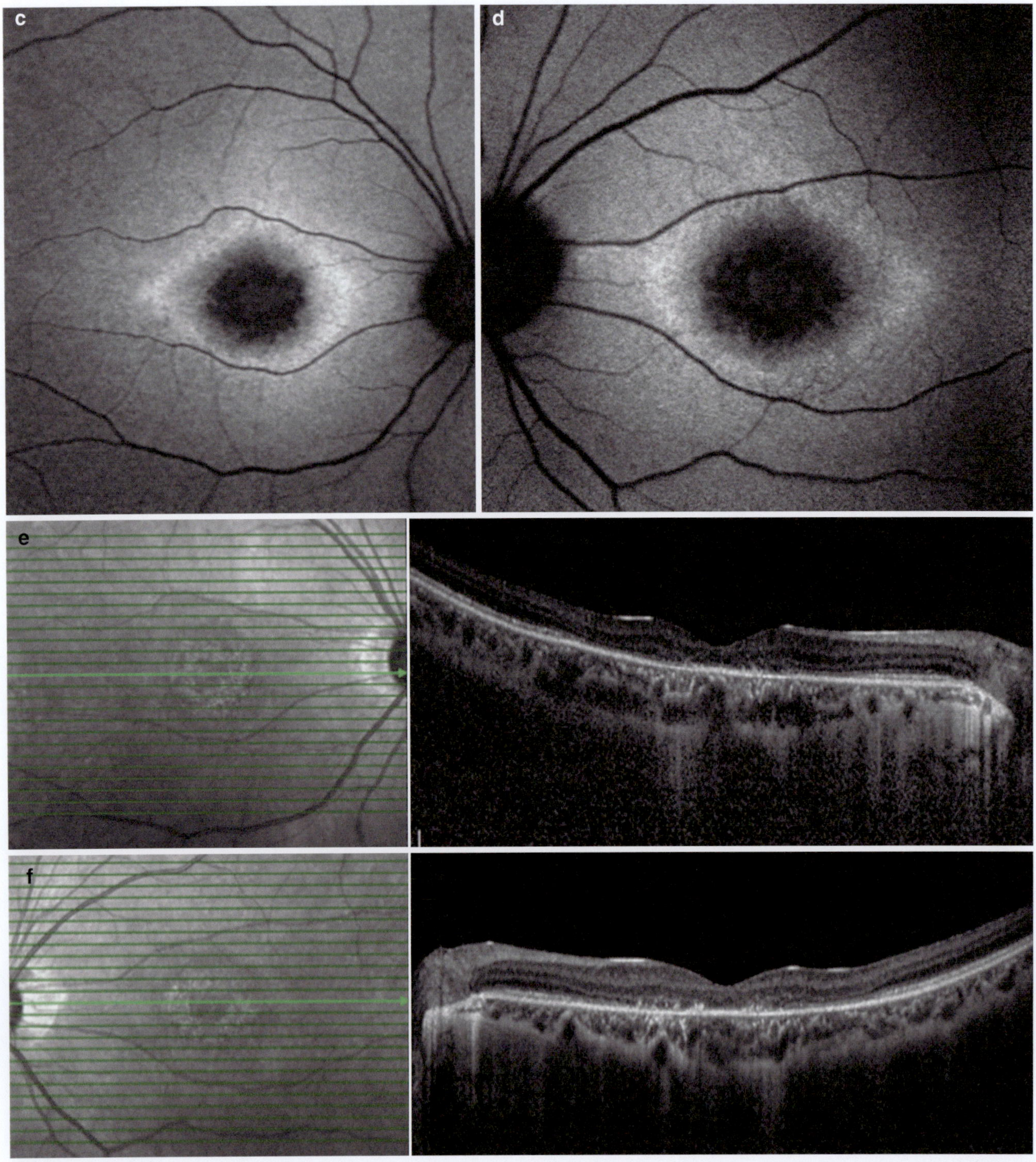

Fig. 4.5 (continued)

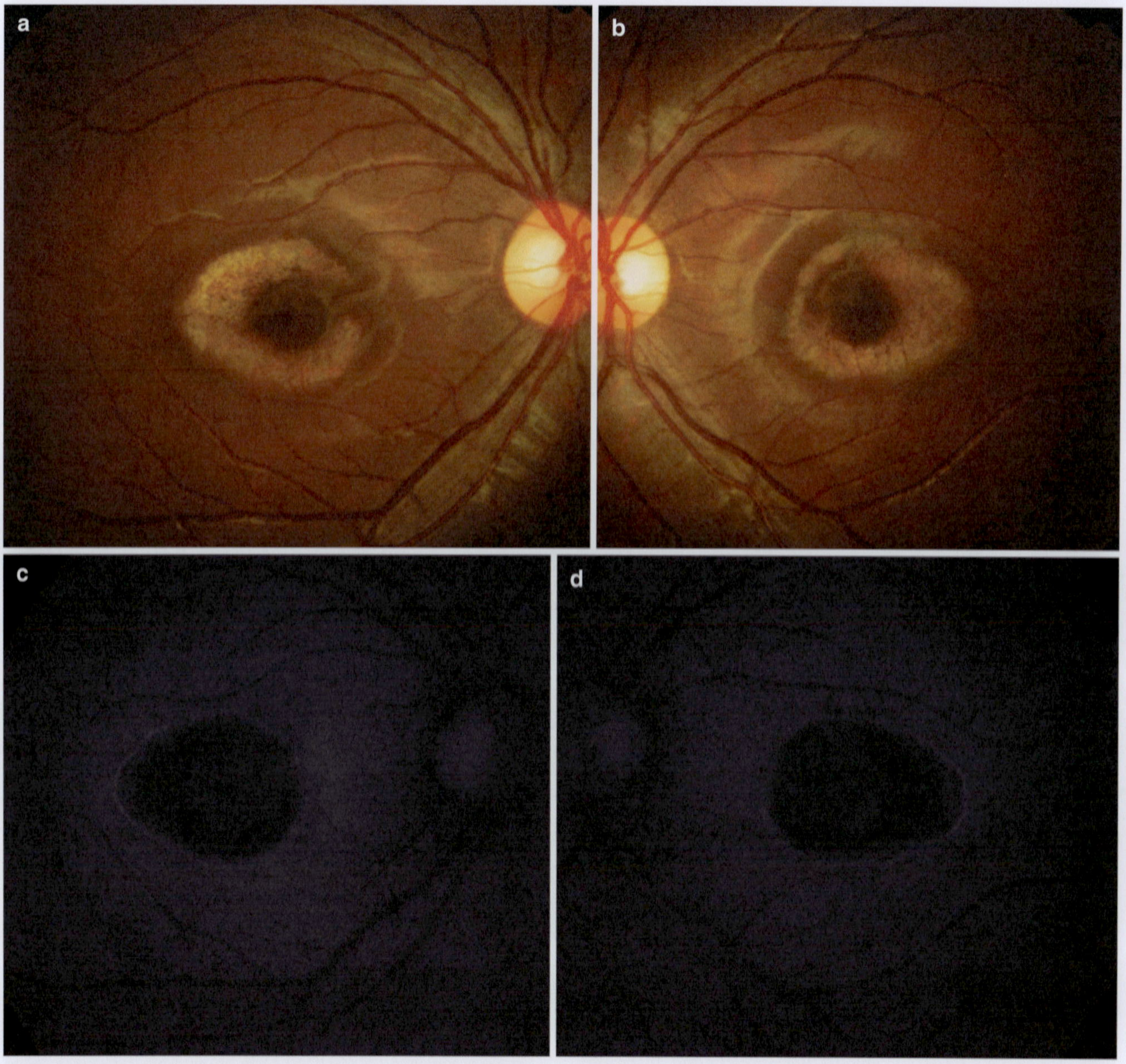

Fig. 4.6 A 12-year-old female with relatively good VA of 6/12 in the right eye and 6/9 in the left eye. (**a**, **b**) Bull's eye maculopathy is also seen in both eyes. Full field ERG was normal, but mfERG was reduced in the central two rings but not delayed. As global cone function is intact, a diagnosis of *benign concentric annular macular dystrophy* was made. (**c**, **d**) FAF shows a central ring of iso-autofluorescence, surrounded by a ring of hypoautofluorescence, then a peripheral ring of hyperautofluorescence, typical of bull's eye lesion. (**e**, **f**) SD-OCT showing EZ disruption corresponding to area of hypoautofluorescence. There is hypertransmission of light into the choroid in areas of atrophy

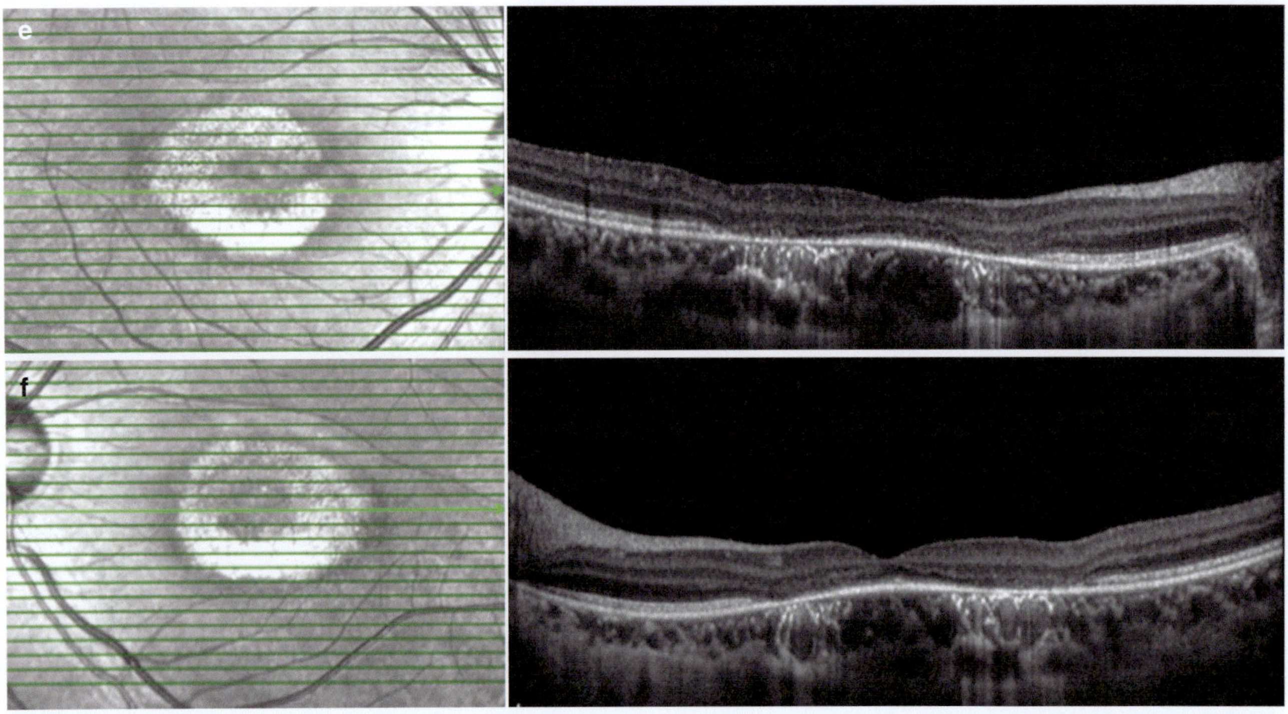

Fig. 4.6 (continued)

Fluorescein angiography may show hyperfluorescence at the macula due to RPE atrophy. However, this finding is not specific to cone/cone-rod dystrophy.

Macular dysfunction can be detected using multifocal electroretinogram (ERG), which can also document the areas of dysfunction topographically. Full-field ERG typically shows poor photopic and 30 Hz flicker responses, with relatively preserved scotopic (rod-derived) responses. Variable disturbance in rod responses may also be seen in later stages (Roosing et al. 2014). ERG is particularly informative as they may be abnormal before distinguishable clinical signs appear. For patients with Bull's eye maculopathy (as in Figs. 4.5 and 4.6), ERG is able to distinguish cone dystrophy from macular dystrophy.

Management and Prognosis

A holistic treatment approach is recommended for patients with cone and CRD. Management is generally conservative and use low vision aids when appropriate. Genetic testing to characterize the mode of inheritance is important for genetic counseling. Current research has been focusing on identifying the genetic basis of cone dystrophies, with the hope that in the future gene therapy might be possible (Roosing et al. 2014).

The clinical course of CRD is more severe than RP, leading to early legal blindness and disability.

References

Hamel CP. Cone rod dystrophies. Orphanet J Rare Dis. 2007;2:7.

Kelsell RE, Gregory-Evans K, Payne AM, et al. Mutations in the retinal guanylate cyclase (RETGC-1) gene in dominant cone-rod dystrophy. Hum Mol Genet. 1998;7(7):1179–84.

Moore AT. Cone and cone-rod dystrophies. J Med Genet. 1992;29(5):289–90.

Payne AM, Downes SM, Bessant DA, et al. A mutation in guanylate cyclase activator 1A (GUCA1A) in an autosomal dominant cone dystrophy pedigree mapping to a new locus on chromosome 6p21.1. Hum Mol Genet. 1998;7(2):273–7.

Robson AG, Webster AR, Michaelides M, et al. "Cone dystrophy with supernormal rod electroretinogram": a comprehensive genotype/phenotype study including fundus autofluorescence and extensive electrophysiology. Retina. 2010;30(1):51–62.

Roosing S, Thiadens AA, Hoyng CB, Klaver CC, den Hollander AI, Cremers FP. Causes and consequences of inherited cone disorders. Prog Retin Eye Res. 2014;42:1–26.

Simunovic MP, Moore AT. The cone dystrophies. Eye (Lond). 1998;12(Pt 3b):553–65.

Wilkie SE, Li Y, Deery EC, et al. Identification and functional consequences of a new mutation (E155G) in the gene for GCAP1 that causes autosomal dominant cone dystrophy. Am J Hum Genet. 2001;69(3):471–80.

Pattern Dystrophy

5

Andrew Tsai, Adrian Koh, Nan-Kai Wang, Ranjana Mathur, and Gemmy C. M. Cheung

Abbreviations

AMD	Age-related macular degeneration
AOVPD	Adult onset vitelliform pattern dystrophy
BPD	Butterfly-shaped pattern dystrophy
CNV	Choroidal neovascularization
EOG	Electrooculography
ERG	Electroretinogram
FA	Fluorescein angiogram
FAF	Fundus autofluorescence
OCT	Optical coherence tomography
ONL	Outer nuclear layer
PD	Pattern dystrophy
RPE	Retinal pigment epithelium
SD-OCT	Spectral domain optical coherence tomography

Introduction

Pattern dystrophy (PD) refers to a group of inherited retinal dystrophies with changes primarily at the level of the retinal pigment epithelium (RPE). The typical features include deposits of yellow, orange, or gray pigment in the macula, associated with mild to moderate visual disturbance. Depending on the pattern of pigment disposition, five subtypes have been described by Gass:

1. Butterfly-shaped pigment dystrophy (Deutman et al. 1970)
2. Adult onset vitelliform pattern dystrophy (peculiar foveomacular dystrophy) (Gass 1974; Epstein and Rabb 1980)
3. Sjogren reticular dystrophy of the RPE (Sjogren 1950)
4. Fundus pulverulentus (Slezak and Hommer 1969)
5. Multifocal pattern dystrophy simulating Stargardt disease

Etiopathogenesis

PDs are most commonly inherited in an autosomal dominant manner. Mutations in peripherin/*RDS* gene (now known as *PRPH2)* have been found to be the most common (Pajic et al. 2006). *PRPH2* encodes for peripherin, a protein with four transmembrane domains that is important for photoreceptor outer receptor function. *PRPH2* assembles into homotetramers and locates in the rim regions of the rhodopsin-containing disk/lamellae of the photoreceptor outer segments, where its putative function is to maintain stability. *PHRP2* also forms heterotetramers with another tetraspanin known as the highly homologous rod outer segment 1 (ROM1) protein (Khan et al. 2016). In disease states, the outer segments become disorganized or fail to form entirely, and the photoreceptors subsequently degenerate (Stuck et al. 2016).

In PDs, the primary defect is presumed to be present in photoreceptor cells, with subsequent damage to RPE and choriocapillaris.

Dominant *PRPH2* mutations have been associated with a variety of retinal phenotypes typically of adult onset and often affect the macula. Phenotypes other than PD include cone-rod dystrophy, retinitis punctata albescens, central areolar choroidal dystrophy, retinitis pigmentosa, fundus

A. Tsai · R. Mathur · G. C. M. Cheung (✉)
Singapore National Eye Centre, Singapore Eye Research Institute, Singapore, Singapore

Duke NUS Graduate Medical School, Singapore, Singapore
e-mail: gemmy.cheung.c.m@snec.com.sg

A. Koh
Singapore National Eye Centre, Singapore Eye Research Institute, Singapore, Singapore

N.-K. Wang
Department of Ophthalmology, Chang Gung Memorial Hospital, Linkou Medical Center, Taoyuan, Taiwan

Department of Medicine, Chang Gung University, College of Medicine, Taoyuan, Taiwan

G. Cheung (ed.), *Hereditary Chorioretinal Disorders*, Retina Atlas, https://doi.org/10.1007/978-981-15-0414-3_5

flavimaculatus, age-related macular degeneration-like late onset maculopathy, and other unspecified autosomal dominant macular dystrophies.

Variable expressivity is also common in *PHRP2* mutations. If one or more of the abovementioned phenotype is present in a family, heterozygous mutations should be suspected.

Clinical Features

Patients commonly present in middle age with disturbance in central vision and may experience macular photostress. The fundus may show a variety of yellow, orange, or gray deposit in the macula. When patients present in advanced age, atrophy of the RPE-photoreceptor complex may develop and result in more severe visual loss. In such cases, pattern dystrophy can be confused with age-related macular degeneration (AMD). Some important differentiating factors include the lack of drusen and high level of symmetry in PD. Rarely, choroidal neovascularization (CNV) can complicate pattern dystrophy (Battaglia Parodi et al. 2003; Marano et al. 1996).

Butterfly-Shaped Pattern Dystrophy (BPD)

The butterfly-shaped pigmentation can be yellow, white, or black. The accumulation of pigment resembles the wings of a butterfly. Generally, the onset of visual symptoms is in the 20s or 30s (Figs. 5.1 and 5.2).

Adult Onset Vitelliform Pattern Dystrophy (AOVPD)

In AOVPD, there are typically symmetric yellowish subretinal lesions at the fovea, or presence of flecks. The vitelliform lesion may be confused with the later stages of Best disease. The yellow foveal lesions may develop a central gray or orange clump of pigment. Later, the foveal lesions may fade, leaving an area of RPE depigmentation (Fig. 5.3).

Sjogren Reticular Dystrophy of the RPE

In reticular dystrophy of the RPE, a network of pigmented lines can be seen in the macula which resembles fishnet with knots or chicken wire. With increasing age, most lesions fade and become replaced by atrophic changes in the RPE. In advanced disease, the network becomes bleached and irregular and small white dots appear in the RPE (Fig. 5.4).

Fundus Pulverulentus

This is the rarest form of PD. Patients typically have mild visual loss associated with prominent, coarse, punctiform mottling of the RPE in the central macula. Some cases are associated with pseudoxanthoma elasticum.

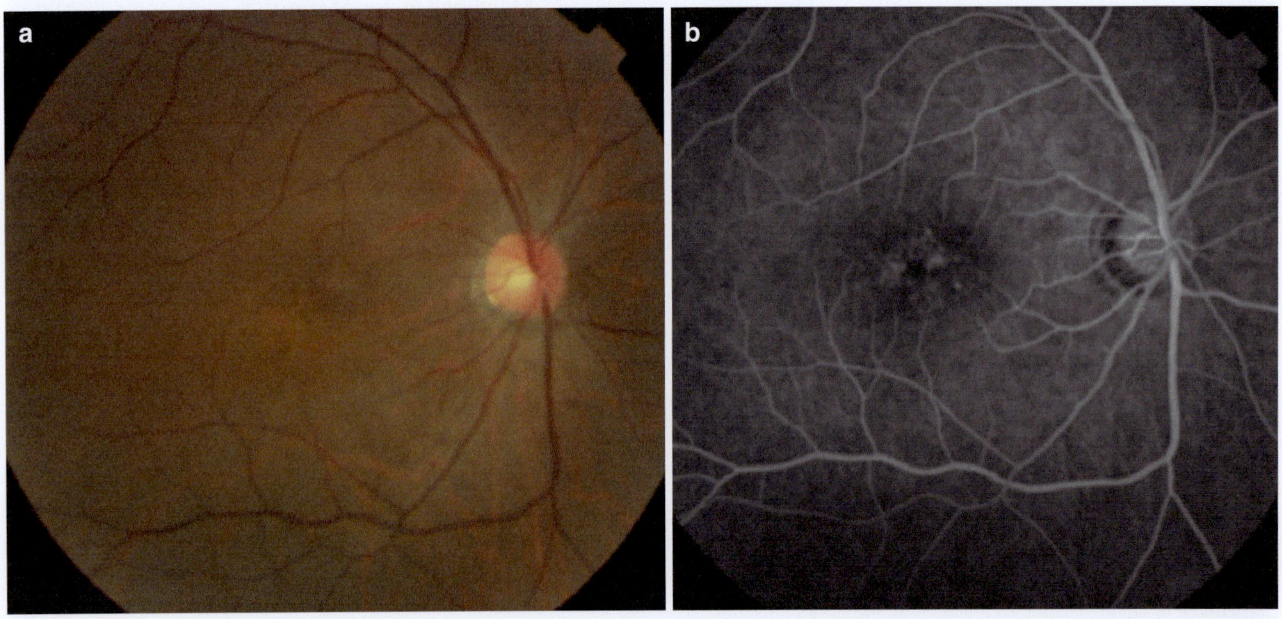

Fig. 5.1 A 40-year-old male with right decreased vision for 3 months. Visual acuity (VA) 6/24 OD (**a**) Color fundus photograph showing yellowish pigment deposition in a shape resembling wings of a butterfly. (**b**) Fluorescein angiogram (FA) showing areas of blocked fluorescence corresponding to the "wings"

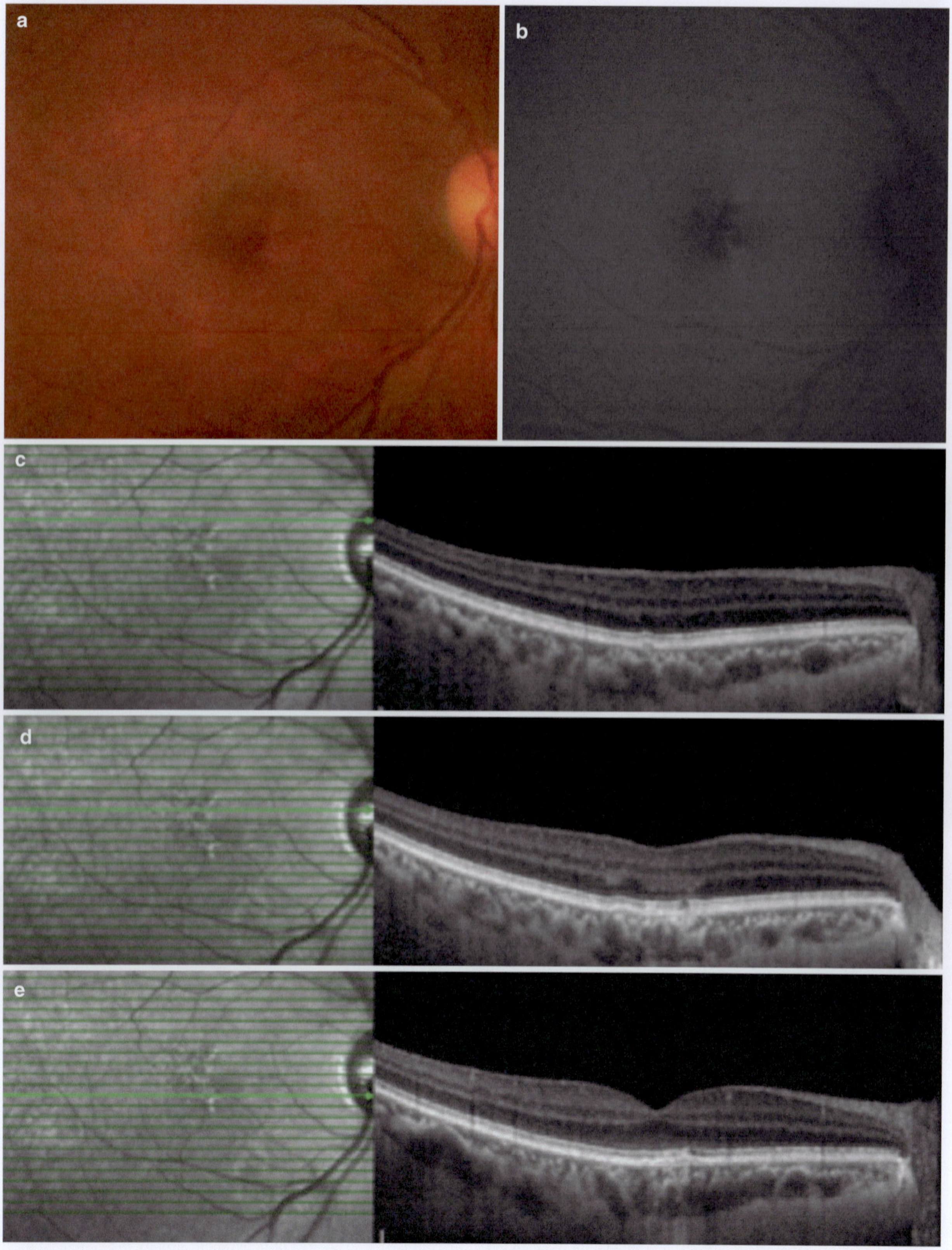

Fig. 5.2 A 50-year-old male with BPD presenting with mild reduced vision. VA 6/9 OD. (**a**) Color fundus photograph showing pigment deposition. (**b**) Fundus autofluorescence (FAF) imaged using a fundus camera showing areas of hyper/hypoautofluorescence corresponding to the pattern of lipofuscin deposition. (**c–e**) Series of spectral domain optical coherence tomography (SD-OCT) showing irregular RPE corresponding to area of hyperautofluorescence likely due to pigment clumping (**e**). The areas of hypoautofluorescence correspond to areas of ellipsoid zone and RPE disruption (**c**, **d**)

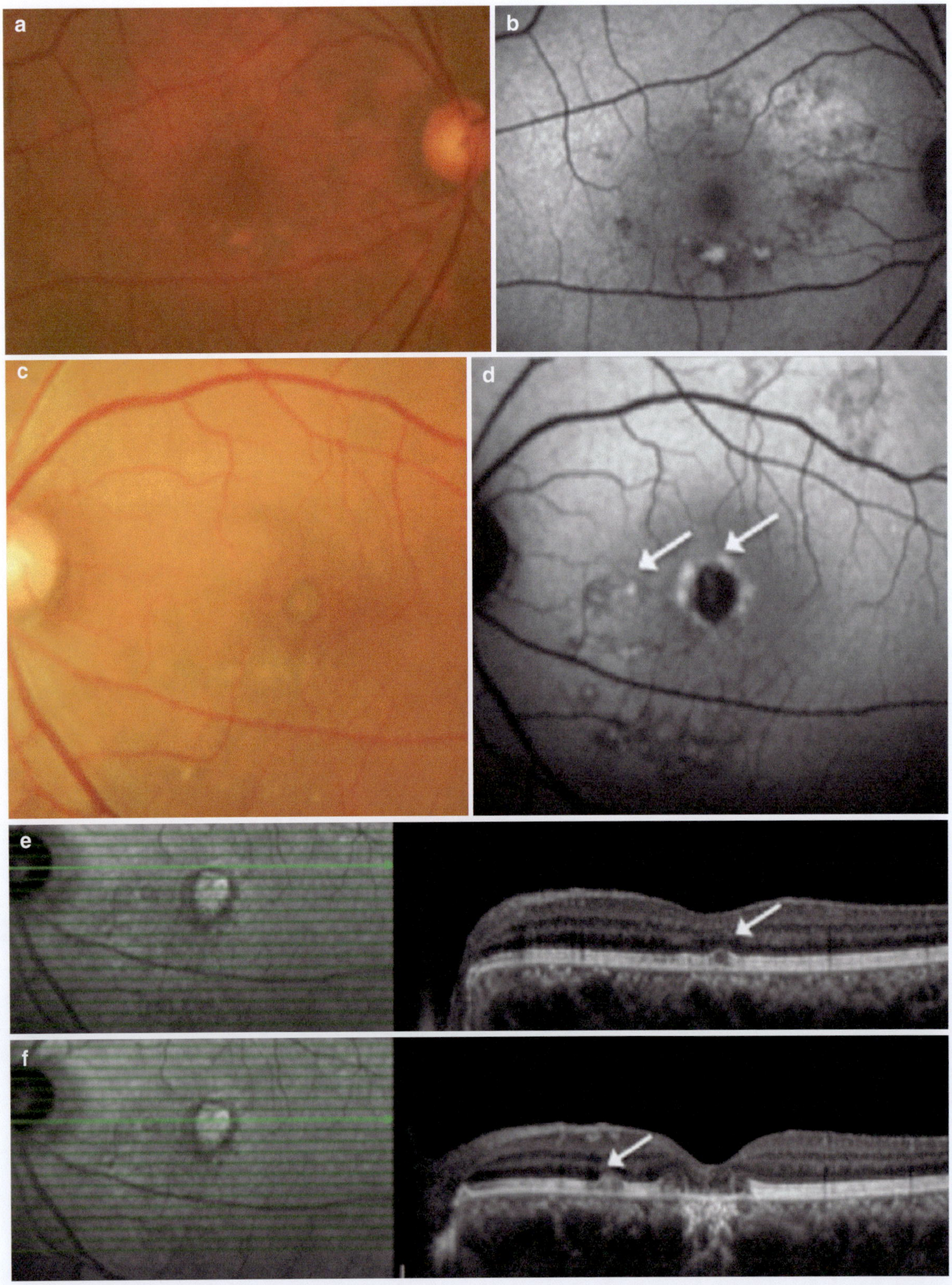

Fig. 5.3 A 43-year-old male with AOVPD presented with reduced left eye vision for 1 year. VA 6/18 OS. (**a**) Multifocal yellowish subretinal deposits surrounded by grayish pigmentary changes. (**b**) FAF shows these areas have hyperautofluorescent cores corresponding to yellow deposits. This is surrounded by hypoautofluorescent areas which are more obvious on FAF compared to color fundus photographs. (**c**, **d**) Later stage of AOFVD with a well-circumscribed yellowish foveal atrophic lesion which appears hypoautofluorescent on FAF. This lesion may be confused with an area of geographic atrophy in age-related macular degeneration. However, the surrounding fleck-like lesions which appear hyperautofluorescent should raise the suspicion that this may be a case of AOFVD. (**e**, **f**) Series of SD-OCT images showing loss of ellipsoid zone, disruption of outer retina, and RPE layer in the fovea area. However, there are areas of possibly early vitelliform lesions (white arrows) which correspond to hyperautofluorescent areas on 3D

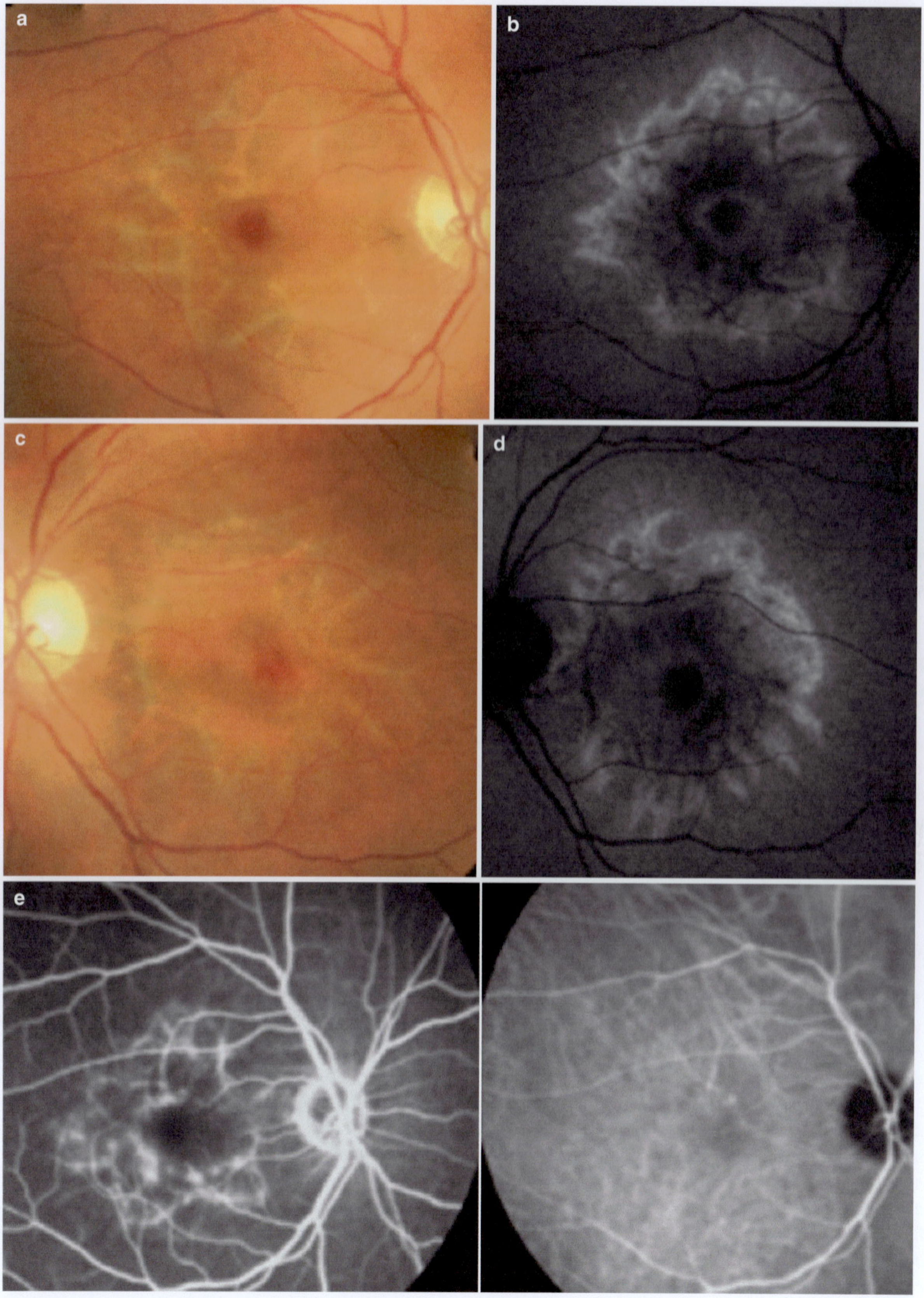

Fig. 5.4 A 56-year-old female who was referred for evaluation of retinal lesions. VA of 6/15 OD and 6/30 OS (proven *RDS* gene mutation). (**a**, **c**) Color fundus photographs showing a prominent reticular network of pale linear lesions at the macula. (**b**, **d**) On FAF, the linear structures appear hypoautofluorescent. However, a wider hyperautofluorescent ring can be seen encompassing the abnormal area. (**e**) The linear structures appear as hyperfluorescent window defects on FA which suggests there is RPE atrophy. The indocyanine green angiogram was unremarkable. (**f**, **g**) SD-OCT shows widespread disruption of the outer retinal layers

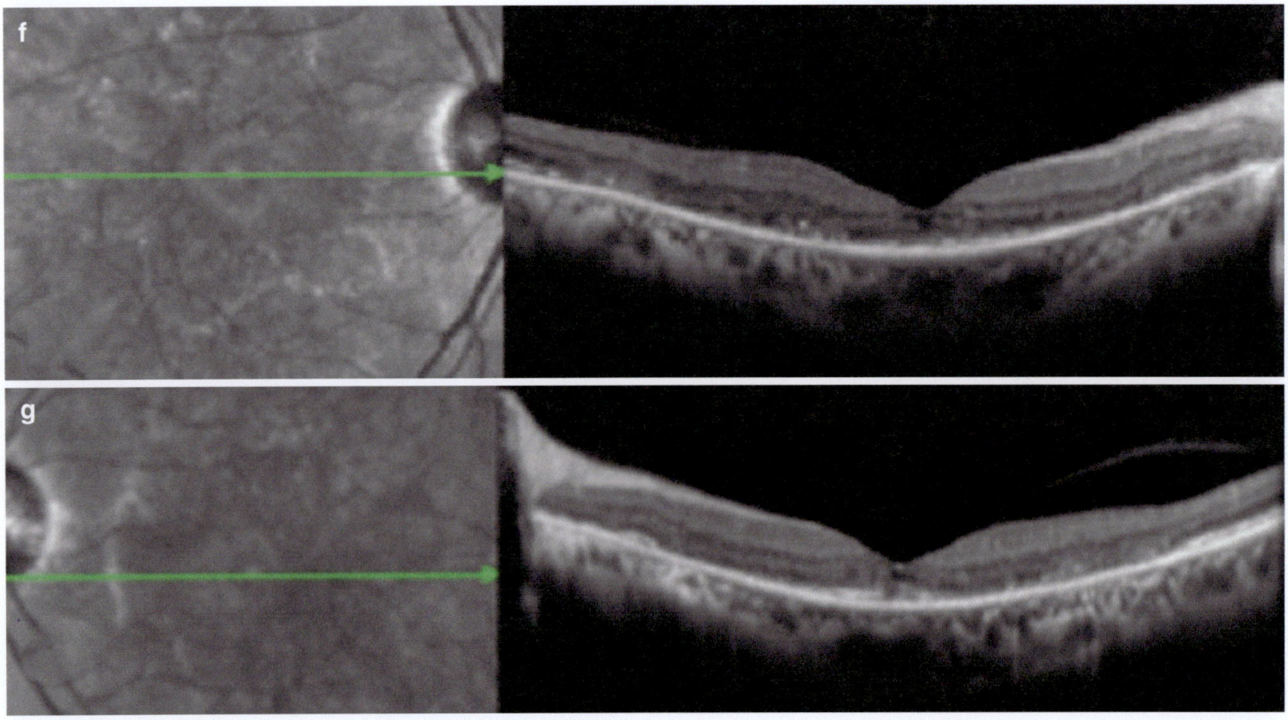

Fig. 5.4 (continued)

Multifocal Pattern Dystrophy Simulating Fundus Flavimaculatus

Occasionally, multifocal pattern dystrophy may also simulate other inherited retinal diseases such as Stargardt disease (Boon et al. 2007). Secondary CNV formation is a possible but rare sequelae of pattern dystrophy (Fig. 5.5). FA in these cases will not show a dark choroid which suggests lipofuscin deposition.

Investigations

On fundus autofluorescence (FAF), lesions in BPD may show increased as well as decreased autofluorescence, with corresponding changes in RPE lipofuscin within the lesion (Boon et al. 2008). The flecks in multifocal pattern dystrophy simulating Stargardt disease exhibit highly increased autofluorescence, with small adjacent zones of decreased autofluorescence. In AOVPD, various autofluorescence patterns described include normal, focal, patchy, ring-like, and linear with inconsistent correlation with visual acuity (Furino et al. 2008; Parodi et al. 2008).

OCT imaging in pattern dystrophy shows a variety of changes (Hannan et al. 2013; Kumar and Kumawat 2018). Features include hyper-reflectivity between the retinal pigment epithelium (RPE)/Bruch's complex and the ellipsoid zone. Ellipsoid zone and outer retinal layer disruption can also be observed. Abnormal focal hyper-reflectivity originating from the RPE toward the outer nuclear layer (ONL) may also be seen.

On FA, a butterfly-shaped defect can be more clearly seen especially when lesions are not clinically obvious. The lesion appears as blocked fluorescence due to pigment deposition, surround by hyperfluoresence (Tuppurainen and Mäntyjärvi 1994). The FA defects are also often more widespread and better manifested than color photographs.

Full-field electroretinogram (ERG) typically shows normal cone and rod amplitudes and implicit times. Some reduction may be seen if there are more extensive changes. EOG light peak to dark trough ratios are frequently normal and only modestly subnormal, in contrast to Best vitelliform macular dystrophy.

Electrophysiology is usually performed for patients with lack of mutations in *PRPH2*, or a fundus appearance which is apparent for more widespread involvement of the photoreceptors.

Management and Prognosis

Most patients with PD retain reasonable vision. Patients should be reassured that the prognosis of maintaining good central vision in one eye until late adulthood is good.

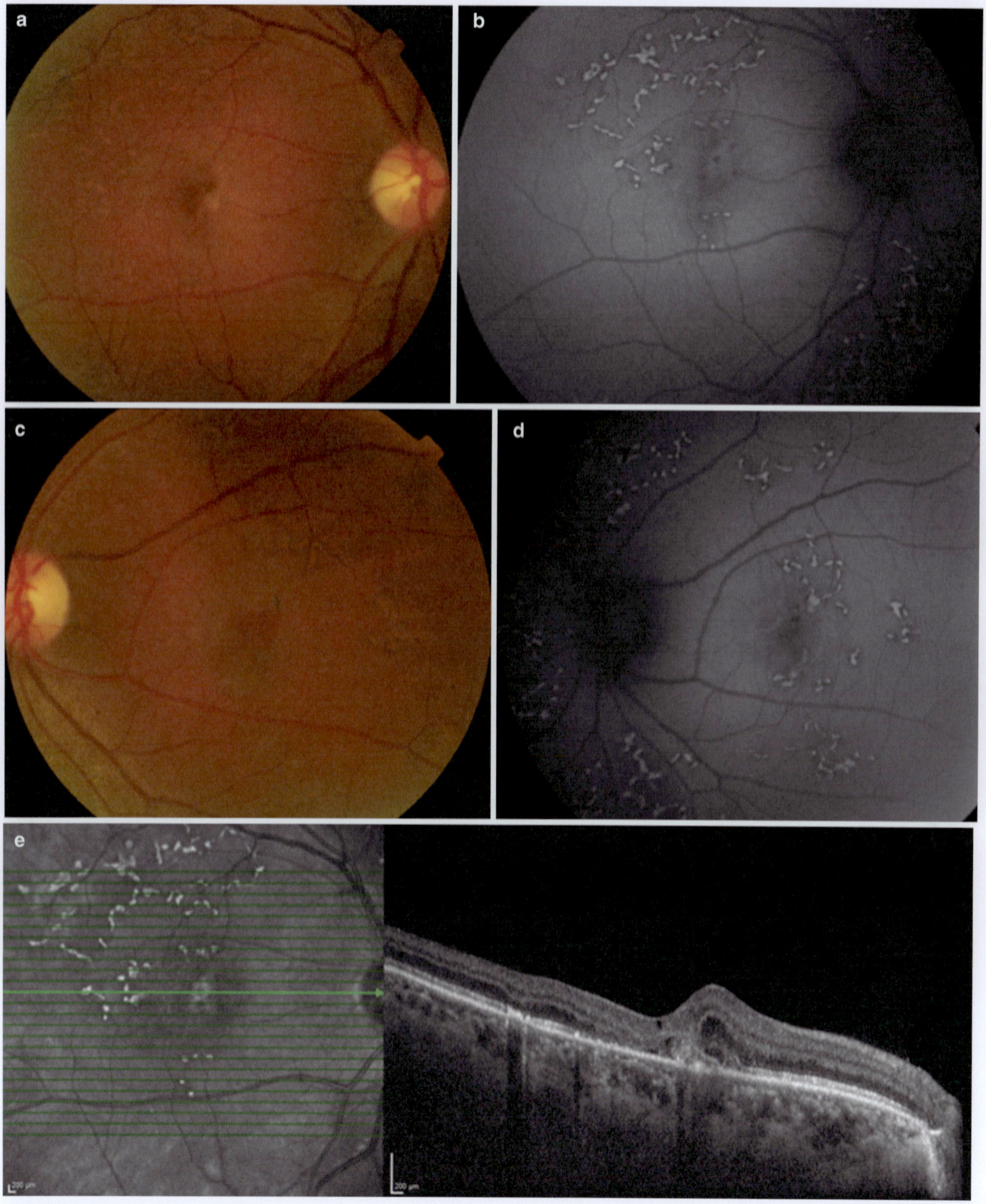

Fig. 5.5 (**a**, **c**) Color fundus photographs showing bilateral macula atrophic changes with yellowish fleck deposition. (**b**, **d**) Fundus AF showing hyperfluorescent areas corresponding to flecks. (**e**, **f**) SD-OCT shows loss of outer retina in both eyes. Retinal edema can be seen in the right resulting from a secondary CNV. (**g**) Early and late phase FA of the right eye demonstrating leakage from CNV. (**h**) FA of left eye showed no leakage. (**i**) Five years after presentation, in addition to yellowish flecks, RPE hyperplasia is seen temporal to the fovea. (**j**) Fundus AF showing hyperfluorescent areas corresponding to flecks and hypofluorescent areas at the fovea corresponding to area of RPE hyperplasia. (**k**) SD-OCT shows a hyperreflective lesion corresponding to a CNV scar. (**l**) Color fundus photograph showing RPE hyperplasia, in addition to flecks. (**m**) Fundus AF showing hypofluorescent area corresponding to area of RPE hyperplasia. (**n**) SD-OCT shows loss of outer retina in the left eye

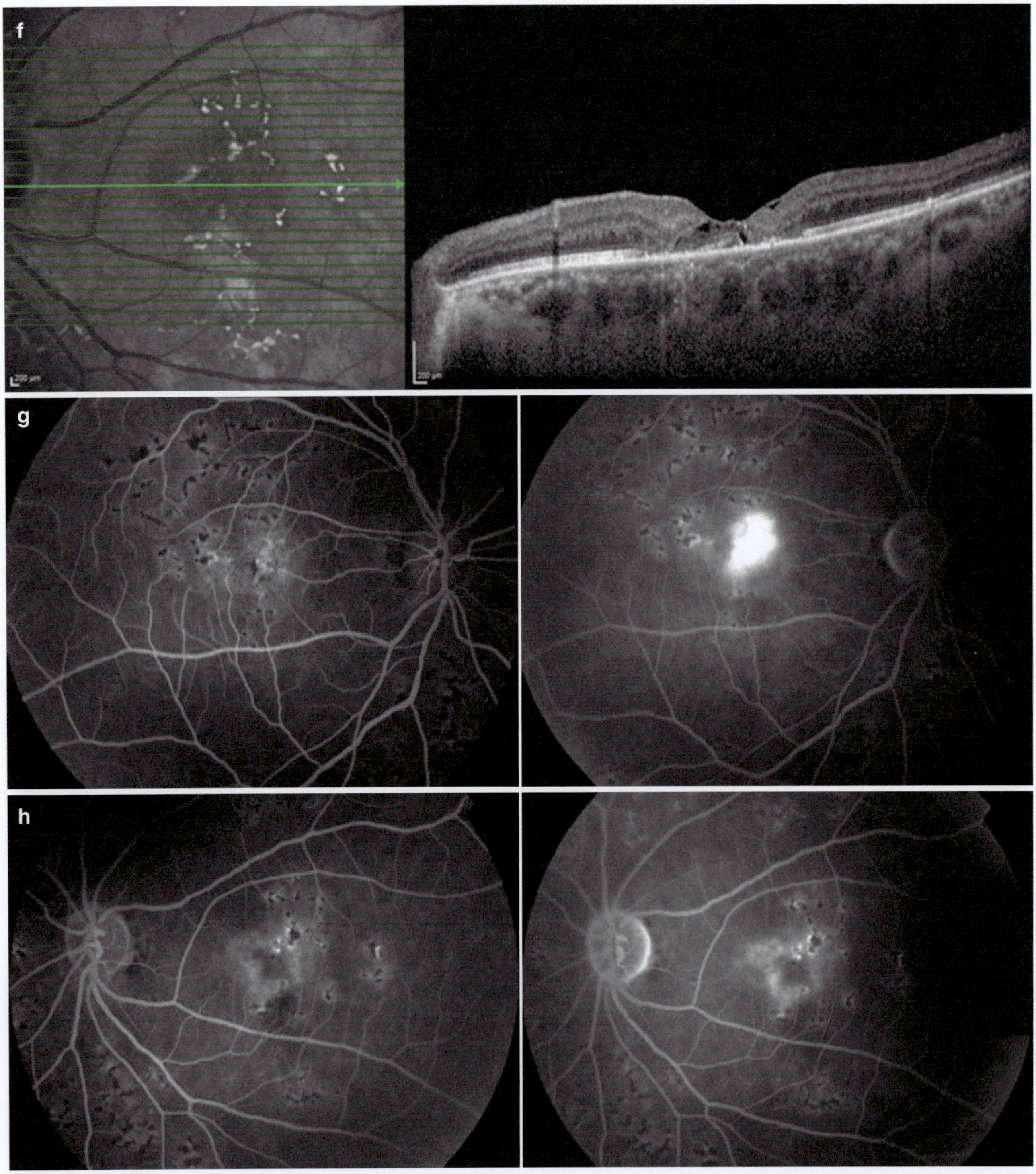

Fig. 5.5 (continued)

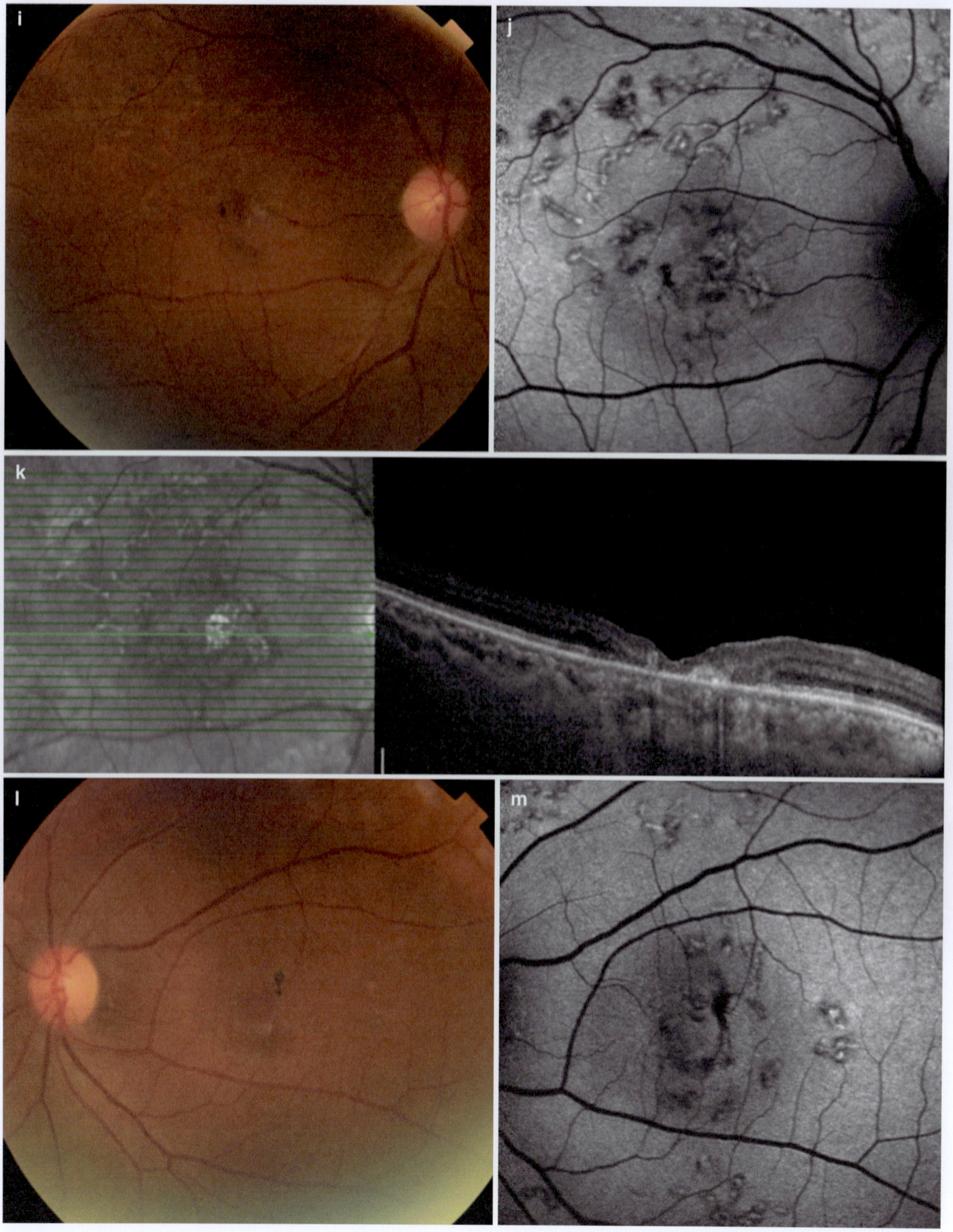

Fig. 5.5 (continued)

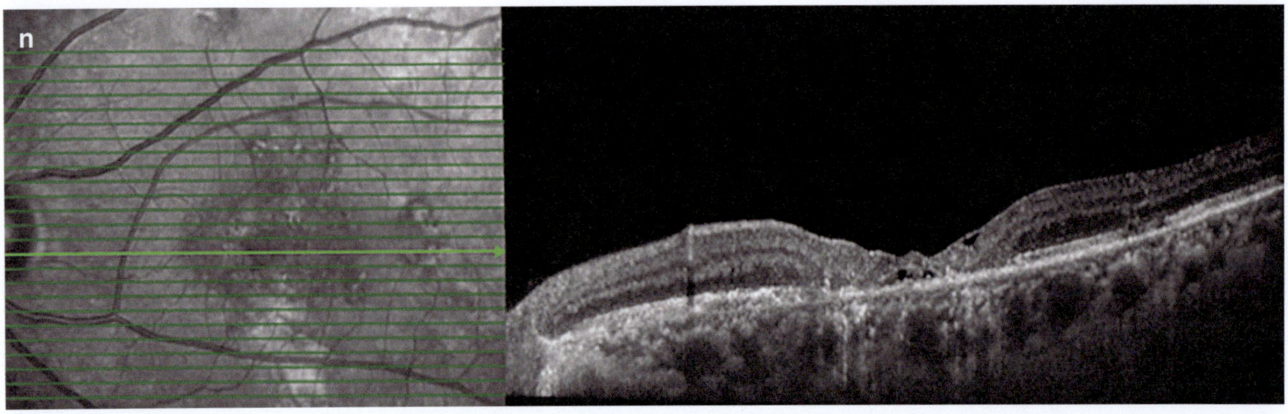

Fig. 5.5 (continued)

In patients who experience difficulty in adapting when moving from a bright light into a dark area, the use of dark glasses when outside may help with symptoms. If CNV develops, anti-vascular endothelial growth factor injections are indicated. However, all patients should also be counseled regarding potential gradual visual deterioration in the long-term and potential implications on driving. It has been reported that about 50% of patients with PD eventually develop geographic atrophy or CNV (Francis et al. 2005).

References

Battaglia Parodi M, Da Pozzo S, Ravalico G. Photodynamic therapy for choroidal neovascularization associated with pattern dystrophy. Retina. 2003;23(2):171–6.

Boon CJ, van Schooneveld MJ, den Hollander AI, et al. Mutations in the peripherin/RDS gene are an important cause of multifocal pattern dystrophy simulating STGD1/fundus flavimaculatus. Br J Ophthalmol. 2007;91(11):1504–11.

Boon CJ, den Hollander AI, Hoyng CB, Cremers FP, Klevering BJ, Keunen JE. The spectrum of retinal dystrophies caused by mutations in the peripherin/RDS gene. Prog Retin Eye Res. 2008;27(2):213–35.

Deutman AF, van Blommestein JD, Henkes HE, Waardenburg PJ, Solleveld-van Driest E. Butterfly-shaped pigment dystrophy of the fovea. Arch Ophthalmol. 1970;83(5):558–69.

Epstein GA, Rabb MF. Adult vitelliform macular degeneration: diagnosis and natural history. Br J Ophthalmol. 1980;64(10):733–40.

Francis PJ, Schultz DW, Gregory AM, et al. Genetic and phenotypic heterogeneity in pattern dystrophy. Br J Ophthalmol. 2005;89(9):1115–9.

Furino C, Boscia F, Cardascia N, Sborgia L, Sborgia C. Fundus autofluorescence, optical coherence tomography and visual acuity in adult-onset foveomacular dystrophy. Ophthalmologica. 2008;222(4):240–4.

Gass JD. A clinicopathologic study of a peculiar foveomacular dystrophy. Trans Am Ophthalmol Soc. 1974;72:139–56.

Hannan SR, de Salvo G, Stinghe A, Shawkat F, Lotery AJ. Common spectral domain OCT and electrophysiological findings in different pattern dystrophies. Br J Ophthalmol. 2013;97(5):605–10.

Khan AO, Al Rashaed S, Neuhaus C, Bergmann C, Bolz HJ. Peripherin mutations cause a distinct form of recessive Leber congenital amaurosis and dominant phenotypes in asymptomatic parents heterozygous for the mutation. Br J Ophthalmol. 2016;100(2):209–15.

Kumar V, Kumawat D. Multimodal imaging in a case of butterfly pattern dystrophy of retinal pigment epithelium. Int Ophthalmol. 2018;38(2):775–9.

Marano F, Deutman AF, Aandekerk AL. Butterfly-shaped pigment dystrophy of the fovea associated with subretinal neovascularization. Graefes Arch Clin Exp Ophthalmol. 1996;234(4):270–4.

Pajic B, Weigell-Weber M, Schipper I, et al. A novel complex mutation event in the peripherin/RDS gene in a family with retinal pattern dystrophy. Retina. 2006;26(8):947–53.

Parodi MB, Iacono P, Pedio M, et al. Autofluorescence in adult-onset foveomacular vitelliform dystrophy. Retina. 2008;28(6):801–7.

Sjogren H. Dystrophia reticularis laminae pigmentosae retinae, an earlier not described hereditary eye disease. Acta Ophthalmol. 1950;28(3):279–95.

Slezak H, Hommer K. [Fundus pulverulentus]. Albrecht Von Graefes Arch Klin Exp Ophthalmol. 1969;178(2):176–82.

Stuck MW, Conley SM, Naash MI. PRPH2/RDS and ROM-1: historical context, current views and future considerations. Prog Retin Eye Res. 2016;52:47–63.

Tuppurainen K, Mäntyjärvi M. The importance of fluorescein angiography in diagnosing pattern dystrophies of the retinal pigment epithelium. Doc Ophthalmol. 1994;87(3):233–43.

Stargardt Macular Dystrophy

6

Veronika Vaclavik

Introduction

ABCA4-associated autosomal recessive Stargardt disease (STGD1; MIM 248200), also known as Stargardt macular dystrophy, is the most common monogenic macular dystrophy in adults and children (Allikmets et al. 1997; Stone et al. 2017). There is an estimated prevalence of 1 in 8000 to 1 in 10,000 (Blacharski 1988). Most common onset of disease symptoms is during childhood or teenage years and is characterized by impairment of central vision that usually progresses to legal blindness (Fishman et al. 1987; Rotenstreich et al. 2003). The peripheral vision is preserved most of the time (Aaberg 1986). Some late and adult onset Stargardt phenotypes are associated with milder missense mutations (Fujinami et al. 2013b; Genead et al. 2009).

Stargardt disease is an autosomal recessive retinal dystrophy, linked to mutations in the *ABCA4* gene (Allikmets et al. 1997), with both sexes equally affected. Over 1000 variants have been identified in the *ABCA4* gene; combinations of variants result in a highly heterogenic phenotype and are predictive of the severity and age of onset of the disease (Cornelis et al. 2017; Zernant et al. 2017). The *ABCA4* gene encodes for a retinal-specific ATP-binding transporter protein. Its dysfunction leads to toxic accumulation of byproducts from the visual cycle in the retinal pigment epithelium and photoreceptor cells, leading to irreversible damage of the outer retinal layers (Allikmets et al. 1997).

There is currently no proven treatment, but there are several axes of intervention being explored, including human clinical trials of gene replacement therapy, stem cell therapy, and pharmacological approaches (Dalkara et al. 2016; Saad and Washington 2016; Schwartz et al. 2015).

V. Vaclavik (✉)
Department of Ophthalmology, Genetic and Rare Disease, Jules Gonin Eye Hospital, University of Lausanne, Lausanne, Switzerland

Department of Ophthalmology, Medical Retina, Hospital Cantonal, HFR, Fribourg, Switzerland
e-mail: veronika.vaclavik@fa2.ch

Clinical Features

Phenotypes of Stargardt disease range from very early-onset panretinal degeneration (Ciccone et al. 2018; Cremers et al. 1998; Lee et al. 2016; Maugeri et al. 2000; Tanaka et al. 2018) to late-onset mild cases, with preserved fovea. This phenotypic variability is due to extensive *ABCA4* disease-associated genetic variation, with more than 1000 definitely or very likely disease-causing variants in the coding sequence and splice site of the *ABCA4* gene (Cornelis et al. 2017).

Early-onset Stargardt *disease* is on the more severe end of *ABCA4*-associated retinal degeneration spectrum and is associated with null or otherwise severe and/or moderate *ABCA4* mutations (Yatsenko et al. 2001). The mean age of onset of symptoms is about 7 years. These patients have a fast decline in visual acuity bilaterally, noticed by themselves or parents or school physicians. The decrease in visual acuity might be initially unexplained, as fundus examination may not reveal any major abnormalities. A normal fundus appearance in affected children was described in 24–33% of cases (Fujinami et al. 2015; Lambertus et al. 2015).

In these early forms, the fundus appearance is characterized by atrophy of the macula, which might be very subtle at the beginning, while the typical yellow flecks can be absent (Lambertus et al. 2015). The lack of typical signs on the retina led to delay in diagnosis of childhood early-onset STGD1 of median 3 years. During that time many unnecessary investigations, such as MRIs or CTs, lumbar punctures as well as mental illness or amblyopia treatments were performed (Bax et al. 2019). Some additional paraclinical (SD-OCT, autofluorescence, full field ERGs) and genetic testing might be therefore necessary to confirm the diagnosis of early-onset STGD1 (Fujinami et al. 2015).

A family with three affected children (Figs. 6.1, 6.2, and 6.3), with an *ABCA4* variants: Allele 1: c.[634C > T], p.(R212C) Allele 2: c.[4539 + 2064C > T;5460 + 1769C > A], is a good illustration of early-onset STGD1 as well as intrafamilial variable phenotype expressivity. The eldest son had reducing visual acuity since his age of 7 years. When aged

G. Cheung (ed.), *Hereditary Chorioretinal Disorders*, Retina Atlas, https://doi.org/10.1007/978-981-15-0414-3_6

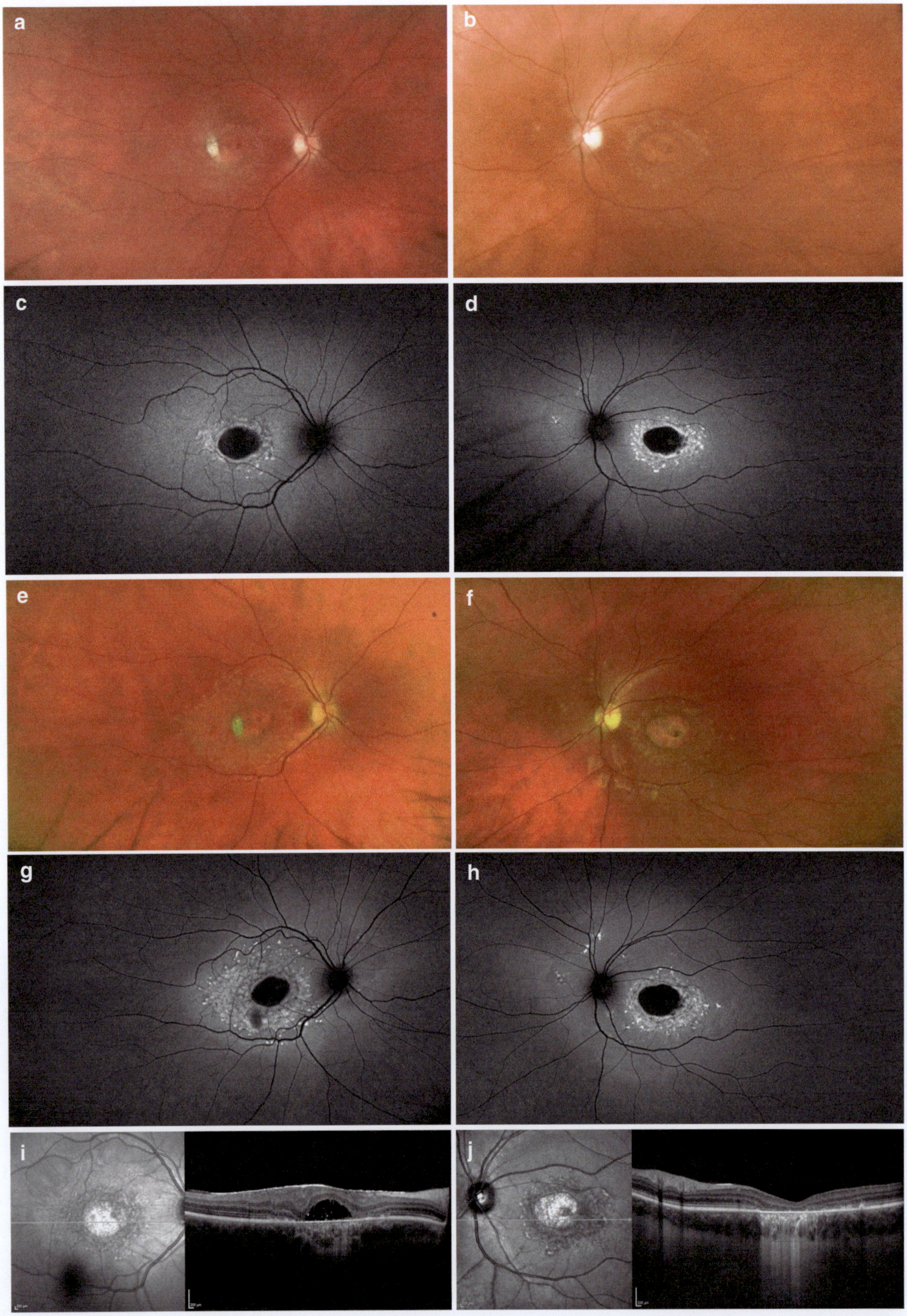

Fig. 6.1 Eldest affected son (family 2, ABCA4 Allele 1: c.[634C > T], p.(R212C) Allele 2: c.[4539 + 2064C > T;5460 + 1769C > A]). (**a**, **b**) Fundus color photos RE and LE, showing central atrophy in both eyes, with a scar temporal to the fovea in the RE. Some flecks can be seen surrounding the atrophy. (**c**, **d**) Autofluorescence RE and LE showing hypofluorescent enlarged central area, surrounded by hyperautofluorescent flecks. The patient was 22 years old, and his VA (eccentrically) was 0.1 in the RE and 0.16 in the LE. (**e**, **f**) Color fundus photos RE and LE, 2 years later, showing concentric extension of flecks that are still within the arcades, at the macula. (**g**, **h**) Autofluorescence imaging RE and LE, 2 years later, showing extension of hyperautofluorescent flecks, extending beyond arcades: some flecks superior to optic nerve can be seen. (**i**, **j**) OCT RE and LE, when the patient was 22 years old, OCT RE showing some cysts, corresponding to the old CNV. Thinning of all subfoveal layers in the LE

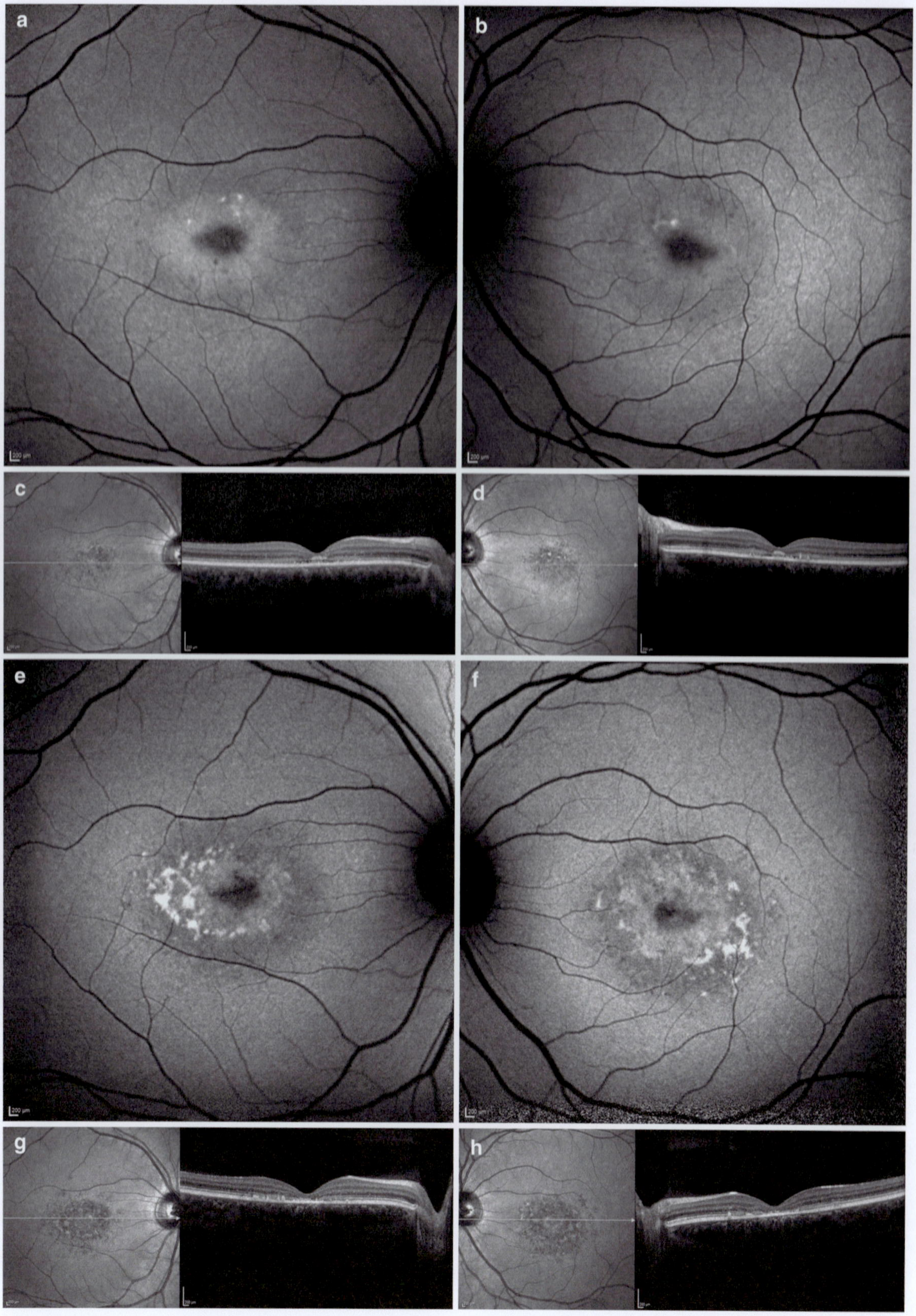

Fig. 6.2 Younger affected sister (family 2, ABCA4 Allele 1: c.[634C > T], p.(R212C) Allele 2: c.[4539 + 2064C > T;5460 + 1769C > A]). (**a**, **b**) Autofluorescence imaging RE and LE, showing hyperautofluorescent ring around an enlarged hypofluorescent central area. Some hyperfluorescent spots, in superior of the fovea, more in RE. (**c**, **d**) OCT LE and RE, showing hyperreflective subfoveal thickening of the external limiting membrane. At this time the patient was 16 years old, and her VA was 0.6 bilaterally. (**e**, **f**) Autofluorescence imaging 4 years later (patient aged 20 years): hyperfluorescent band enlarged, hyperautofluorescent flecks enraged in number and size. (**g**, **h**) OCT RE and LE 4 years later: thinning of layer, absence of ellipsoid layer, and external limiting membrane in the subfoveal area. The VA dropped to 0.16

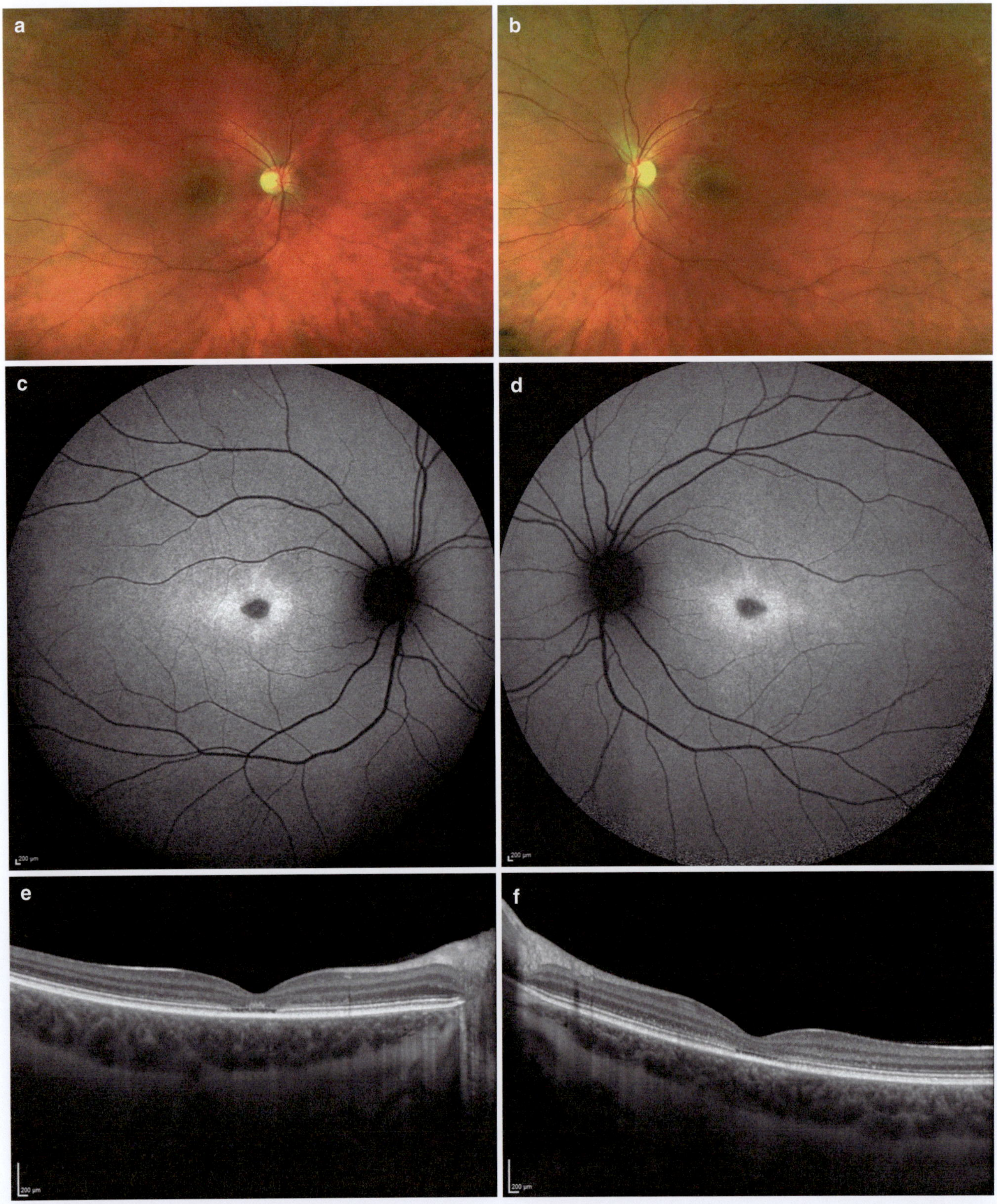

Fig. 6.3 Youngest affected sister (family 2, ABCA4 Allele 1: c.[634C > T], p.(R212C) Allele 2: c.[4539 + 2064C > T;5460 + 1769C > A]). (**a**, **b**) Color fundus photo RE and LE, showing normal appearance of fundus. (**c**, **d**) Autofluorescence imaging RE and LE, showing hyper-fluorescent halo surrounding an enlarged hypofluorescent foveal area. (**e**, **f**) OCT RE and LE, showing subfoveal "cystic space" due to interrupted ellipsoid layer. Her BCVA was 0.5 bilaterally

11 years, his Snellen VA was 0.2 bilaterally, no flecks were visible on AF imaging. When he was 22 years, a CNV complicated his enlarging central atrophy (Fig. 6.1i), and some flecks were noticed on AF (Fig. 6.1c, d). The flecks increased in number and extended 2 years later (Fig. 6.1g, h). A younger sister had a milder phenotype, with a Snellen visual acuity of 0.6 bilaterally aged 16 years. The AF image showed enlarged hypofluorescent central area, surrounded by a hyperfluorescent ring and a few flecks (Fig. 6.2a, b). The OCT showed hyperreflective subfoveal thickening of the band representing the external limiting membrane (Fig. 6.2c, d). Four years later, her VA dropped to 0.16, with more flecks on AF (Fig. 6.2e, f) and thinning of layers on OCT: disrupted ellipsoid and external limiting membrane layer (Fig. 6.2g, h). The youngest affected sister came, aged 12 years, with reducing VA for 2–3 years. Her BCVA was 0.5 bilaterally, with enlarged hypofluorescence on AF, surrounded by hyperfluorescent ring (Fig. 6.3c, d). Her fundus examination was within normal limits, some small atrophy could be seen at the fovea (Fig. 6.3a, b). The OCTs showed subfoveal interrupted ellipsoid layer, with the appearance of "cystic space" (Fig. 6.3e, f).

The natural course of early-onset STGD1 can extend beyond macula to diffuse chorioretinal atrophy, some stay limited to the macula, depending on the severity of *ABCA4* mutations.

Intermediate-Onset (or Adult Onset) Stargardt

The mean age of onset is young adulthood. At presentation, the fundus shows typical yellow-white flecks, with central atrophy. Figure 6.4 shows progression of central atrophy of a patient with variants in *ABCA4*: 1: c.[634C > T], p.R212C, 2: c.[1937 + 393 T > C]. He started losing his VA in his 30s and then developed photophobia in his mid-40s. The AF imaging showed central atrophy surrounded by hyperfluorescent flecks when he was 50 years old (Fig. 6.4c, d). The VA at this time was 0.1 bilaterally, eccentric. Nine years later the area of atrophy enlarged, and hyperfluorescent flecks became confluent (Fig. 6.4e, f).

Very widespread flecks at presentation can also be seen. The diagnosis of STGD1 was established when the patient was 15 years old, the first AF imaging showed widespread flecks and enlarged hypofluorescent area at macula (Fig. 6.5a, b). His VA was 0.4 in his right eye and 0.3 in the left. Two years later, more flecks appeared at the posterior pole, with centrifugal expansion, while hypofluorescent area enlarged (Fig. 6.5e, f). The vision dropped to 0.2 bilaterally. The OCTs showed thinning of the retina, with interrupted ellipsoid layer—enlarging over the period of 2 years (Fig. 6.5c, d, g, h). The screening of *ABCA4* gene showed variants: Allele 1: c.[5087G > A], p.(S1696N) Allele 2: c.[1957G > A], p.(R653C).

Late-Onset Stargardt

STGD1 can be diagnosed as late as 50 years. In these cases, it is often associated with foveal sparing and a better prognosis and some specific missense variants are often associated (Fujinami et al. 2013a; Yatsenko et al. 2001). Historically the late-onset STGD1 has been found to have one mutant allele only, while the second allele has not been found. Several recent reports described that the second allele in many of those cases harbored a hypomorphic p N1868I (c.5603A > T) *ABCA4* variant (Collison and Fishman 2018; Zernant et al. 2017). This variant was consistently associated with foveal sparing, late-onset STGD1, when the opposing ABCA4 allele carried a deleterious mutation (Zernant et al. 2017).

Figure 6.6 illustrates a patient with variants in *ABCA4* (c.[2971G > C], G991R exon 20; c.[3899G > A], R1300Q exon 27). She started to notice reducing vision since she was 50 years old. The AF imaging showed foveal sparing and some surrounding hyperfluorescent flecks. The visual acuity was 0.8 in the right eye and 0.3 in the left.

Paraclinic Testing (Imaging and ERGs)

Electrophysiological assessment, including full-field, pattern, and multifocal ERG, can be helpful. Some authors established classification of three established subtypes, according to their electrophysiology (Lois et al. 2001). Group 1 was classified as severe pattern ERG abnormality, with otherwise normal rod and cone function. Group 2 was classified as severe pattern ERG abnormality, with additional generalized loss of cone function. Group 3 was additional generalized loss of both cone and rod function. In the original publication, it was thought that these groups have prognostic value, with Group 1 having a better prognosis, with a more localized disease. However, further studies demonstrated that 22% of patients from Group 1 showed progression to Group 2 or 3, while 47% patients from Group 2 progressed to Group 3 (Fujinami et al. 2013b).

Autofluorescence imaging enables imaging of RPE lipofuscin distribution in vivo, using properties of lipofuscin, and related metabolites, A2E (Delori et al. 1995). AF is more useful in the diagnosis of STGD1 disease than fluorescein angiography, previously used to identify the "dark choroid," observed in 80% of STGD1 due to blockage of underlying choroidal fluorescence by "lipofuscin-overloaded" RPE (Fishman et al. 1999). AF can identify fundus changes before they are clinically obvious on ophthalmoscopy—such as early atrophy and flecks (Wabbels et al. 2006). An abnormally increased AF signal derives from excessive lipofuscin accumulation, while reduced signal translate and absent or

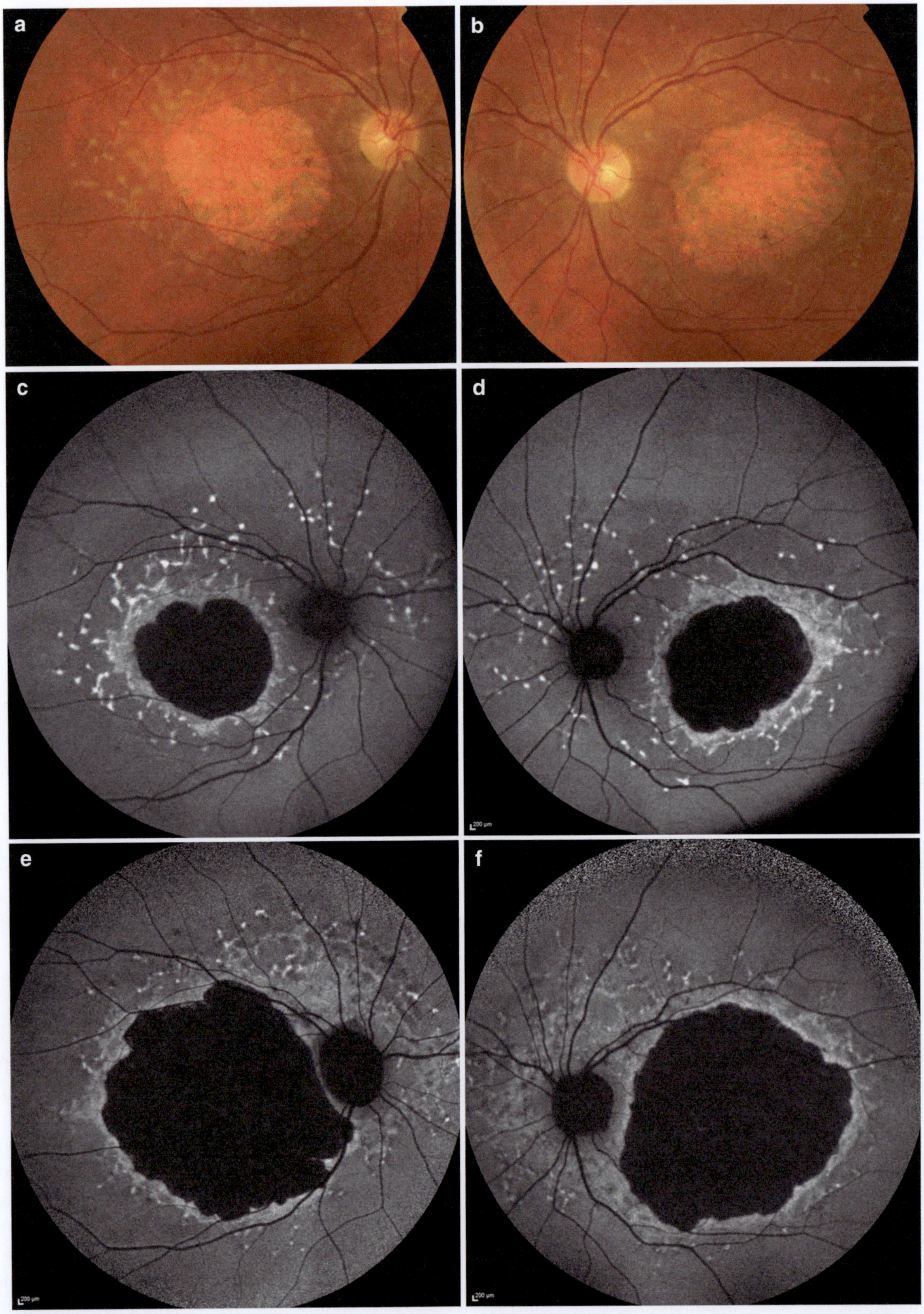

Fig. 6.4 Family 1 ABCA4 Allele 1: c.[634C > T], p.R212C Allele 2: c.[1937 + 393 T > C]. (**a**, **b**) Color fundus photo RE and LE, showing central atrophy and flecks all over the posterior pole. (**c**, **d**) Autofluorescent images of RE and LE, showing large central hypofluorescent atrophy and hyperfluorescent flecks extending beyond the optic nerve. The patient was 50 years old, and his BCVA (excentric) was 0.07 in the RE and 0.1 in the LE. (**e**, **f**) Autofluorescent images RE and LE, 9 years later, showing enlarged central hypofluorescent area of atrophy and further increase of hyperfluorescent flecks, becoming confluent

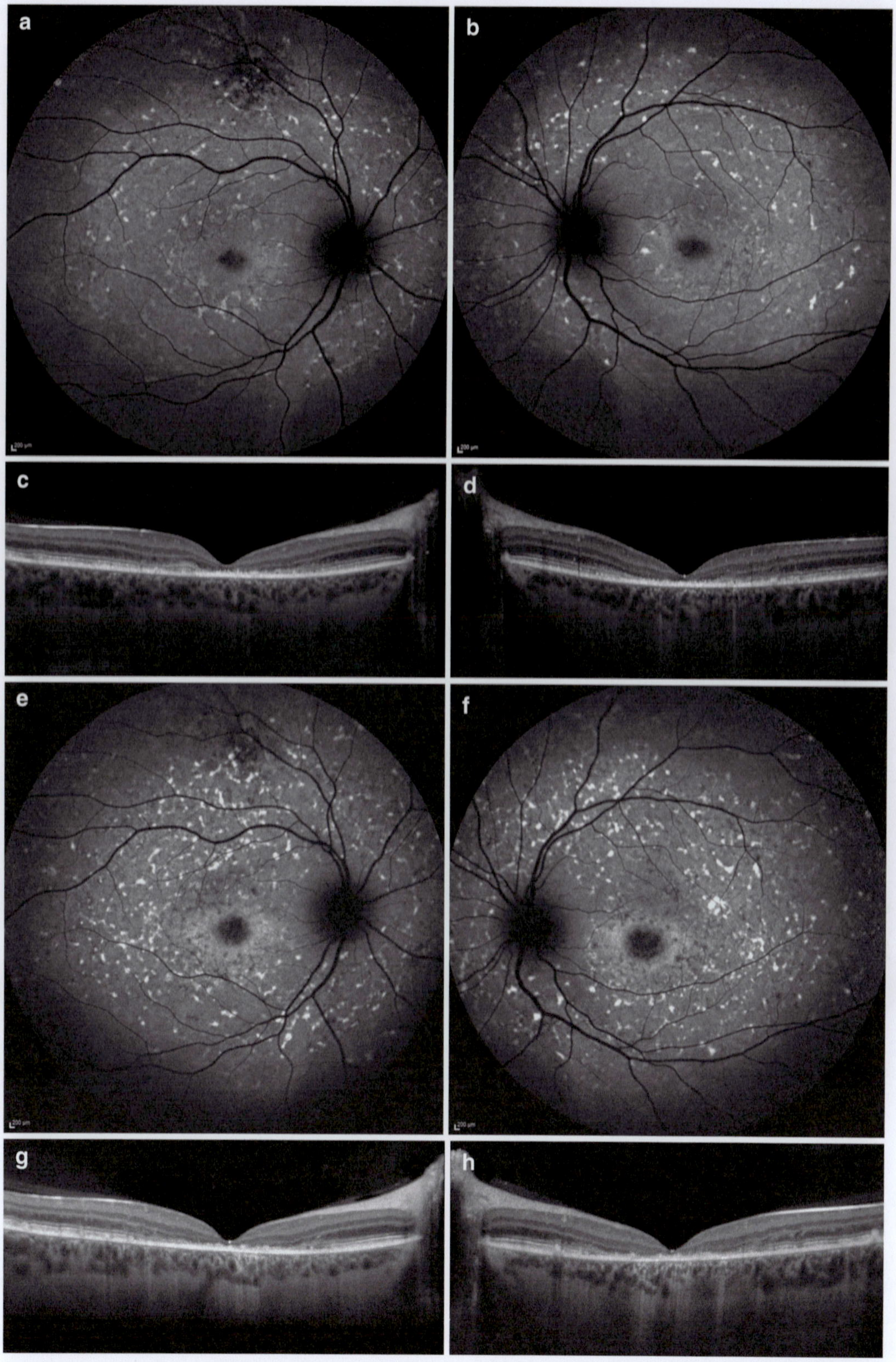

Fig. 6.5 Family 3, ABCA4 Allele 1: c.[5087G > A], p.(S1696N) Allele 2: c.[1957G > A], p.(R653C). (**a**, **b**) Autofluorescence images RE and LE, showing widespread hyperfluorescent flecks on the posterior pole and enlarged hypofluorescent central area. The patient was 15 years old, and his BCVA was 0.4 RE and 0.3 LE. (**c**, **d**) OCT images RE and LE, showing thinning of the retina (absent ellipsoid layer). (**e**, **f**) Autofluorescent images RE and LE 2 years later, showing increased density of flecks, some becoming confluent; further enlargement of central hypofluorescent area. (**g**, **h**) OCT RE and LE, 2 years later, showing enlarged area of thin retina (absent ellipsoid layer). The VA dropped to 0.2 bilaterally

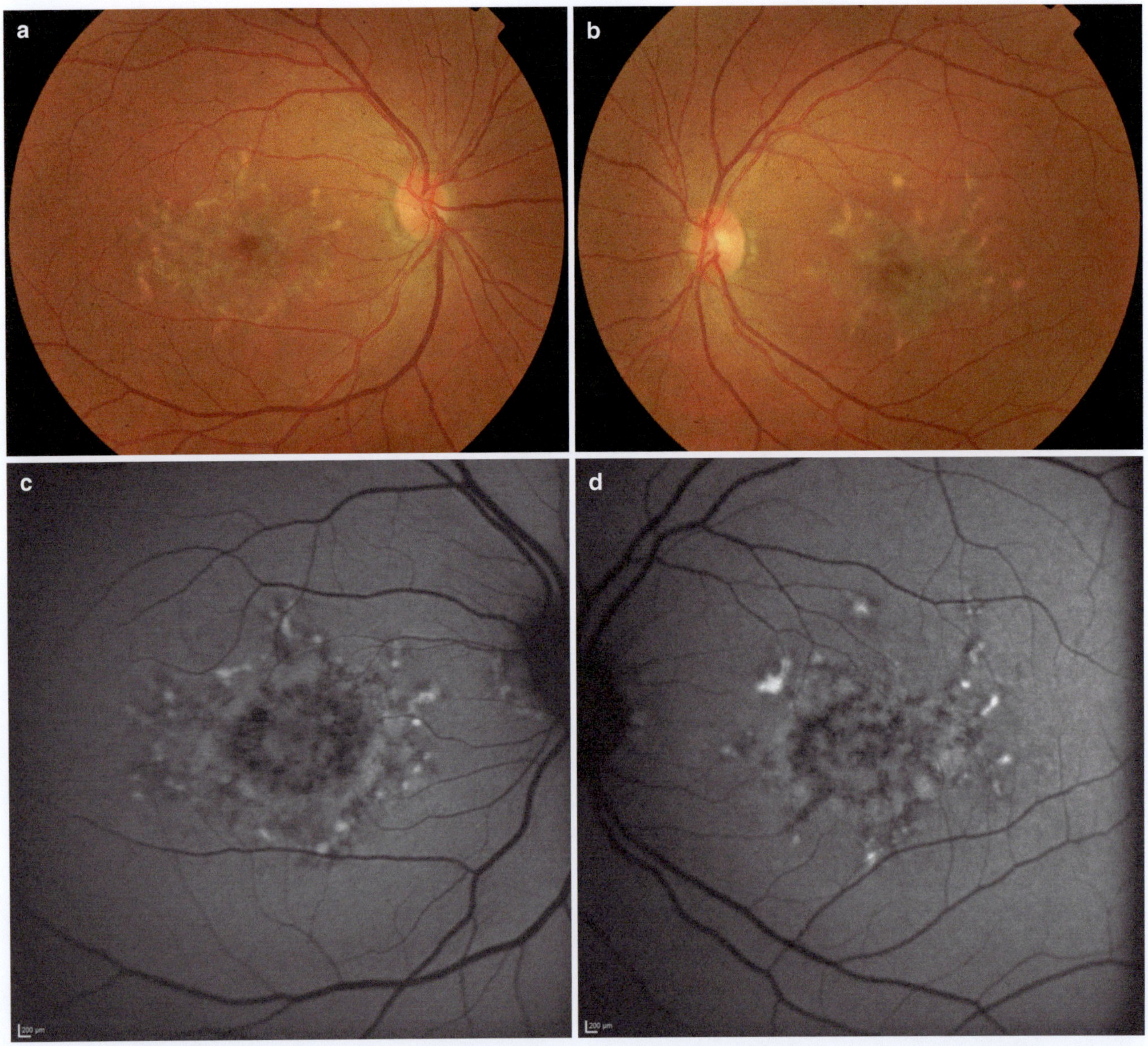

Fig. 6.6 Family 4, ABCA4 c.[2971G > C], G991R exon 20; c.[3899G > A], R1300Q exon 27. (**a**, **b**) Color fundus photo RE and LE, showing confluent flecks, bilaterally. (**c**, **d**) Autofluorescence images RE and LE, showing preserved fovea surrounded by hypofluorescent ring, and some confluent flecks. The patient is 51 years old, her VA is 0.8 RE, 0.3 LE

reduced RPE lipofuscin density or RPE/photoreceptor loss (Smith et al. 2009). SD-OCT provides high-resolution cross-sectional images and allows early detection. The earliest OCT abnormality described in children is external limiting membrane thickening (Fig. 6.2c, d), which precede development of atrophy (Chen et al. 2011). An OCT angiography study (Muller et al. 2018) was helpful in distinguishing between STGD1 patients and AMD patients: at the choroidal flow signal, the STGD1 patients had a more pronounced rarefaction of the choriocapillaris flow signal as compared to AMD patients.

Molecular Genetics

Stargardt disease was mapped to the long arm of chromosome 1 in 1993 (Kaplan et al. 1993) and was later shown to be caused by variants in the *ABCA4* gene, consisting of 50 exons (Allikmets et al. 1997). *ABCA4* gene encodes the adenosine triphosphate (ATP)-binding cassette transporter type A4 (*ABCA4* (MIM: 601691)), a transmembrane protein located at the rims of disc membranes of rod and cone outer segments, that transport vitamin A derivatives in the visual cycle (Allikmets et al. 1997).

Besides STGD1, variants in *ABCA4* gene are also associated with cone-rod dystrophy (ar CRD (MIM: 604116)), bull's eye maculopathy, rod-cone dystrophy, and panretinal dystrophies (Cremers et al. 1998; Duncker et al. 2015).

STGD1 is inherited in an autosomal recessive fashion. Biallelic variants in *ABCA4* gene can be identified in about 80% of patients with STGD1 (Schulz et al. 2017; Zernant et al. 2017), and 30% of cases with arCRD (Maugeri et al. 2000) after sequencing coding regions and flanking splice sites. The genotype–phenotype correlation is challenging due to highly polymorphic nature and large number of variants. In general, missense variants are associated with later onset, milder disease, while null alleles are associated with more severe, earlier onset. Some missense variants can also have severe functional effects similar to null: pLeu541Pro, p. Ala1038Val, and pArg1640Trp (Wiszniewski et al. 2005). Some missense variants seem to be more frequently associated in the mildest phenotype, foveal sparing-STGD1, including pArg2030Gln (Fujinami et al. 2013b).

In remaining STGD1 patients with missing *ABCA4* variants, it has been hypothesized that the majority of missing variants reside in intronic regions of the gene. Several groups demonstrated such deep-intronic variants (Albert et al. 2018; Bauwens et al. 2015; Braun et al. 2013) and proved pathogenicity of some (Albert et al. 2018).

Pathogenesis and Animal Models

The visual cycle consists of recycling of all-trans retinal back to 11-cis retinal (Travis et al. 2007). All-trans retinal is released from light-activated rhodopsin or cone opsin into rod and cone outer segments, transported to the disc surface by ABCA4, after forming a complex N-retinylidene-phosphatidylethanolamine (N-ret-PE). The lack of removal of N-ret-PE from photoreceptor outer segment results in accumulation of bisretinoid compounds and toxic levels of A2PE in photoreceptor membranes (Sparrow et al. 2012). A2PE is hydrolyzed to form a highly toxic metabolite A2E which accumulate in the RPE cells, as component of lipofuscin, leading to RPE dysfunction and death, followed by photoreceptor dysfunction/loss (Sparrow and Boulton 2005).

A STGD1 mouse model (ABCA4 knockout) has significant limitations: as a nocturnal animal, the morphology of mouse eye differs from humans, including the lack of macula.

More recently a dog model showing clinical signs similar to human STGD1 has been studied. A novel form of retinal degeneration in Labrador retriever become available. The whole-genome sequencing of this dog model identified a loss of function mutation in the ABCA4 gene. This finding may enable to develop a canine model for human STGD1 (Makelainen et al. 2019).

Clinical Management/Possibilities of Intervention

Several clinical trials are being conducted for STGD1, with different therapeutic strategies:

1. Gene replacement therapy by delivering the full ABCA4 cDNA (6.8 kb) via lentiviral vector, since the size of ABCA4 exceeded the previous adeno-associated virus (AAV) vector capacities (ClinicalTrials.gov: NCT01367444 and NCT01736592). Currently a Phase I/II is ongoing, with no safety concerns in the first three cohorts of subjects with relatively severe disease.
2. Subretinal transplantation of human embryonic stem cell-derived RPE cells (hESC-RPE) (ClinicalTrials.gov: NCT02445612 and NCT02941991), considering the fact that RPE cell loss is believed to precede photoreceptor cell loss.
3. Administration of a chemically modified vitamin A, taken orally, that will enter the visual cycle but not dimerize: C20-D3-retinylacetate (NCT02402660), in Phase II.
4. Modulation of ABCA4 pre-mRNA splicing by using antisense oligonucleotides (AONs), in order to rescue a splicing defect, in vitro study (Albert et al. 2018).

References

Aaberg TM. Stargardt's disease and fundus flavimaculatus: evaluation of morphologic progression and intrafamilial co-existence. Trans Am Ophthalmol Soc. 1986;84:453–87.

Albert S, et al. Identification and rescue of splice defects caused by two neighboring deep-intronic ABCA4 mutations underlying Stargardt disease. Am J Hum Genet. 2018;102:517–27. https://doi.org/10.1016/j.ajhg.2018.02.008.

Allikmets R, et al. A photoreceptor cell-specific ATP-binding transporter gene (ABCR) is mutated in recessive Stargardt macular dystrophy. Nat Genet. 1997;15:236–46. https://doi.org/10.1038/ng0397-236.

Bauwens M, et al. An augmented ABCA4 screen targeting noncoding regions reveals a deep intronic founder variant in Belgian Stargardt patients. Hum Mutat. 2015;36:39–42. https://doi.org/10.1002/humu.22716.

Bax NM, Lambertus S, Cremers FPM, Klevering BJ, Hoyng CB. The absence of fundus abnormalities in Stargardt disease. Graefes Arch Clin Exp Ophthalmol. 2019;257:1147–57. https://doi.org/10.1007/s00417-019-04280-8.

Blacharski P. Fundus flavimaculatus. In: Retinal dystrophies and degenerations; 1988. p. 135–59.

Braun TA, et al. Non-exomic and synonymous variants in ABCA4 are an important cause of Stargardt disease. Hum Mol Genet. 2013;22:5136–45. https://doi.org/10.1093/hmg/ddt367.

Chen Y, et al. Cone photoreceptor abnormalities correlate with vision loss in patients with Stargardt disease. Invest Ophthalmol Vis Sci. 2011;52:3281–92. https://doi.org/10.1167/iovs.10-6538.

Ciccone L, Lee W, Zernant J, Tanaka K, Schuerch K, Tsang SH, Allikmets R. Hyperreflective deposition in the background of advanced Stargardt disease. Retina. 2018;38:2214–9. https://doi.org/10.1097/IAE.0000000000001841.

Collison FT, Fishman GA. Visual acuity in patients with Stargardt disease after age 40. Retina. 2018;38:2387–94. https://doi.org/10.1097/IAE.0000000000001903.

Cornelis SS, et al. In silico functional meta-analysis of 5,962 ABCA4 variants in 3,928 retinal dystrophy cases. Hum Mutat. 2017;38:400–8. https://doi.org/10.1002/humu.23165.

Cremers FP, et al. Autosomal recessive retinitis pigmentosa and cone-rod dystrophy caused by splice site mutations in the Stargardt's disease gene ABCR. Hum Mol Genet. 1998;7:355–62. https://doi.org/10.1093/hmg/7.3.355.

Dalkara D, Goureau O, Marazova K, Sahel JA. Let there be light: gene and cell therapy for blindness. Hum Gene Ther. 2016;27:134–47. https://doi.org/10.1089/hum.2015.147.

Delori FC, Staurenghi G, Arend O, Dorey CK, Goger DG, Weiter JJ. In vivo measurement of lipofuscin in Stargardt's disease—fundus flavimaculatus. Invest Ophthalmol Vis Sci. 1995;36:2327–31.

Duncker T, Tsang SH, Lee W, Zernant J, Allikmets R, Delori FC, Sparrow JR. Quantitative fundus autofluorescence distinguishes ABCA4-associated and non-ABCA4-associated bull's-eye maculopathy. Ophthalmology. 2015;122:345–55. https://doi.org/10.1016/j.ophtha.2014.08.017.

Fishman GA, Farber M, Patel BS, Derlacki DJ. Visual acuity loss in patients with Stargardt's macular dystrophy. Ophthalmology. 1987;94:809–14. https://doi.org/10.1016/s0161-6420(87)33533-x.

Fishman GA, Stone EM, Grover S, Derlacki DJ, Haines HL, Hockey RR. Variation of clinical expression in patients with Stargardt dystrophy and sequence variations in the ABCR gene. Arch Ophthalmol. 1999;117:504–10. https://doi.org/10.1001/archopht.117.4.504.

Fujinami K, et al. A longitudinal study of Stargardt disease: quantitative assessment of fundus autofluorescence, progression, and genotype correlations. Invest Ophthalmol Vis Sci. 2013a;54:8181–90. https://doi.org/10.1167/iovs.13-12104.

Fujinami K, et al. Clinical and molecular analysis of Stargardt disease with preserved foveal structure and function. Am J Ophthalmol. 2013b;156:487–501.e481. https://doi.org/10.1016/j.ajo.2013.05.003.

Fujinami K, et al. Clinical and molecular characteristics of childhood-onset Stargardt disease. Ophthalmology. 2015;122:326–34. https://doi.org/10.1016/j.ophtha.2014.08.012.

Genead MA, Fishman GA, Stone EM, Allikmets R. The natural history of Stargardt disease with specific sequence mutation in the ABCA4 gene. Invest Ophthalmol Vis Sci. 2009;50:5867–71. https://doi.org/10.1167/iovs.09-3611.

Kaplan J, et al. A gene for Stargardt's disease (fundus flavimaculatus) maps to the short arm of chromosome 1. Nat Genet. 1993;5:308–11. https://doi.org/10.1038/ng1193-308.

Lambertus S, et al. Early-onset Stargardt disease: phenotypic and genotypic characteristics. Ophthalmology. 2015;122:335–44. https://doi.org/10.1016/j.ophtha.2014.08.032.

Lee W, et al. Complex inheritance of ABCA4 disease: four mutations in a family with multiple macular phenotypes. Hum Genet. 2016;135:9–19. https://doi.org/10.1007/s00439-015-1605-y.

Lois N, Holder GE, Bunce C, Fitzke FW, Bird AC. Phenotypic subtypes of Stargardt macular dystrophy-fundus flavimaculatus. Arch Ophthalmol. 2001;119:359–69. https://doi.org/10.1001/archopht.119.3.359.

Makelainen S, et al. An ABCA4 loss-of-function mutation causes a canine form of Stargardt disease. PLoS Genet. 2019;15:e1007873. https://doi.org/10.1371/journal.pgen.1007873.

Maugeri A, et al. Mutations in the ABCA4 (ABCR) gene are the major cause of autosomal recessive cone-rod dystrophy. Am J Hum Genet. 2000;67:960–6. https://doi.org/10.1086/303079.

Muller PL, et al. Choroidal flow signal in late-onset Stargardt disease and age-related macular degeneration: an OCT-Angiography Study. Invest Ophthalmol Vis Sci. 2018;59:AMD122–31. https://doi.org/10.1167/iovs.18-23819.

Rotenstreich Y, Fishman GA, Anderson RJ. Visual acuity loss and clinical observations in a large series of patients with Stargardt disease. Ophthalmology. 2003;110:1151–8. https://doi.org/10.1016/S0161-6420(03)00333-6.

Saad L, Washington I. Can vitamin a be improved to prevent blindness due to age-related macular degeneration, Stargardt disease and other retinal dystrophies? Adv Exp Med Biol. 2016;854:355–61. https://doi.org/10.1007/978-3-319-17121-0_47.

Schulz HL, et al. Mutation spectrum of the ABCA4 gene in 335 Stargardt disease patients from a multicenter German cohort-impact of selected deep Intronic variants and common SNPs. Invest Ophthalmol Vis Sci. 2017;58:394–403. https://doi.org/10.1167/iovs.16-19936.

Schwartz SD, et al. Human embryonic stem cell-derived retinal pigment epithelium in patients with age-related macular degeneration and Stargardt's macular dystrophy: follow-up of two open-label phase 1/2 studies. Lancet. 2015;385:509–16. https://doi.org/10.1016/S0140-6736(14)61376-3.

Smith RT, Gomes NL, Barile G, Busuioc M, Lee N, Laine A. Lipofuscin and autofluorescence metrics in progressive STGD. Invest Ophthalmol Vis Sci. 2009;50:3907–14. https://doi.org/10.1167/iovs.08-2448.

Sparrow JR, Boulton M. RPE lipofuscin and its role in retinal pathobiology. Exp Eye Res. 2005;80:595–606. https://doi.org/10.1016/j.exer.2005.01.007.

Sparrow JR, Gregory-Roberts E, Yamamoto K, Blonska A, Ghosh SK, Ueda K, Zhou J. The bisretinoids of retinal pigment epithelium. Prog Retin Eye Res. 2012;31:121–35. https://doi.org/10.1016/j.preteyeres.2011.12.001.

Stone EM, et al. Clinically focused molecular investigation of 1000 consecutive families with inherited retinal disease. Ophthalmology. 2017;124:1314–31. https://doi.org/10.1016/j.ophtha.2017.04.008.

Tanaka K, et al. The rapid-onset chorioretinopathy phenotype of ABCA4 disease. Ophthalmology. 2018;125:89–99. https://doi.org/10.1016/j.ophtha.2017.07.019.

Travis GH, Golczak M, Moise AR, Palczewski K. Diseases caused by defects in the visual cycle: retinoids as potential therapeutic agents. Annu Rev Pharmacol Toxicol. 2007;47:469–512. https://doi.org/10.1146/annurev.pharmtox.47.120505.105225.

Wabbels B, Demmler A, Paunescu K, Wegscheider E, Preising MN, Lorenz B. Fundus autofluorescence in children and teenagers with hereditary retinal diseases. Graefes Arch Clin Exp Ophthalmol. 2006;244:36–45. https://doi.org/10.1007/s00417-005-0043-2.

Wiszniewski W, Zaremba CM, Yatsenko AN, Jamrich M, Wensel TG, Lewis RA, Lupski JR. ABCA4 mutations causing mislocalization are found frequently in patients with severe retinal dystrophies. Hum Mol Genet. 2005;14:2769–78. https://doi.org/10.1093/hmg/ddi310.

Yatsenko AN, Shroyer NF, Lewis RA, Lupski JR. Late-onset Stargardt disease is associated with missense mutations that map outside known functional regions of ABCR (ABCA4). Hum Genet. 2001;108:346–55. https://doi.org/10.1007/s004390100493.

Zernant J, et al. Frequent hypomorphic alleles account for a significant fraction of ABCA4 disease and distinguish it from age-related macular degeneration. J Med Genet. 2017;54:404–12. https://doi.org/10.1136/jmedgenet-2017-104540.

7 North Carolina Macular Dystrophy

Leslie Small, Kent Small, and Fadi Shaya

North Carolina macular dystrophy (NCMD) is a congenital, developmental abnormality of the macula. It was first described in families living in western North Carolina by Lefler, Wadsworth, and Sidbury in 1971 and initially called autosomal dominant macular degeneration and aminoaciduria (Lefler et al. 1971). Subsequently this disease became known as the Lefler Wadsworth Sidbury syndrome. However, the aminoaciduria was later found to not consistently manifest in the affected family members, making this a misnomer in that it is not a syndrome at all. J Donald M. Gass, MD named NCMD after the founder effect of this initial family in his textbook *Stereoscopic Atlas of Macular Diseases: Diagnosis and Treatment* (Gass 1997). However, NCMD has now been described in many unrelated families from the United States, the United Kingdom, France, Germany, Korea, and Belize (Small 1998; Reichel et al. 1998; Pauleikhoff et al. 1997).

Due in part to the great phenotypic variability, several names have been attributed to the disease including dominant macular degeneration and aminoaciduria, dominant progressive foveal dystrophy, central areolar pigment epithelial dystrophy, central pigment epithelial and choroidal degeneration, Caldera maculopathy, and NCMD. All of these published "unique diseases" were found by Small et al. to be merely branches of the original NCMD family (Small 1989; Hermsen and Judisch 1984; Fetkenhour et al. 1976; Leveille et al. 1982). The Human Genome Organization (HUGO) Gene Nomenclature Committee (HGNC) named it MCDR1 (MC = macula, D = dystrophy, R = retina, 1 = first macular disease mapped in the human genome). Additionally, due to the varied phenotypical appearance, MCDR1 was originally believed to be a progressive disease, hence the name dominant progressive foveal dystrophy. However, Small and colleagues reexamined the original Lefler Wadsworth Sidbury family almost two decades later and found that the disease in fact was not progressive but a developmental disorder that presented with a highly variable expressivity (Small 1989; Small et al. 1991a). Patients are born with the disease, and it does not progress from less severe to more severe grades. Some progression and vision loss, however, can occur namely from the development of choroidal neovascularization (Small et al. 1991a).

Therefore, a grading system was assigned by Small, rather than a staging system which implies progression and was established to describe the expression of the disease(Small et al. 1991a):

- Grade 1: good visual acuity (20/20–20/30) with bilateral yellow specks in the central macula.
- Grade 2: good to moderate visual acuity (20/25–20/200), with bilateral confluent yellow specks in the macula.
- Grade 3: moderate to poor visual acuity (20/20—count fingers) with bilateral excavated lesions of the macula. The grade 3 disease has been misdiagnosed in several patients as congenital toxoplasmosis. The variable expressivity has caused NCMD to have several phenocopies. These include AMD (drusen), Best disease, idiopathic CNVM, and toxoplasmosis (Small et al. 1991a) (Figs. 7.1, 7.2, 7.3, and 7.4).

What is surprising about NCMD for most clinicians is the level of preserved vision despite the severe macular appearances. It is important to note that about half of the patients are asymptomatic. Therefore, the absence of the history of other affected family members may not be useful in correctly diagnosing MCDR1. In other words, the absence of a "positive family history" does not rule this disease out in the differential diagnoses. Of note, full-field electroretinography (ff ERG), electro-oculogram (EOG), dark adaptation, and color vision are normal in patients with MCDR1 (Small 1989).

L. Small (✉)
University of California, San Francisco, USA

K. Small · F. Shaya
Molecular Insight Research Foundation,
Glendale, CA, USA

G. Cheung (ed.), *Hereditary Chorioretinal Disorders*, Retina Atlas, https://doi.org/10.1007/978-981-15-0414-3_7

About one third of the patients have a coloboma-like excavation of the macula that has a well-demarcated area of RPE and absence of choriocapillaris and surrounding subretinal fibrosis that tends to result in shelving on the temporal edge compared to smooth sloping on the nasal edge. Patients tend to use the nasal edge for fixation, causing a positive angle kappa with strabismus appearance. A few patients have had strabismus surgery for this as a child with marginal benefit (personal communication Kent W Small).

Because of the large North Carolina family initially ascertained by Small et al., it was apparent that the size was sufficient for genetic linkage studies in order to map the gene location in the human genome. This was achieved by Small et al. by using LINKAGE ANALYSIS (Small et al. 1991b).

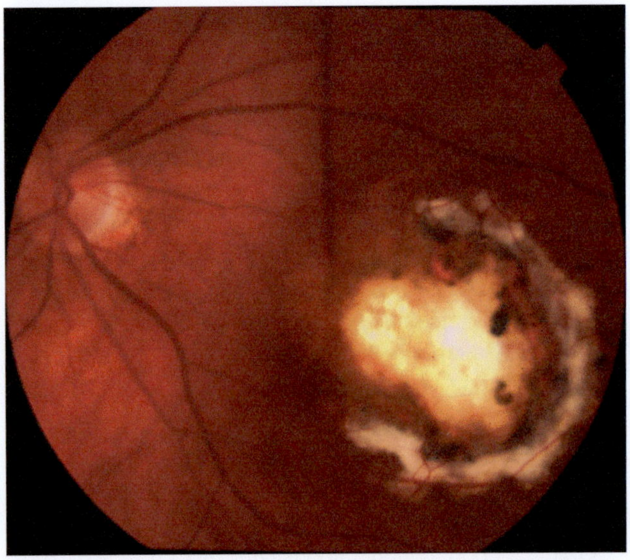

Fig. 7.1 Left eye, 35-year-old male, grade 3 lesion with 20/20 visual acuity. Previously, this patient was misdiagnosed with toxoplasmosis

The studies began with the then state-of-the-art genetic markers, RFLPs (restriction length polymorphisms). Later Small et al. were the first in ophthalmology to use the new PCR (polymerase chain reaction)-based genetic marker ("CA repeats," microsatellites) developed by Jim Weber, PhD, in Marshfield Wisconsin. These markers were more efficient and highly informative.

After having excluded most of the human genome, linkage was finally obtained to chromosome 6q16. The Human Genome Organization (HUGO) named it *MCDR1*; mc = macula, d = dystrophy, r = retina, 1 = first one mapped in the Human Genome. Over the decades, many more families with the NCMD phenotype were ascertained through national and international collaborations. The peak logarithm of odds (LOD) score (a score indicating significance of genetic linkage) was 40.01, one of the highest ever obtained in human genetics and narrowed the genetic distance to 870 kb (Small 1998). All NCMD families had mapped to the same chromosome six locus until Edwin Stone et al. found a Danish family with NCMD phenotype that mapped to chromosome 5, documenting the only known instance of genetic heterogeneity for NCMD (Rosenberg et al. 2010).

A classical positional cloning strategy was engaged using the newest techniques that were coming out of the Human Genome Project focused on only the 880 kb region, using YACs (yeast artificial chromosomes), BACs (bacterial artificial chromosomes), PACs (P1 artificial chromosomes), even the Fugu cDNA library. By 2001, Small et al. had sequenced all known expressed sequences (genes) and some of the promoters including an unnamed zinc finger. At that point, it became apparent that the mutations causing NCMD would be atypical and likely in a non-coding region.

Eventually, a new efficient and cheaper sequencing technology became commercially available called NEXGEN

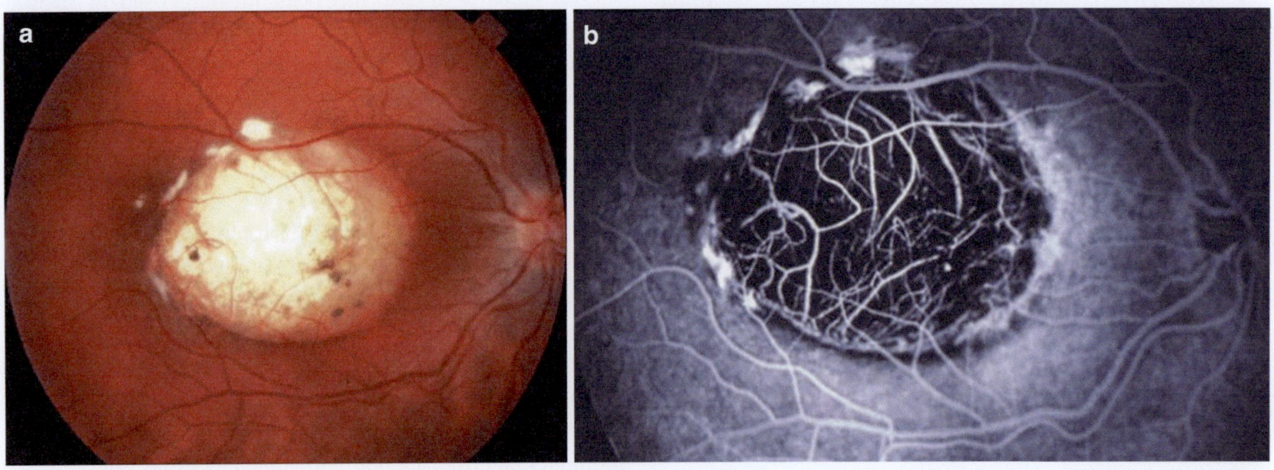

Fig. 7.2 (**a**) Fundus photo right eye, 21-year-old male, 20/40 visual acuity: courtesy of Dr. Thomas Rice. (**b**) Corresponding fluorescein angiography of (**a**)

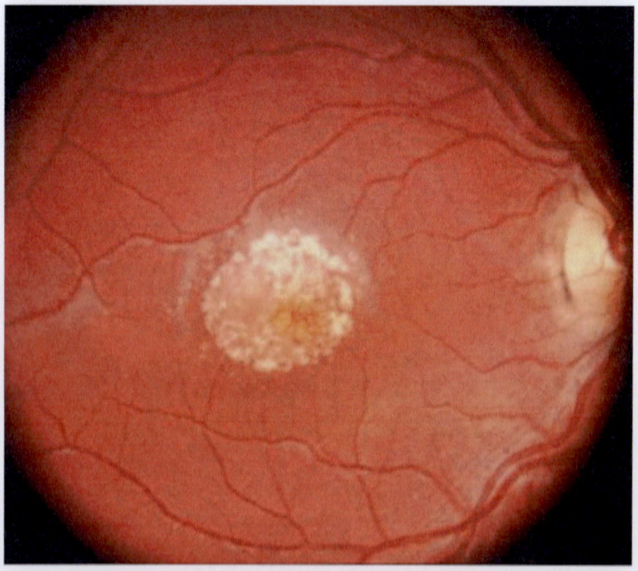

Fig. 7.3 Fundus photo right eye, 6-year-old girl, 20/50 VA grade 2 NCMD with confluent drusen

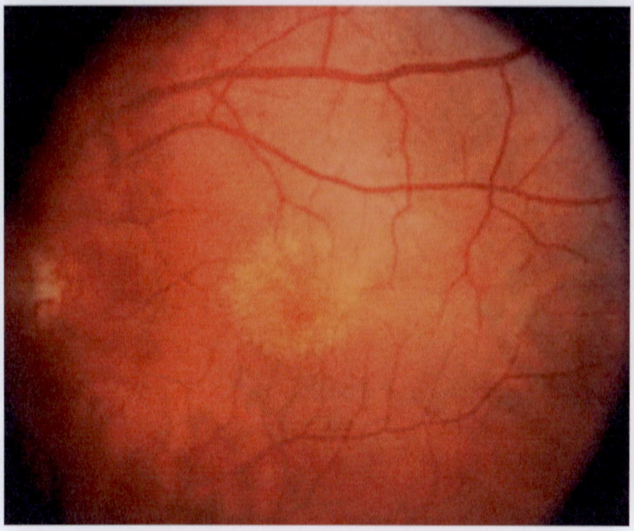

Fig. 7.4 Fundus photo left eye, 32-year-old male, 20/25 visual acuity, grade1 NCMD

sequencing. The volume of data generated with the method was extensive. Sorting through and analyzing this data required sophisticated algorithms and expertise provided by Edwin Stone, MD, PhD, and Adam DeLuca, PhD, at University of Iowa. In 11 of Small's largest and most complete NCMD families, with additional sequencing, five different mutations were found. Three point mutations were found in a non-coding region in a regulatory region known as a DNASE 1 hypersensitivity binding site. This site is 20 kb away from the nearest gene *PRDM13* which is a retinal transcription factor. A fourth mutation found was a large duplication that involved *PRDM13*. The fifth mutation was a duplication on chromosome 5 involving another transcription factor IRX1 in the Danish family (Small et al. 2016, 2017).

These findings were called "one of the most important studies in the past several decades" by Richard Weleber in an editorial (Weleber 2016). Several issues make these findings so noteworthy. NCMD is rare but is found worldwide in over 40 families studied by Small et al. with mutations found in over half to date in the United States, Europe, Central America, and China. It appears that overexpression of PRDM13 and IRX1 are the cause of the NCMD phenotype. These are new pathways to explore in macular diseases, and it appears that PRDM13 and IRX1 are important in the embryogenesis of the macula (Small et al. 2016; Cipriani et al. 2017). Understanding/manipulating these genes could help us learn to control, grow, and/or develop new maculae. IRX1 has recently been found to be expressed in the 19-week human embryonic maculae (Cipriani et al. 2017).

There is a single point mutation (Chr6:99593030) in most of the American families. A majority of these families studied also have the same haplotype in this region, suggesting a common founder. The same is true for most British, French, German, and Dutch families with the single point mutation Chr6:99593111, which is also in the non-coding DNASE1 hypersensitivity binding site affecting the expression of *PRDM13*. Additionally, most of the Europeans tested have the same haplotype again suggesting a common founder. PRDM13 is expressed in GABAergic amacrine cells (Watanabe et al. 2015). A knockout mouse of this gene has a mild retinal phenotype with apparent increased retinal sensitivity (Watanabe et al. 2015). Since mice do not have maculae and because NCMD is due to overexpression of PRDM13, this mouse model would not be expected to mimic NCMD. Although amacrine cells contribute to the oscillatory potentials of the full-field electroretinogram, no such abnormalities have been found in NCMD patients studied.

Others have confirmed two overlapping duplications in the DNASE1 hypersensitivity binding site which regulates the transcription factor IRX1 (Cipriani et al. 2017). *IRX1* is a member of the Iroquois homeobox gene family. Members of this family appear to play multiple roles during pattern formation of vertebrate embryos (Bosse et al. 1997). Iro/Irx genes have generally been thought to act as patterning genes that perform "early" functions in neural development and are also thought to have redundant functions. Irx genes also possess important "late" functions in terminal differentiation of neurons in vertebrates. IRX5 regulates the expression of some of the genes that define terminally differentiated OFF cone bipolar cells and demonstrate that mammalian Irx genes also possess regulatory functions in neuronal differentiation (Cheng et al. 2005).

References

Bosse A, Zulch A, Becker MB, et al. Identification of the vertebrate Iroquois homeobox gene family with overlapping expression during early development of the nervous system. Mech Dev. 1997;69:169–81.

Cheng CW, Chow RL, Lebel M, et al. The Iroquois homeobox gene, Irx5, is required for retinal cone bipolar cell development. Dev Biol. 2005;287:48–60.

Cipriani V, Silva RS, Arno G, et al. Duplication events downstream of IRX1 cause North Carolina macular dystrophy at the MCDR3 locus. Sci Rep. 2017;7:7512.

Fetkenhour CL, Gurney N, Dobbie JG, Choromokos E. Central areolar pigment epithelial dystrophy. Am J Ophthalmol. 1976;81:745–53.

Gass JDM. Stereoscopic atlas of macular diseases: diagnosis and treatment. St. Louis: Mosby; 1997.

Hermsen VM, Judisch GF. Central areolar pigment epithelial dystrophy (with 1 color plate). Ophthalmologica. 1984;189:69–72.

Lefler WH, Wadsworth JA, Sidbury JB Jr. Hereditary macular degeneration and amino-aciduria. Am J Ophthalmol. 1971;71:224–30.

Leveille AS, Morse PH, Kiernan JP. Autosomal dominant central pigment epithelial and choroidal degeneration. Ophthalmology. 1982;89:1407–13.

Pauleikhoff D, Sauer CG, Muller CR, Radermacher M, Merz A, Weber BH. Clinical and genetic evidence for autosomal dominant North Carolina macular dystrophy in a German family. Am J Ophthalmol. 1997;124:412–5.

Reichel M, Kelsell R, Fan J, et al. Phenotype of a British North Carolina macular dystrophy family linked to chromosome 6q. Br J Ophthalmol. 1998;82:1162–8.

Rosenberg T, Roos B, Johnsen T, et al. Clinical and genetic characterization of a Danish family with North Carolina macular dystrophy. Mol Vis. 2010;16:2659–68.

Small KW. North Carolina macular dystrophy, revisited. Ophthalmology. 1989;96:1747–54.

Small KW. North Carolina macular dystrophy: clinical features, genealogy, and genetic linkage analysis. Trans Am Ophthalmol Soc. 1998;96:925–61.

Small KW. Indentifying the genetic mutation for North Carolina dystrophy. Retina Physician. 2017;29–32.

Small KW, Killian J, McLean WC. North Carolina's dominant progressive foveal dystrophy: how progressive is it? Br J Ophthalmol. 1991a;75:401–6.

Small KW, Weber JL, Hung WY, Vance J, Roses A, Pericak-Vance M. North Carolina macular dystrophy: exclusion map using RFLPs and microsatellites. Genomics. 1991b;11:763–6.

Small KW, DeLuca AP, Whitmore SS, et al. North Carolina macular dystrophy is caused by dysregulation of the retinal transcription factor PRDM13. Ophthalmology. 2016;123:9–18.

Watanabe S, Sanuki R, Sugita Y, et al. Prdm13 regulates subtype specification of retinal amacrine interneurons and modulates visual sensitivity. J Neurosci Off J Soc Neurosci. 2015;35:8004–20.

Weleber RG. Dysregulation of retinal transcription factor PRDM13 and North Carolina macular dystrophy. Ophthalmology. 2016;123:2–4.

Choroideremia

8

Ian M. MacDonald, Natalia Binczyk, Alina Radziwon, and Ioannis Dimopoulos

The Phenotype

Affected Males

Males affected by choroideremia (CHM) experience progressive choroidal and retinal degeneration, which results in clinical symptoms of varying severity. The classical disease manifestations include decreased night vision in childhood and progressive visual field constriction, starting in the first or second decades of life. Visual acuity (VA) may be well preserved until middle age or later, but blindness may occur in the eighth or ninth decades of life (Aleman et al. 2017; Khan et al. 2016).

Carrier Females

Although carrier females are typically asymptomatic, they may at times present with severe symptoms similar to those of affected males. This may be due to lyonization or the random X-chromosome inactivation in the female embryo that results in silencing of the functional allele (Wuthisiri et al. 2013; Fahim and Daiger 2016). Curiously, the *CHM* gene in humans has been shown to escape inactivation in some cell lines from females and also demonstrate variable levels of expression (Carrel and Willard 1999).

Diagnoses That Overlap Choroideremia and Contiguous Gene Syndromes

Several diseases may present with findings similar to CHM including retinitis pigmentosa (RP), gyrate atrophy, and Usher syndrome. RP is a group of disorders that presents with autosomal dominant, recessive, and X-linked patterns of inheritance. Similar to CHM patients, RP patients may present with preserved central visual acuity, constricted visual fields, and nyctalopia. Fundus examination of these patients may reveal extensive pigment clumping, arteriolar narrowing, vitreous cells, and optic nerve pallor, all of which are not typical of CHM (Lee et al. 2003).

Gyrate atrophy has an autosomal recessive pattern of inheritance and bears a similar presentation to CHM: visual field constriction, progressive visual loss, and chorioretinal atrophy in the midperipheral fundus (Kim et al. 2013). Gyrate atrophy results from mutations in the *OAT* gene encoding ornithine amino transferase, which leads to toxic levels of plasma ornithine; as such, the diagnosis of gyrate atrophy can be confirmed by demonstrating increased serum or plasma concentrations of ornithine (MacDonald et al. 1993). Clinically, gyrate atrophy can be distinguished from CHM by the presence of hyperpigmentation of remaining RPE and the lobular loss of the RPE and choroid.

Usher syndrome is a group of genetic conditions involving both congenital hearing loss and adolescent-onset RP. Fundus exam may detect chorioretinal degeneration in the mid-periphery (Lee et al. 2003). Although the majority of CHM cases are non-syndromic, contiguous gene mutations that include Xq21 may rarely cause syndromic cases of CHM. For instance, a large mutation spanning Xq21.2, and the adjacent *POU3F4* and *ZNF711* genes may result in CHM accompanied by hearing loss and intellectual impairment (Simunovic et al. 2016). Recessive mutations in *RPE65* may also give a similar appearance to CHM; the onset of visual impairment in these cases occurs much earlier than CHM (Hull et al. 2016; Zhu et al. 2017).

Diagnostic and Research Testing

Typical diagnostic testing includes visual acuity measures, visual field testing, dilated funduscopy, electroretinography (ERG), optical coherence tomography (OCT), and fundus

I. M. MacDonald (✉) · N. Binczyk · A. Radziwon · I. Dimopoulos
Department of Ophthalmology and Visual Sciences, University of Alberta, Edmonton, AB, Canada
e-mail: macdonal@ualberta.ca

G. Cheung (ed.), *Hereditary Chorioretinal Disorders*, Retina Atlas, https://doi.org/10.1007/978-981-15-0414-3_8

autofluorescence imaging (FAF). Additional information may be gleaned from tests typically generally performed in a research setting, such as optical coherence tomography angiography (OCTA), adaptive optics—scanning laser ophthalmoscopy (AO-SLO), and microperimetry testing.

Visual Acuity

In a cross-sectional study of 115 CHM patients, 84% of patients younger than 60 years of age had a VA of 20/40 or better, 33% of patients older than 60 years had a VA of 20/200 or worse, while VA of counting fingers or worse did not occur until the seventh decade of life (Roberts et al. 2002). The best corrected visual acuity (BCVA) in CHM patients decreases symmetrically between both eyes and declines most rapidly when the degeneration encroaches on the central retina (Seitz et al. 2015). The 5-year rate of change for visual acuity in CHM patients is equivalent to reading one less line on the Lighthouse chart (Roberts et al. 2002). In contrast, visual acuity in carrier females is usually unaffected (Thobani et al. 2010; Wuthisiri et al. 2013; Ma et al. 2017). While changes in visual acuity are well characterized, they are not typically diagnostic; other abnormalities as outlined below can often be detected much earlier.

Visual Field

Males with CHM start experiencing visual field loss in the first or second decades of life, leading to tunnel vision with as little as 5–10° of remaining central area and eventually progressing to blindness (Pameyer et al. 1960). In contrast, visual fields in carrier females are often normal but cases of scotomas, an enlarging blind spot, and mild to moderate restrictions to the visual fields have been reported (Thobani et al. 2010; Wuthisiri et al. 2013).

Fundus Exam

The earliest changes observed on fundus photography in the affected males are widespread pigmentary disturbances at the level of the retinal pigment epithelium (RPE), especially in the mid-peripheral retina, between the major vascular arcades and the equator (Fig. 8.1a) (Khan et al. 2016). These areas of pigmentary change eventually progress to diffuse areas of chorioretinal atrophy (Fig. 8.1b). RPE mottling can also involve the macula early on (Lee et al. 2003). In carrier females, the clinician may appreciate areas of mid-peripheral depigmentation, RPE clumping, and patchy peripheral pigmentary changes also described as “moth-eaten” in appearance (Thobani et al. 2010; Wuthisiri et al. 2013; Wu et al. 2018) (Fig. 8.2).

Electrophysiology

The ERG is an objective and highly sensitive assessment of cone and rod function, based on corneal electrode recording of retinal responses to standardized flashes of light. In affected males, the ERG may initially show a pattern of rod-cone dysfunction and over-time, the ERG may not be recordable to all stimuli, consistent with the underlying pathology of progressive retinal degeneration (Wuthisiri et al. 2013). In contrast to affected males, the ERG findings are abnormal in only 15% of CHM carriers (Thobani et al. 2010).

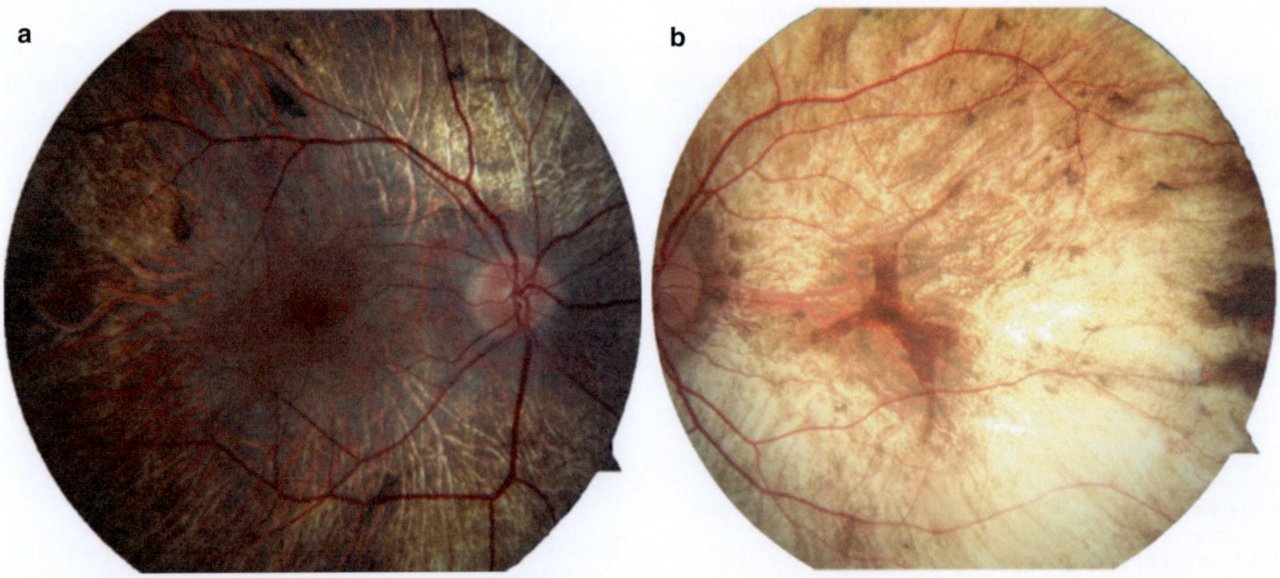

Fig. 8.1 Fundus photograph of the right eye of a non-Caucasian male with choroideremia (**a**) and left eye of a Caucasian male (**b**)

Optical Coherent Tomography

The OCT uses infrared light for noninvasive imaging of ocular structures. In affected males, the earliest abnormalities revealed by OCT imaging (Fig. 8.3) are loss of the photoreceptor outer segment (POS) and the ellipsoid zone (EZ) (Aleman et al. 2017). There may be a decrease in the central choroidal thickness (Fig. 8.3) with advancing age (Khan et al. 2016). The subfoveal retinal thickness may increase above normal in younger individuals and subsequently decline below normal with increasing age (Duncan et al. 2002). Intraretinal edema and outer retinal tubulations (Fig. 8.4) may be seen at transition zones between healthy and atrophic tissues (Khan et al. 2016). The migration of the transition zones centripetally with age has been reported to coincide with a decline in VA (Aleman et al. 2017). Additionally, cystic macular edema (CME) has been reported to occur in at least one eye in 62.5% CHM patients (Genead and Fishman 2011). In carrier females, the OCT may show abnormalities in the RPE integrity primarily outside the macular region (Thobani et al. 2010). Abnormalities in the ellipsoid zone have also been reported (Ma et al. 2017).

Fundus Autofluorescence

FAF stimulates emission of light from lipofuscin in metabolically active RPE, thus facilitating objective mapping of viable retinal pigmented epithelium (RPE). In affected males, there may be a reduction in retained macular autofluorescence (Fig. 8.5), with the more severely affected eye progressing at a slower rate than the fellow eye (Khan et al. 2016).

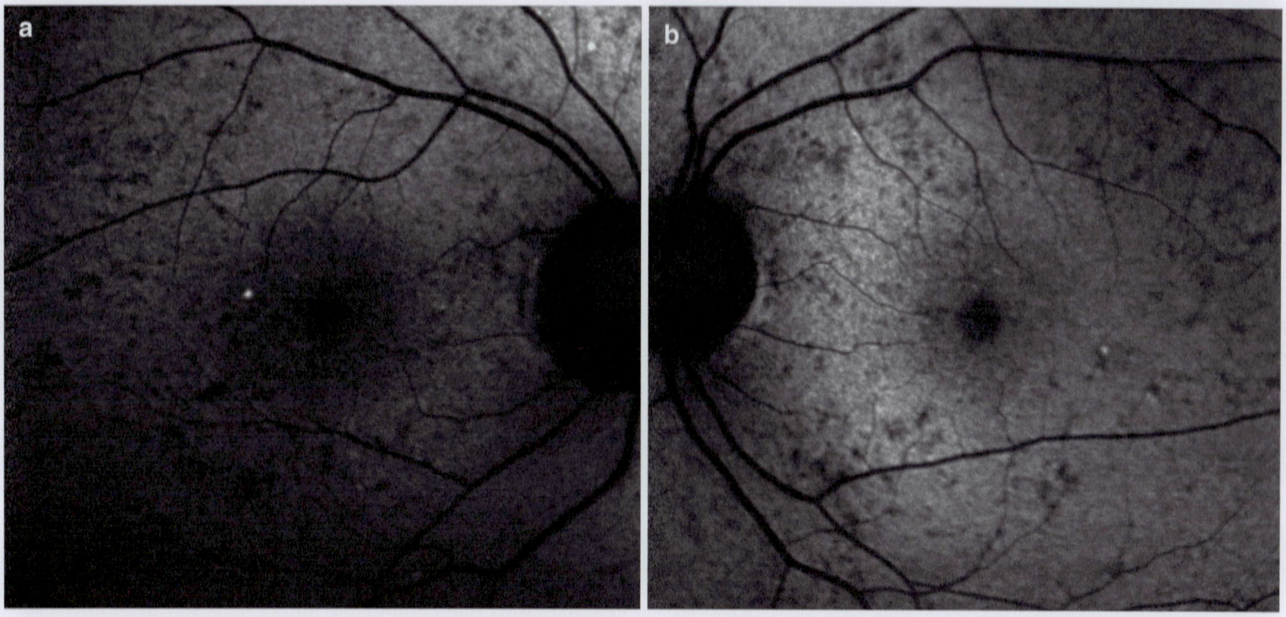

Fig. 8.2 Fundus autofluorescence images of the right eye (**a**) and left eye (**b**) of a female choroideremia carrier demonstrating scattered areas of decreased autoflouresence

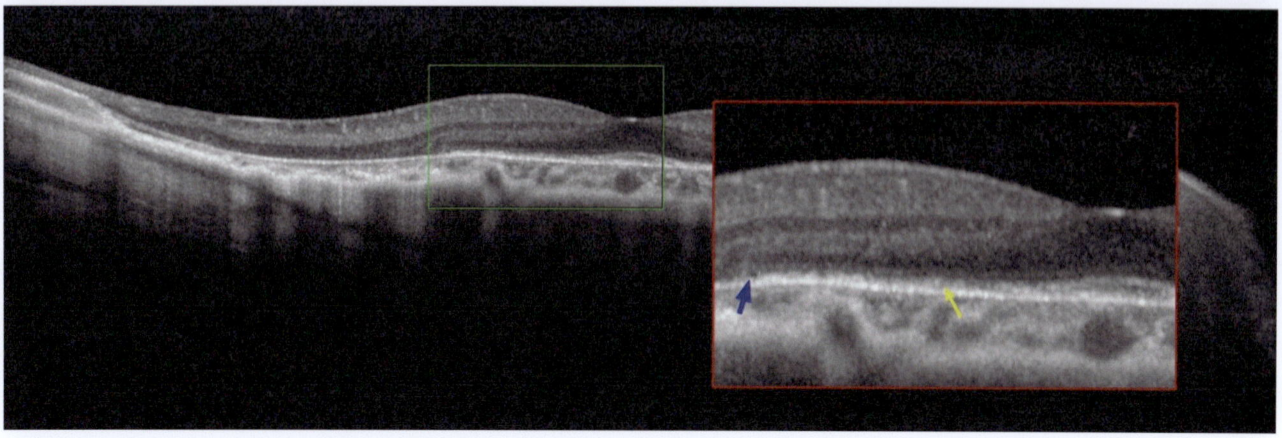

Fig. 8.3 Spectral domain OCT imaging revealing the boundary loss of ellipsoid zone (blue arrow) and loss of photoreceptors (yellow arrow)

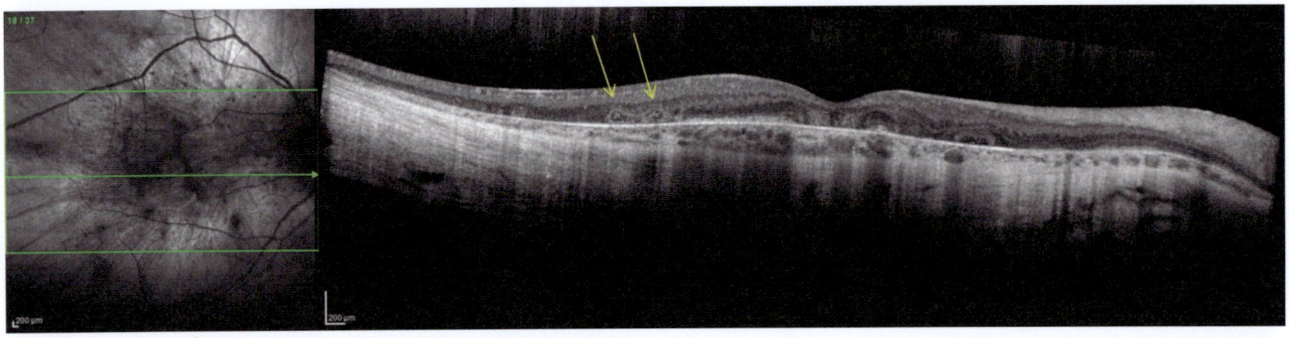

Fig. 8.4 Spectral domain OCT imaging. Arrows indicate retinal tubulations

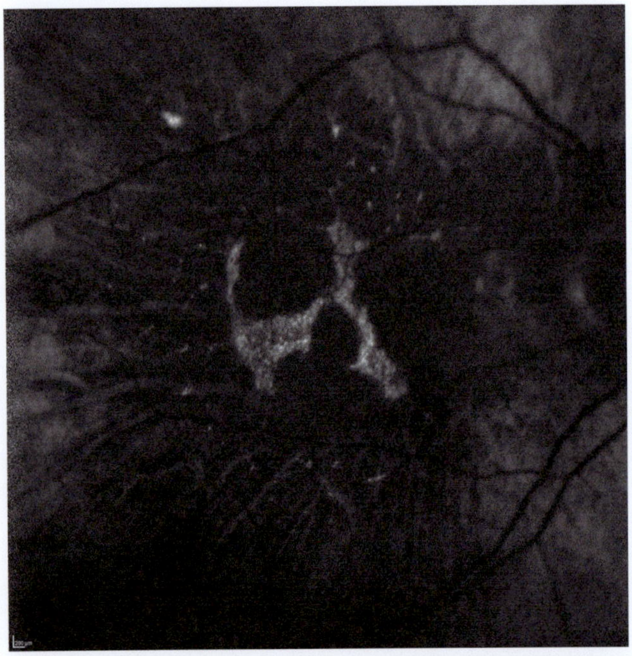

Fig. 8.5 Irregular area of retained fundus autofluorescence

Others, however, showed symmetry in the rate of change on FAF imaging between both eyes (Seitz et al. 2015). Although there are no FAF patterns that confirm the carrier state, FAF can be used to differentiate CHM from RP and ocular albinism (OA) carrier states (Wuthisiri et al. 2013). In CHM carrier state, the clinician may expect to see a "speckled" pattern of hypo- or hyperfluorescence areas on FAF (Fig. 8.2), in contrast to the "radially oriented line" pattern of hypo- and hyperfluorescence in carriers of RP or OA (Wu et al. 2018).

Optical Coherent Tomography: Angiography

The exact role of the choroid in CHM pathogenesis remains unclear. Several lines of evidence suggest a strong correlation between neuroretinal thinning on OCT and choriocapillaris loss on fluorescein angiography (Affortit-Demoge et al. 2009). Subfoveal choroidal thickness can also serve as a prognostic indicator of visual acuity (Abbouda et al. 2017). More recently, newer technologies such as OCT-angiography (OCT-A) have been utilized to better characterize the natural history of choroid degeneration relative to its overlying layers. OCT-A distinguishes between moving and stationary structures by analyzing changes in contrast in repeated high-speed OCT scans (Schachat 2018). Recent studies suggest that degeneration of the choriocapillaris appears to generally follow that of the RPE/photoreceptor complex (Jain et al. 2016; Kato et al. 2017). In carriers, there are no obvious abnormalities (Ma et al. 2017).

AO-SLO and Microperimetry

In vivo markers of photoreceptor structure can be extremely useful to determine subclinical disease progression and evaluate the safety and efficacy of experimental therapies for CHM. Adaptive optics combined with scanning laser ophthalmoscopy (AOSLO) is an emerging technology used to visualize the cone cell mosaic and density at the "single-cell" level (Roorda 2010). AOSLO has provided evidence of cone density loss in choroideremia that is independent of age and present even at early disease stages with no macular involvement (Nabholz et al. 2016). These findings have important implications from a clinical standpoint as both cones and rods appear to be targeted by experimental therapies (Dimopoulos et al. 2015; Nabholz et al. 2016).

Fundus-driven perimetry (microperimetry) has gradually replaced conventional perimetry in choroideremia research, emerging as a principal outcome measure for clinical trials. The main advantage of its adaptation is the eye tracking and continuous fundus projection technology it employs, allowing for higher accuracy and reliability in sensitivity measures (Acton and Greenstein 2013). In addition, it can be used to correlate functional measures with underlying anatomical structures. In a study of 10 CHM carriers, 50% of study subjects showed focal areas of threshold abnormalities on microperimetry (Thobani et al. 2010). Microperimetry could theoretically detect disease progression earlier than conventional perimetry; however, recent studies reveal comparable test-retest variability (Dimopoulos et al. 2016).

Etiology and Pathogenesis

Choroideremia is a monogenic disorder caused by mutations in the *CHM* gene (OMIM: 300390) that spans over 150 kb of Xq21.2 on the long arm of the X chromosome (Cremers et al. 1990). Fifteen exons are transcribed to produce a 3642 base pair mRNA which encodes the 653 amino acid Rab escort protein 1 (REP1) (van Bokhoven et al. 1994). REP1 plays a critical role in the processes of intracellular vesicle trafficking through its interaction with Rab geranylgeranyl transferase in a complex that serves to transfer lipid groups onto small GTPases known as Ras-associated binding proteins (Rabs) (Seabra et al. 1993). REP-2, a homologue encoded by the retrogene *CHML* (CHM-like), functions similarly and appears to compensate for the absence of REP-1 in all tissues except the eye (Cremers et al. 1994). A total loss of REP activity is presumed to be lethal in humans (van den Hurk et al. 1997). *CHM* mRNA and the REP1 protein are both broadly expressed across different tissues and cell types throughout the body and choroideremia's presentation as an isolated ophthalmic disease is therefore not the result of the protein's activity that is specific to the light sensing function of the eye (Bernstein and Wong 1998; Keiser et al. 2005). Conversely, it is the functionality of Rabs, which number over 70 and are involved in multiple processes including vesicle formation, tethering, motility, fusion, recycling, and signaling, and whose activity is predicated on their activation by REPs, that determine which type of tissue will be affected (Corbeel and Freson 2008). A lack of systemic symptoms does not result from tissue- or cell-specific expression of REP-1, but rather from the differing affinities of the two escort proteins for their Rab targets, which themselves are varyingly expressed across cells or tissues. Investigators have suggested Rab27a, Rab27b, and Rab38 as possible major contributors to choroideremia; these molecules function in melanosome transport within the retinal pigment epithelium (RPE) and possess a low affinity for REP-2 (Kohnke et al. 2013; Seabra et al. 1995).

The mutation spectrum of this monogenic disorder is characterized by loss-of-function changes in *CHM* that abrogate REP1 activity (McTaggart et al. 2002; Simunovic et al. 2016). The LOVD Retinal and Hearing Impairment Genetic Mutation Database (https://grenada.lumc.nl/LOVD2/Usher_montpellier/home.php) reports nearly 300 disease-causing variants, dominated by transitions and transversions leading to protein truncation, splice defects, indels, and large deletions ranging from a single exon to the full gene (Fokkema et al. 2011). Missense mutations altering REP1 structure or function (Esposito et al. 2011; Sergeev et al. 2009), promoter defects (Radziwon et al. 2017), transposon insertions (Van Den Hurk et al. 2003), partial gene duplications (Chi et al. 2013), deep intronic variant causing cryptic splicing (Carss et al. 2017), and other variations are infrequently found. There is no evidence suggesting that any correlation between genotype and phenotype exists: visual acuity, onset and progression of symptoms, and visual field were found to be unrelated to mutation type (Freund et al. 2016; Simunovic et al. 2016). Large deletions extending beyond *CHM* and into neighboring genes *POU3F4* and *ZNF711* have, however, been linked to a syndromic presentation that includes deafness and developmental delay typical of a contiguous gene syndrome (Iossa et al. 2015; Tarpey et al. 2009).

While a clinical evaluation made by an ophthalmologist with expertise in inherited retinal disease bears a high likelihood of accuracy, molecular confirmation is nevertheless the most direct method of diagnosis. Sanger sequencing of exons and intron/exon junctions together with deletion and duplication analysis has been shown to uncover the causative mutation in a large majority of cases (Simunovic et al. 2016). Most disease-causing variants are truncating mutations or frameshifts and can be presumed to be pathogenic based on genotype alone, but analysis of protein or mRNA derived from the patient may be required with variants of unknown significance, or when no mutation is found (Furgoch et al. 2014). Molecular genotyping brings the additional advantage of establishing carrier status in females who may present with a subtle phenotype, difficult to determine conclusively, especially early in children before symptoms are present, and qualify for interventions such as gene therapy trials currently underway. The increasing availability and affordability of next-generation sequencing, disease panels, and other high-throughput techniques may eventually replace this candidate gene approach based on presentation and a "best guess" by the clinician. These methods may also more readily differentiate choroideremia phenocopies such as some cases of retinitis pigmentosa or a rare form of dominant *RPE65* disease (Hull et al. 2016; Zhu et al. 2017).

Choroideremia is characterized by progressive degeneration of the retinal pigment epithelium (RPE), photoreceptors, and choroid that begins at an early age. Despite several decades of active research and an understanding of the abnormalities underlying CHM, the pathology and pathogenesis of the disease have not been fully revealed. Whether a specific cell type or tissue is the initial site of degeneration that leads to secondary loss of a dependent layer or whether several targets degenerate simultaneously remains unknown. Mouse models appear to indicate that a deficiency of REP1 causes cell-autonomous and intrinsic problems in photoreceptors and the RPE and that both can be considered the leading and principal sites of disease (Tolmachova et al. 2006, 2010).

Spectral-domain optical coherence tomography (SD-OCT) also points to early structural thinning of the RPE, anomalies in the photoreceptor interdigitation zone band, suggesting loss of outer segments and loss of the ellipsoid zone as primary events, but the precise sequence of morphological changes remains unknown (Aleman et al. 2017; Sun et al. 2016). Though promising gene therapy trials investigating delivery of the *CHM* gene product through subfoveal injection are currently underway (MacLaren et al. 2014), at present, no proven treatment exists to halt or abate the progressive retinal degeneration that characterizes CHM.

Management

Medical Management

Given that one third of CHM mutations are premature stop codons, novel pharmacotherapies are being tested that could provide functional rescue of REP1 through translational bypass. Ataluren (PTC124), a small molecule drug with this mechanism of action, was recently tested on preclinical nonsense mutation models of the disease: the chm^{ru848} zebrafish and primary human CHM fibroblasts (Moosajee et al. 2016). The onset of retinal degeneration was delayed, with partial restoration of prenylation and rep1 protein expression. Following the example of other genetic conditions (aniridia, cystic fibrosis, muscular dystrophy), a clinical trial of this drug for CHM could be possible in the future (Dimopoulos et al. 2017).

Surgical Management

A common feature of many rod-cone dystrophies—including CHM—is the development of posterior subcapsular cataract (Heckenlively 1982). The prevalence though does not seem to be higher in CHM than the general population. Cataract surgery in CHM patients does not add any additional risk of intra- or postoperative complications (Edwards et al. 2015). Similarly, full-thickness macular holes can rarely develop in a small percentage of patient with end-stage CHM. Surgical correction seems to be effective in establishing anatomic closure (Zinkernagel et al. 2013).

Experimental Therapies (AAV-2-Mediated Gene Therapy)

Following success of gene augmentation trials for Leber congenital amaurosis (LCA) (Pierce and Bennett 2015), choroideremia became the second genetic ocular disorder to be considered for gene therapy (Dimopoulos et al. 2015). The first phase of human clinical trials enrolled primarily subjects with advanced disease stages to establish safety of subfoveal gene delivery in this group of patients. Currently, only adeno-associated virus type 2 (AAV-2) vectors have been used that carry a copy of the human REP1 cDNA (Barnard et al. 2014). Initial 6-month results from the first trial conducted at the University of Oxford suggested improvement in both rod and cone function for two out of six treated subjects (MacLaren et al. 2014). Long-term follow-up of these subjects showed sustained visual acuity gain at 3.5 years (Edwards et al. 2016). Although promising, the current published experience of gene replacement in CHM still has limited information to determine efficacy (Dimopoulos et al. 2017). Larger studies will now focus on enrolling younger individuals to assess preservation of both functional and structural outcomes. Alternative vector and delivery methods are also under development to avoid the consequences of delivering gene therapy to the subretinal space (Duncan 2017).

References

Abbouda A, Lim WS, Sprogyte L, et al. Quantitative and qualitative features of spectral-domain optical coherence tomography provide prognostic indicators for visual acuity in patients with choroideremia. Ophthalmic Surg Lasers Imaging Retina. 2017;48:711–6.

Acton JH, Greenstein VC. Fundus-driven perimetry (microperimetry) compared to conventional static automated perimetry: similarities, differences, and clinical applications. Can J Ophthalmol. 2013;48:358–63.

Affortit-Demoge A, Querques G, Angulo-Bocco C, et al. Optical coherence tomography features of x-linked choroideremia. Retin Cases Brief Rep. 2009;3:180–2.

Aleman TS, Han G, Serrano LW, et al. Natural history of the central structural abnormalities in choroideremia: a prospective cross-sectional study. Ophthalmology. 2017;124:359–73.

Barnard AR, Groppe M, MacLaren RE. Gene therapy for choroideremia using an adeno-associated viral (AAV) vector. Cold Spring Harb Perspect Med. 2014;5:a017293.

Bernstein SL, Wong P. Regional expression of disease-related genes in human and monkey retina. Mol Vis. 1998;4:24.

Carrel L, Willard HF. Heterogeneous gene expression from the inactive X chromosome: an X-linked gene that escapes X inactivation in some human cell lines but is inactivated in others. Proc Natl Acad Sci U S A. 1999;96:7364–9.

Carss KJ, Arno G, Erwood M, et al. Comprehensive rare variant analysis via whole-genome sequencing to determine the molecular pathology of inherited retinal disease. Am J Hum Genet. 2017;100:75–90.

Chi JY, MacDonald IM, Hume S. Copy number variant analysis in CHM to detect duplications underlying choroideremia. Ophthalmic Genet. 2013;34:229–33.

Corbeel L, Freson K. Rab proteins and Rab-associated proteins: major actors in the mechanism of protein-trafficking disorders. Eur J Pediatr. 2008;167:723–9.

Cremers FP, van de Pol DJ, van Kerkhoff LP, et al. Cloning of a gene that is rearranged in patients with choroideraemia. Nature. 1990;347:674–7.

Cremers FP, Armstrong SA, Seabra MC, et al. REP-2, a Rab escort protein encoded by the choroideremia-like gene. J Biol Chem. 1994;269:2111–7.

Dimopoulos IS, Chan S, MacLaren RE, et al. Pathogenic mechanisms and the prospect of gene therapy for choroideremia. Expert Opin Orphan Drugs. 2015;3:787–98.

Dimopoulos IS, Tseng C, MacDonald IM. Microperimetry as an outcome measure in choroideremia trials: reproducibility and beyond. Invest Ophthalmol Vis Sci. 2016;57:4151–61.

Dimopoulos IS, Radziwon A, St Laurent CD, et al. Choroideremia. Curr Opin Ophthalmol. 2017;28:410–5.

Duncan JL. Visual consequences of delivering therapies to the subretinal space. JAMA Ophthalmol. 2017;135:242–3.

Duncan JL, Aleman TS, Gardner LM, et al. Macular pigment and lutein supplementation in choroideremia. Exp Eye Res. 2002;74:371–81.

Edwards TL, Groppe M, MacLaren RE. Outcomes following cataract surgery in choroideremia. Eye (Lond). 2015;29:460–4.

Edwards TL, Jolly JK, Groppe M, et al. Visual acuity after retinal gene therapy for choroideremia. NEJM. 2016;374:1996–8.

Esposito G, De Falco F, Tinto N, et al. Comprehensive mutation analysis (20 families) of the choroideremia gene reveals a missense variant that prevents the binding of REP1 with Rab geranylgeranyl transferase. Hum Mutat. 2011;32:1460–9.

Fahim AT, Daiger SP. The role of X-chromosome inactivation in retinal development and disease. Adv Exp Med Biol. 2016;854:325–31.

Fokkema IF, Taschner PE, Schaafsma GC. LOVD v.2.0: the next generation in gene variant databases. Hum Mutat. 2011;32:557–63.

Freund PR, Sergeev YV, MacDonald IM. Analysis of a large choroideremia dataset does not suggest a preference for inclusion of certain genotypes in future trials of gene therapy. Mol Genet Genomic Med. 2016;4:344–58.

Furgoch MJB, Mewes-Arès J, Radziwon A. Molecular genetic diagnostic techniques in choroideremia. Mol Vis. 2014;20:535–44.

Genead MA, Fishman GA. Cystic macular oedema on spectral-domain optical coherence tomography in choroideremia patients without cystic changes on fundus examination. Eye (Lond). 2011;25:84–90.

Heckenlively J. The frequency of posterior subcapsular cataract in the hereditary retinal degenerations. Am J Ophthalmol. 1982;93:733–8.

Hull S, Mukherjee R, Holder GE, et al. The clinical features of retinal disease due to a dominant mutation in RPE65. Mol Vis. 2016;22:626–35.

Iossa S, Costa V, Corvino V, et al. Phenotypic and genetic characterization of a family carrying two Xq21.1–21.3 interstitial deletions associated with syndromic hearing loss. Mol Cytogenet. 2015;8:18. eCollection 2015.

Jain N, Jia Y, Gao SS, et al. Optical coherence tomography angiography in choroideremia: correlating choriocapillaris loss with overlying degeneration. JAMA Ophthalmol. 2016;134:697–702.

Kato M, Maruko I, Koizumi H, et al. Optical coherence tomography angiography and fundus autofluorescence in the eyes with choroideremia. BMJ Case Rep. 2017;2017:217682.

Keiser NW, Tang W, Wei Z, et al. Spatial and temporal expression patterns of the choroideremia gene in the mouse retina. Mol Vis. 2005;11:1052–60.

Khan KN, Islam F, Moore AT, et al. Clinical and genetic features of choroideremia in childhood. Ophthalmology. 2016;123:2158–65.

Kim SJ, Lim DH, Kim JH, et al. Gyrate atrophy of the choroid and retina diagnosed by ornithine-delta-aminotransferase gene analysis: a case report. Korean J Ophthalmol. 2013;27:388–91.

Kohnke M, Delon C, Hastie ML, et al. Rab GTPase prenylation hierarchy and its potential role in choroideremia disease. PLoS One. 2013;8(12):e81758.

Lee TK, McTaggart KE, Sieving PA, et al. Clinical diagnoses that overlap with choroideremia. Can J Ophthalmol. 2003;38:364–72.

Ma KK, Lin J, Boudreault K, et al. Phenotyping choroideremia and its carrier state with multimodal imaging techniques. Retin Cases Brief Rep. 2017;11(Suppl 1):S178–81.

MacDonald IM, Hume S, Chan S, et al. Choroideremia. *GeneReviews(R)*. Seattle, WA: University of Washington, Seattle. GeneReviews is a registered trademark of the University of Washington, Seattle. All rights reserved. doi: NBK1337 [bookaccession]; 1993.

MacLaren RE, Groppe M, Barnard AR, et al. Retinal gene therapy in patients with choroideremia: initial findings from a phase 1/2 clinical trial. Lancet (London, England). 2014;383:1129–37.

McTaggart KE, Tran M, Mah DY, et al. Mutational analysis of patients with the diagnosis of choroideremia. Hum Mutat. 2002;20:189–96.

Moosajee M, Tracey-White D, Smart M, et al. Functional rescue of REP1 following treatment with PTC124 and novel derivative PTC-414 in human choroideremia fibroblasts and the nonsense-mediated zebrafish model. Hum Mol Genet. 2016;25:3416–31.

Nabholz N, Lorenzini MC, Bocquet B, et al. Clinical evaluation and cone alterations in choroideremia. Ophthalmology. 2016;123:1830–2.

Pameyer JK, Waardenburg PJ, Henkes HE. Choroideremia. Br J Ophthalmol. 1960;44:724–38.

Pierce EA, Bennett J. The status of RPE65 gene therapy trials: safety and efficacy. Cold Spring Harb Perspect Med. 2015;5:a017285.

Radziwon A, Arno G, Wheaton D, et al. Single-base substitutions in the CHM promoter as a cause of choroideremia. Hum Mutat. 2017;38:704–15.

Roberts MF, Fishman GA, Roberts DK, et al. Retrospective, longitudinal, and cross sectional study of visual acuity impairment in choroideraemia. Br J Ophthalmol. 2002;86:658–62.

Roorda A. Applications of adaptive optics scanning laser ophthalmoscopy. Optom Vis Sci. 2010;87:260–8.

Schachat AP. Optical coherence tomography. In: Ryan's retina, 6th edn. Edinburgh; New York: Elsevier; 2018.

Seabra MC, Brown MS, Goldstein JL. Retinal degeneration in choroideremia: deficiency of Rab geranylgeranyl transferase. Science. 1993;259:377–81.

Seabra MC, Ho YK, Anant JS. Deficient geranylgeranylation of Ram/Rab27 in choroideremia. J Biol Chem. 1995;270:24420–7.

Seitz IP, Zhour A, Kohl S, et al. Multimodal assessment of choroideremia patients defines pre-treatment characteristics. Graefes Arch Clin Exp Ophthalmol. 2015;253:2143–50.

Sergeev YV, Smaoui N, Sui R, et al. The functional effect of pathogenic mutations in Rab escort protein 1. Mutat Res. 2009;665:44–50.

Simunovic MP, Jolly JK, Xue K, et al. The spectrum of CHM gene mutations in choroideremia and their relationship to clinical phenotype. Invest Ophthal Vis Sci. 2016;57:6033–9.

Sun LW, Johnson RD, Williams V, et al. Multimodal imaging of photoreceptor structure in choroideremia. PLoS One. 2016;11:e0167526.

Tarpey PS, Smith R, Pleasance E, et al. A systematic, large-scale resequencing screen of X-chromosome coding exons in mental retardation. Nat Genet. 2009;41:535–43.

Thobani A, Anastasakis A, Fishman GA. Microperimetry and OCT findings in female carriers of choroideremia. Ophthalmic Genet. 2010;31:235–9.

Tolmachova T, Anders R, Abrink M, et al. Independent degeneration of photoreceptors and retinal pigment epithelium in conditional knockout mouse models of choroideremia. J Clin Invest. 2006;116:386–94.

Tolmachova T, Wavre-Shapton ST, Barnard AR, et al. Retinal pigment epithelium defects accelerate photoreceptor degeneration in cell type-specific knockout mouse models of choroideremia. Invest Ophthalmol Vis Sci. 2010;51:4913–20.

van Bokhoven H, van den Hurk JA, Bogerd L, et al. Cloning and characterization of the human choroideremia gene. Hum Mol Genet. 1994;3:1041–6.

van den Hurk JA, Schwartz M, van Bokhoven H, et al. Molecular basis of choroideremia (CHM): mutations involving the Rab escort protein-1 (REP-1) gene. Hum Mutat. 1997;9:110–7.

Van Den Hurk J, Van De Pol D, et al. Novel types of mutation in the choroideremia (CHM) gene: a full-length L1 insertion and an intronic mutation activating a cryptic exon. Hum Genet. 2003;113:268–75.

Wu AL, Wang JP, Tseng YJ, et al. Multimodal imaging of mosaic retinopathy in carriers of hereditary X-linked recessive diseases. Retina (Philadelphia, Pa.). 2018;38(5):1047–57.

Wuthisiri W, Lingao MD, Capasso JE, Levin AV. Lyonization in ophthalmology. Curr Opin Ophthalmol. 2013;24:389–97.

Zhu L, Cheng J, Zhou B, et al. Diagnosis for choroideremia in a large Chinese pedigree by next-generation sequencing (NGS) and non-invasive prenatal testing (NIPT). Mol Med Rep. 2017;15:1157–64.

Zinkernagel MS, Groppe M, MacLaren RE. Macular hole surgery in patients with end-stage choroideremia. Ophthalmology. 2013;120:1592–6.

Malattia Leventinese

9

Veronika Vaclavik

Introduction

Malattia Leventinese (ML), also known as dominant radial drusen (DRD) or Doyne honeycomb retinal dystrophy (DHRD) (O'Neill 2009) or autosomal dominant drusen (ADD) is the first histopathologically and clinically described maculopathy of Mendelian inheritance. Malattia Leventinese (ML) was first described in patients living in the Leventine Valley in canton Ticino of southern Switzerland in 1925 (Vogt 1925). In the nineteenth century in England, Doyne reported Doyne honeycomb retinal dystrophy (DRHD) (Doyne 1899). In four sisters, he observed white deposits in a honeycomb pattern at the macula and nasally to the disc. In his original report, he believed that these white spots were exudates in the choroid and named the disease "honeycomb choroiditis." Many years later, Waardenburg (1948) and Forni and Babel (1962) concluded, following histopathological studies, that features of Leventinese disease might be similar to those of Doyne honeycomb choroiditis.

Due to their phenotypic variability and previous histopathological findings (Forni and Babel 1962), ML and DHRD were considered separate entities until 1999, when a missense mutation (Arg345Trp) in the gene *EFEMP1* (EGF-containing fibrillin-like extracellular matrix protein 1) was discovered to be causative for both conditions, confirming that ML and DHRD are the same disorder (Stone et al. 1999).

Although originally recognized in England and Switzerland, families affected with autosomal radial drusen have been identified in Czechoslovakia (Dusek et al. 1982; Streicher and Krcmery 1976) and the United States (Gass 2012).

Characteristic clinical findings consist of macular drusen: large confluent, small radial, or a combination of both (Figs. 9.1 and 9.2). Drusen can spare the fovea and be present in perifo-

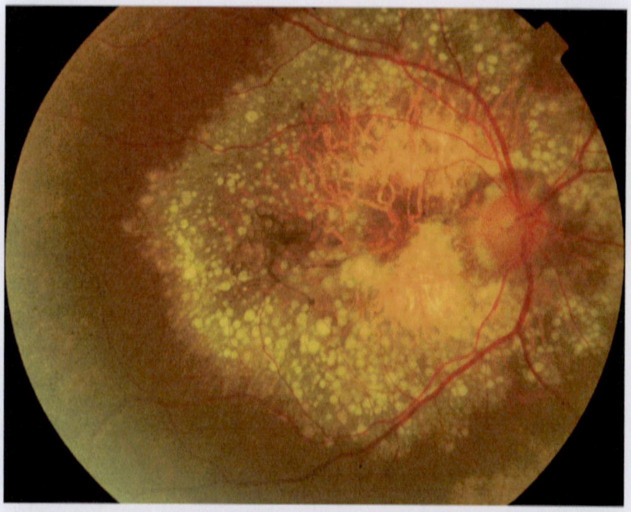

Fig. 9.1 Family 1—Right fundus color of a 66-year-old female, with macular soft drusen and juxta and peripapillary drusen. Scaring at the fovea. Visual acuity: hand movement

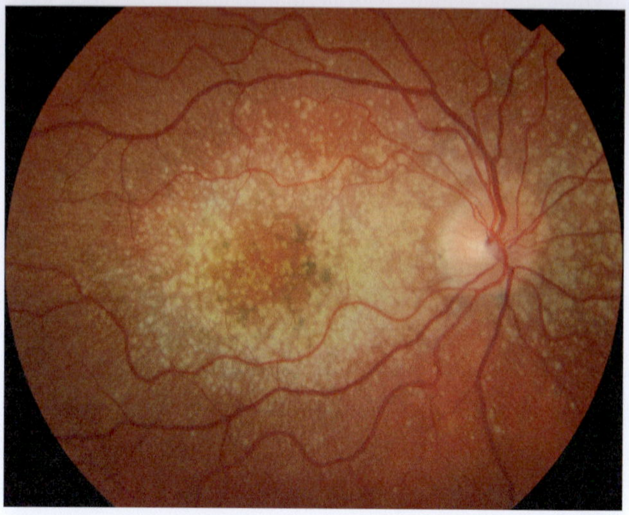

Fig. 9.2 Family 2—Right fundus color of a 31-year-old male, with macular soft drusen, small radial drusen, juxta and peripapillary drusen. Visual acuity: 1.0

V. Vaclavik (✉)
Department of Ophthalmology, Genetic and Rare Disease, Jules Gonin Eye Hospital, University of Lausanne, Lausanne, Switzerland

Department of Ophthalmology, Medical Retina, Canton Hospital, HFR, Fribourg, Switzerland
e-mail: veronika.vaclavik@fa2.ch

G. Cheung (ed.), *Hereditary Chorioretinal Disorders*, Retina Atlas, https://doi.org/10.1007/978-981-15-0414-3_9

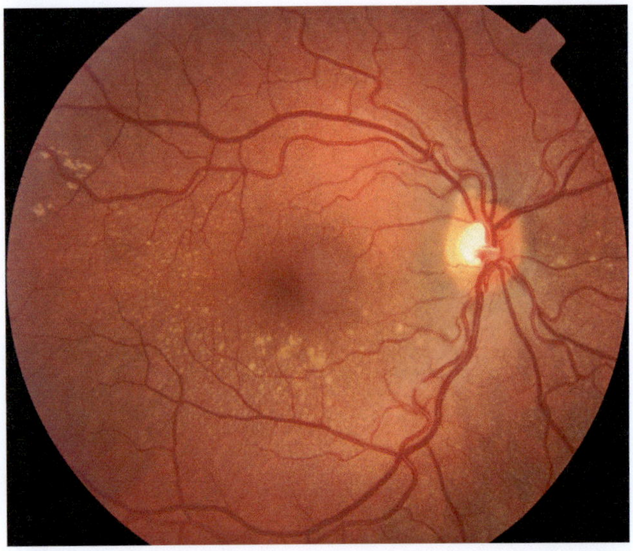

Fig. 9.3 Family 3—Right fundus color of a 30-year-old female, with some perifoveal soft drusen (mainly in the inferior part), 1 juxtapapillary and several peripapillary drusen. Visual acuity: 1.25

veal and peripapillary area (Fig. 9.3). Juxtapupillary drusen are present in most cases and can be isolated finding (Fig. 9.4e, f).

Clinical Features

The onset of symptoms is typically at the age of 30–50 years; however, childhood cases with severe visual loss have also been reported (Evans et al. 1997). Although both ML and DHRD (or ADD) were reported to be autosomal dominant with full penetrance (Evans et al. 1997; Piguet et al. 1995), a case of non-penetrance in a 62-year-old mutation positive, asymptomatic patient with normal fundus appearance have been reported (Michaelides et al. 2006; Scarpatetti et al. 1978) illustrating the variability of disease phenotypic expressivity.

Disease severity varies with the evidence of interocular, intrafamilial (Fig. 9.4), and interfamilial variability (Fig. 9.5) in visual loss and natural history. It has also been reported in more recent reports of British, Japanese, Chinese, and Indian pedigrees (Fu et al. 2007; Michaelides et al. 2006; Takeuchi et al. 2010; Zhang et al. 2014).

Main clinical findings include early onset small radial drusen and larger drusen at the posterior pole and also nasal to the optic nerve head (Fig. 9.2). A distinct phenotypic feature with only juxtapapillary drusen as an isolated sign, with normal macula (Fig. 9.4e, f) can be observed. The small drusen display a pathognomonic radial distribution converging toward the fovea (Gregory et al. 1996; Piguet et al. 1995). In Doyne honeycomb retinal dystrophy, the radial distribution of drusen was a rare finding (Evans et al. 1997; Pearce 1968) and was originally used to distinguish Malattia Leventinese from Doyne honeycomb dystrophy. Drusen can be first noticed in asymptomatic teenager or young adult. They might remain few in numbers, with no progression, the patient keeping his 1.0 vision until late 50s (Figs. 9.6 and 9.7) or 60s (Figs. 9.5, 9.8, and 9.9). Sometimes they increase in number and size, some become soft and round, confluent, and merge to form multiple solid plaques displaying a honeycomb pattern at the level of Bruch's membrane (Evans et al. 1997; Forni and Babel 1962; Piguet et al. 1995).

Early visual symptoms include reduced central vision, photophobia, slow dark adaptation, paracentral scotomas, and metamorphopsias (Gerber et al. 2003; Haimovici et al. 2002; Michaelides et al. 2006). Color vision loss is a later finding (Michaelides et al. 2006). Symptomatic patients report very gradual deterioration over many years (Fig. 9.10). Mild cases are characterized by normal visual acuity and the presence of small, discrete drusen at the macula; in some cases, the macula is normal and only some drusen deposited at the optic disc margin are observed (Michaelides et al. 2006; Zhang et al. 2014). In the later stages of the disease and in severe cases, central vision deteriorates and absolute scotomas can develop predominantly as result of retinal pigment epithelium atrophy or scaring (Fig. 9.11) (Evans et al. 1997; Héon et al. 1996). Subretinal neovascular membrane can develop but is a very uncommon complication (Michaelides et al. 2006; Sohn et al. 2011; Takeuchi et al. 2010; Zhang et al. 2014), which is sometimes associated with a subretinal hemorrhage, as the presenting symptom of the disease (Pager et al. 2001). The neovascular membrane, if present, can lead to severe vision loss in younger patients, in their 30s to 40s (Querques et al. 2013; Sohn et al. 2011; Zech et al. 1999; Zhang et al. 2014) and, rarely, can be bilateral (Zhang et al. 2014). In some cases, hyperplasia of the retinal pigment epithelium and subretinal fibrous metaplasia can occur (Matsumoto and Traboulsi 2001; Zech et al. 1999)

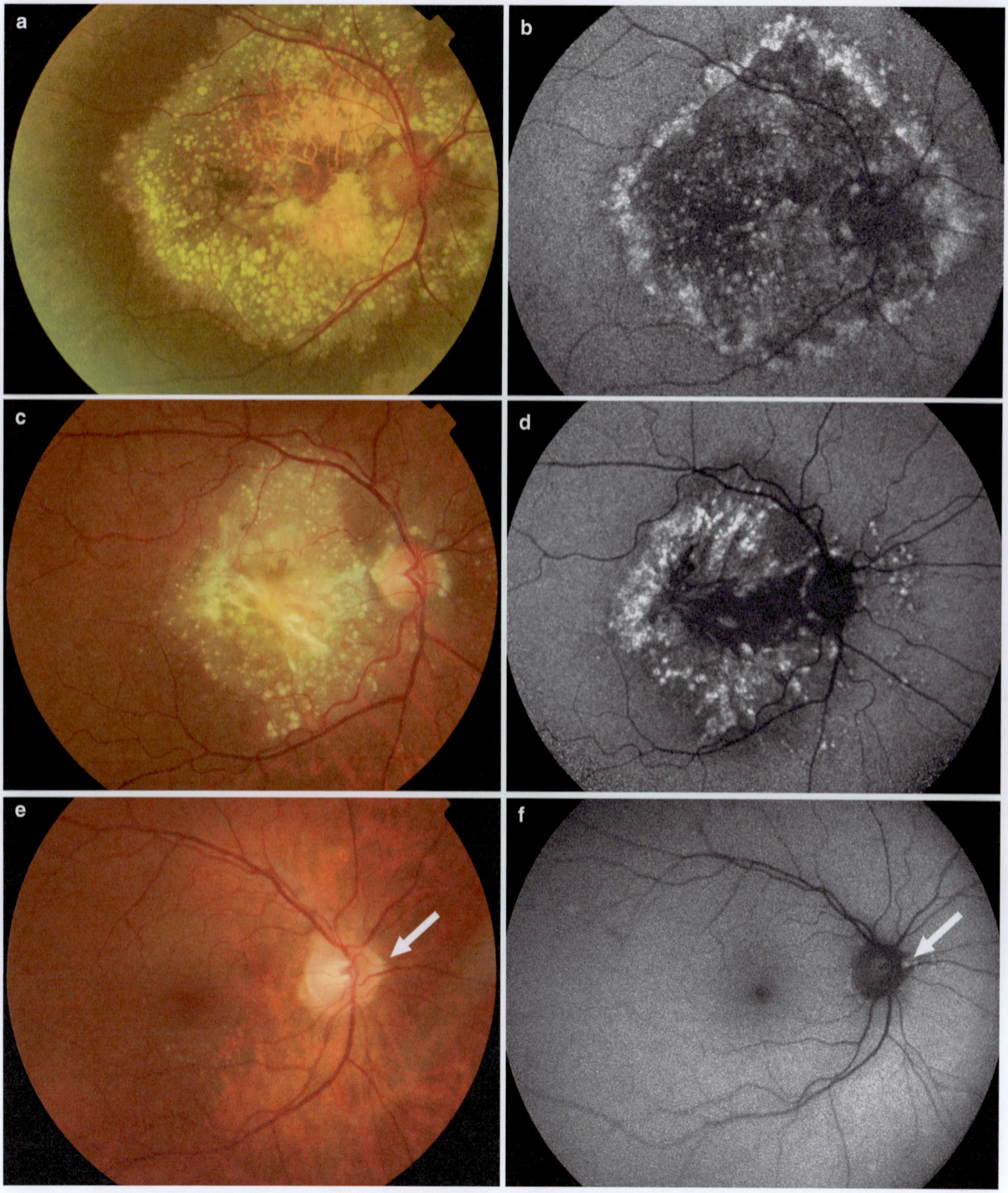

Fig. 9.4 Family 1—Affected mother (**a**, **b**) and two affected daughters (**c**, **d**, **e**, **f**). (**a**) Fundus color RE of the 64-year-old mother showing confluent macular and peripapillary drusen, some foveal scaring, and juxtapapillary drusen. Visual acuity: hand movement. (**b**) RE fundus autofluorescence, hypofluorescence corresponding to scaring and areas of atrophy, hyperautofluorescence corresponding to confluent and isolated drusen. (**c**) Fundus color RE of 39-year-old daughter, confluent drusen, and hyperpigmented area of fibrosis; juxta and peripapillary drusen. Visual acuity 0.1. (**d**) FAF RE hypoautofluorescence corresponding to central scar, hyperautofluorescence of drusen. (**e**) Fundus color RE of 36-year-old sister: only some juxtapapillary drusen and a few at the posterior pole. Her visual acuity 0.8; she is myopic (−10D). (**f**) FAF RE of the same patient: hyperautofluorescence of juxtapapillary drusen

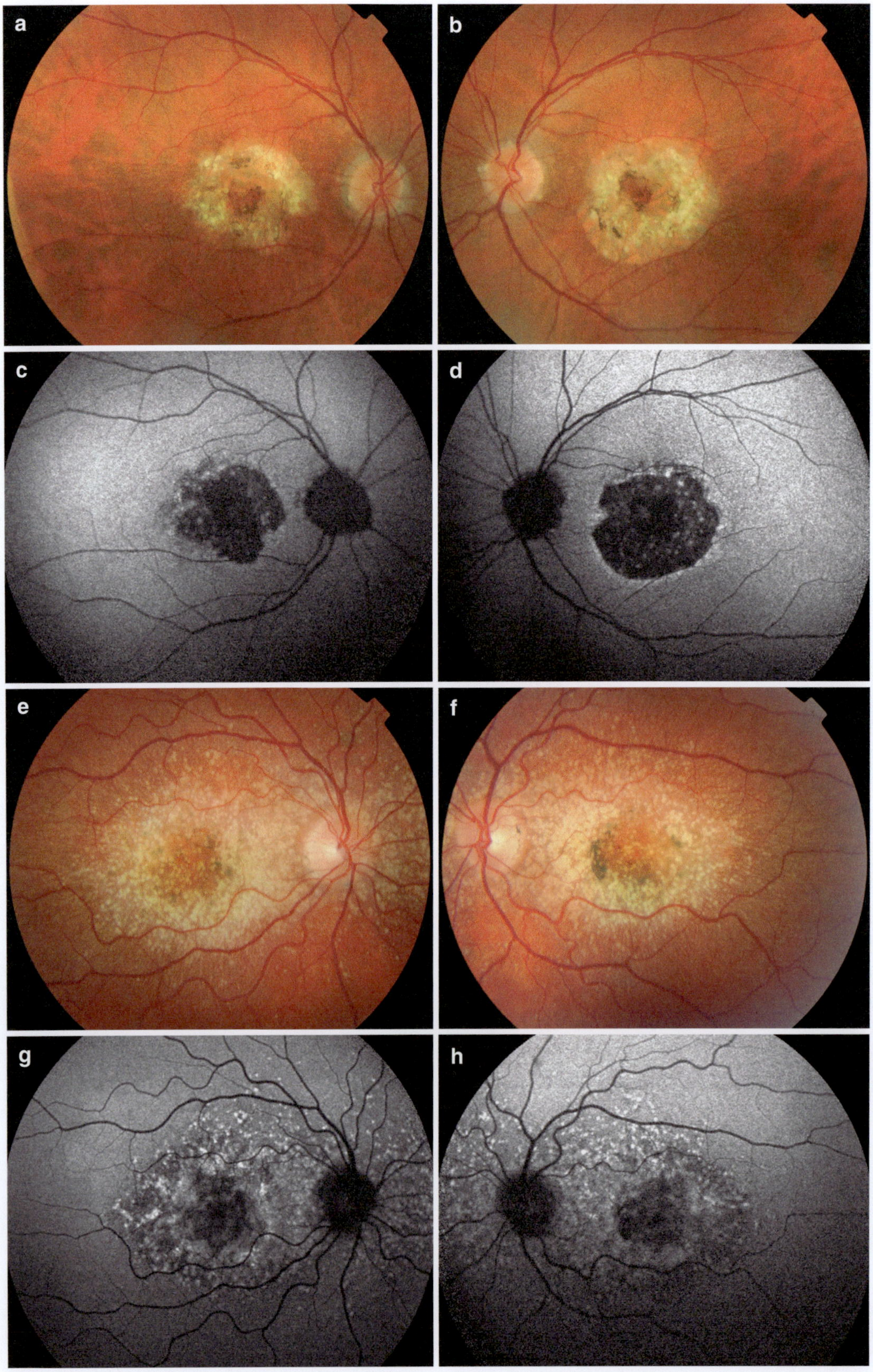

Fig. 9.5 Family 2—61-year-old father (**a**, **b**, **c**, **d**) and his affected 31-year-old son (**c**, **d**, **e**, **f**). (**a**, **b**) Fundus color right and left eye showing confluent macular drusen some foveal scaring and juxtapapillary drusen; visual acuity is 0.8 RE, 1.0 LE. (**c**, **d**) FAF RE and LE hypofluorescence corresponding to scaring and areas of atrophy, hyperautofluorescence corresponding to confluent drusen. (**e**, **f**) Fundus color LE and RE of the son, showing confluent drusen and small radial drusen. Some hyperpigmented areas. Numerous peri- and juxtapapillary drusen Visual acuity is 1.0 in both eyes. (**g**, **h**) FAF RE and LE: some hypoautofluorescence corresponding to beginning of central scar, hyperautofluorescence of drusen

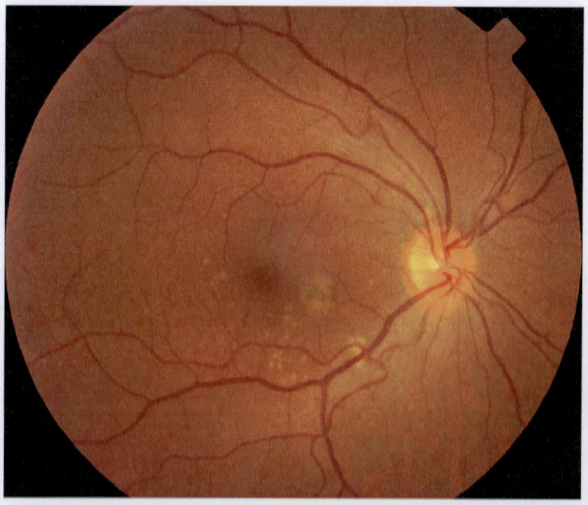

Fig. 9.6 Family 3—55-year-old mother. Fundus color showing few soft macular drusen not involving the fovea, some peripapillary drusen. Visual acuity is 1.0

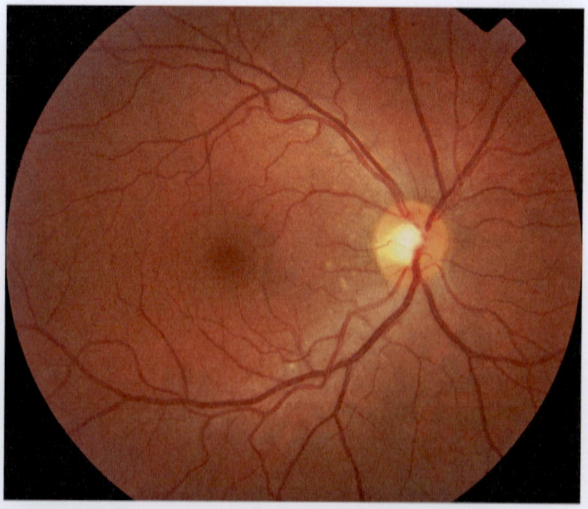

Fig. 9.7 Family 3—32-year-old daughter. Fundus color showing very few macular drusen not involving the fovea, mainly in the inferior part of the retina. Visual acuity is 1.0

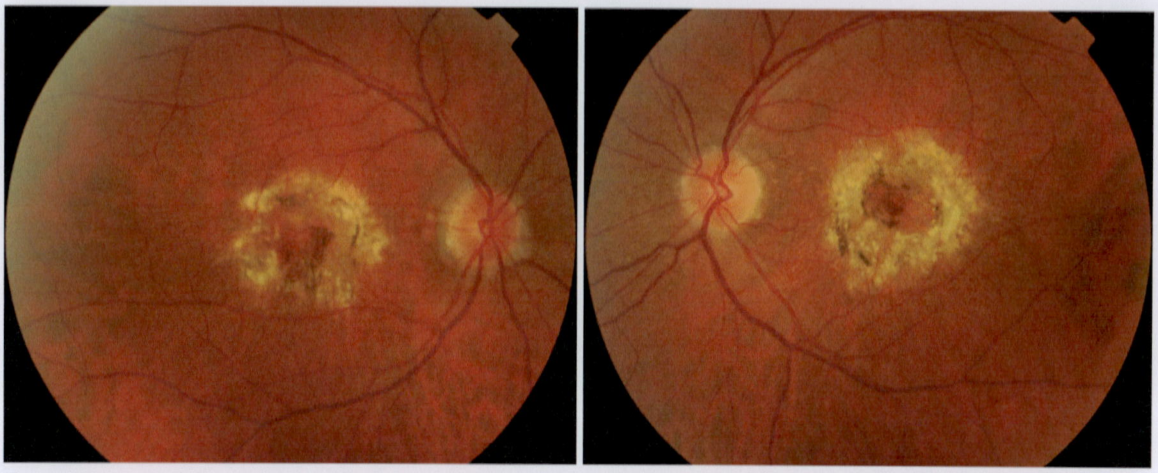

Fig. 9.8 Family 2—father (Photo taken at when 56 years old) (see also Fig 9.5). Fundus color showing confluent macular drusen partly involving the fovea. Juxtapapillary drusen. Corrected visual acuity is 1.0 in both eyes

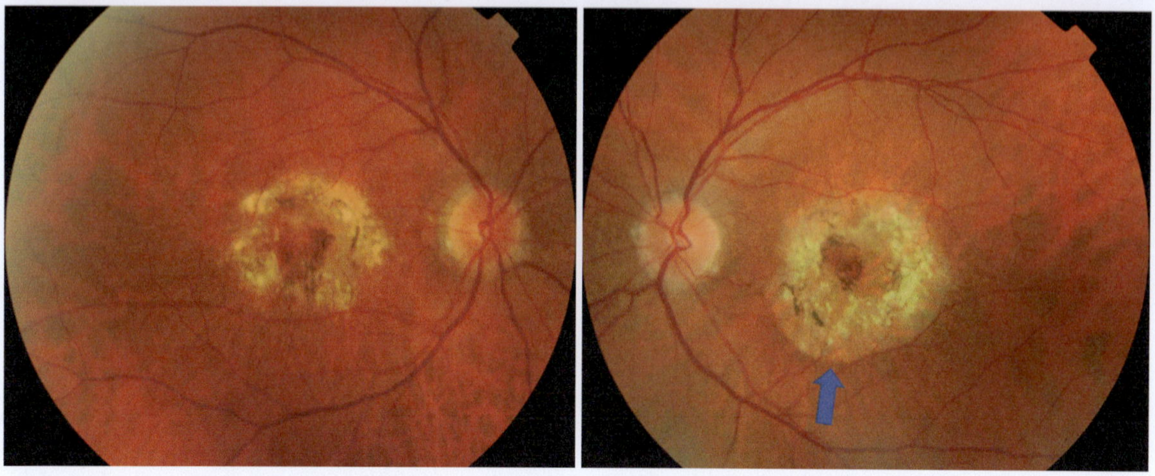

Fig. 9.9 Family 2—Follow-up 5 years later of the same father (now 61 years old—also Fig. 9.5). Fundus color showing the concentric expansion of confluent macular drusen. The arrow showing expansion of drusen and corresponding atrophy. Very mild expansion of juxtapapillary drusen. The visual acuity dropped to 0.8 RE, remaining at 1.0 LE

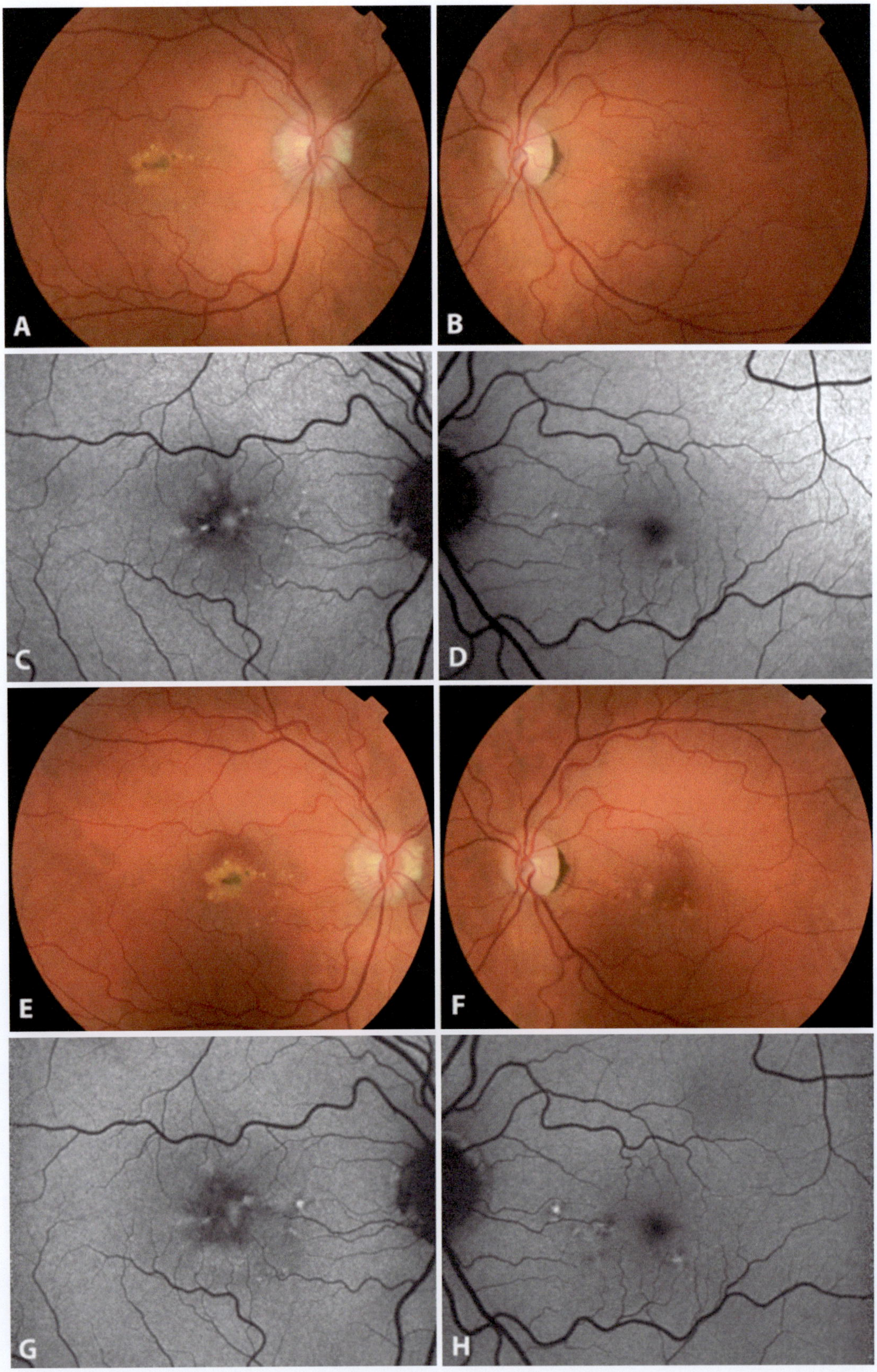

Fig. 9.10 Family 4—3 years follow-up of 47 years old affected patient from a large dominant pedigree. (**a**, **b**) Fundus color showing foveal confluent macular drusen, as well as juxtapapillary drusen. Visual acuity is 1.0 bilaterally, but the patient was complaining of metamorphopsias in the RE. A neovascular membrane was suspected at that time. (**c**, **d**) FAF showing some hyperfluorescent drusen at the fovea RE, and perifoveal drusen LE. (**e**, **f**) Fundus color of same patient 3 years later, very comparable to the previous one. Visual acuity is 1.0 bilaterally, and persistent complaint of metamorphopsia. (**g**, **h**) FAF of same patient, 3 years later, confirming mild progression: some new hyperfluorescent dots (drusen) or existing hyperfluorescent dots becoming larger

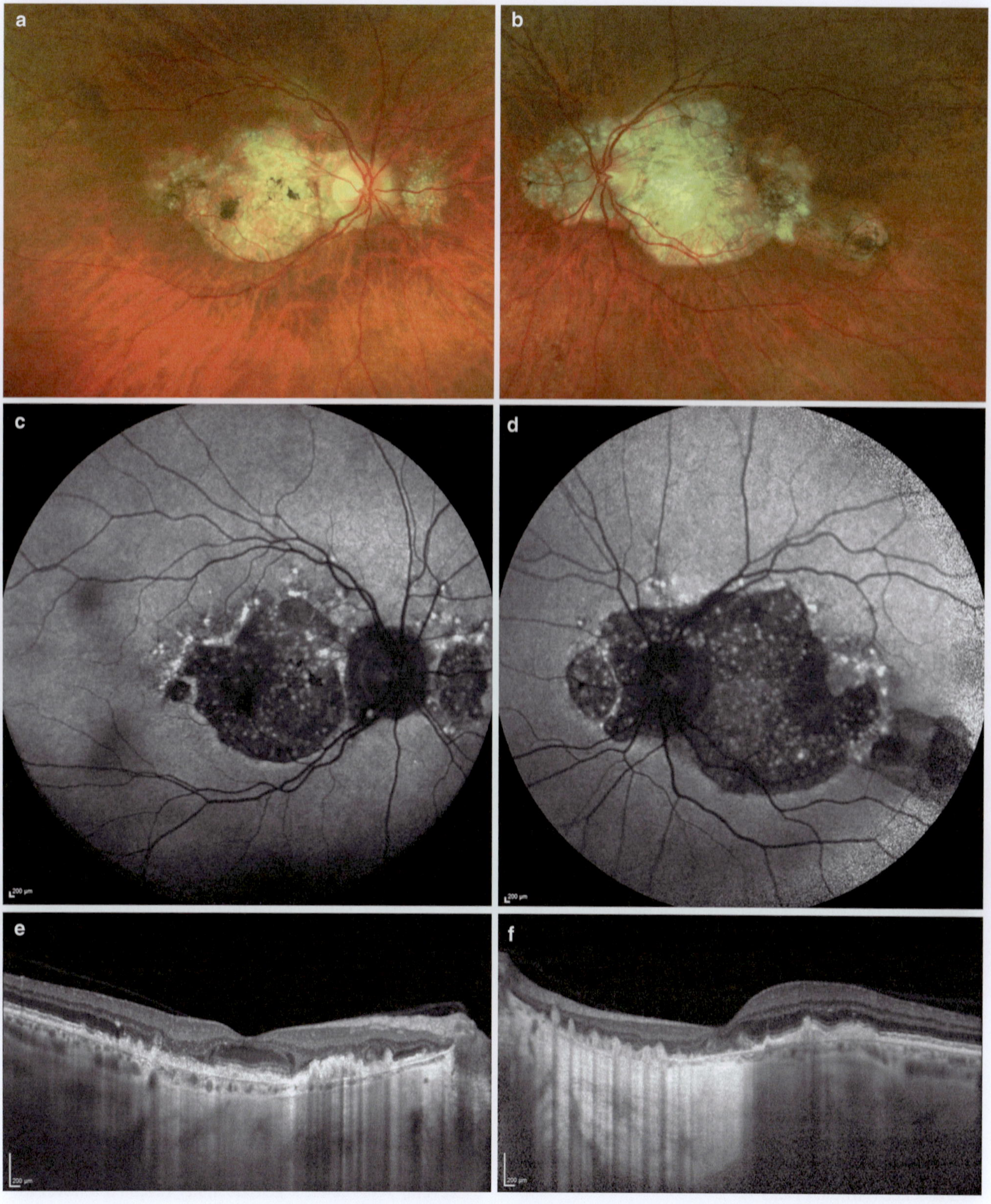

Fig. 9.11 Family 5—56-year-old affected female from a large pedigree. (**a**, **b**) Fundus color showing the large area of subretinal fibrous metaplasia and atrophy and the macula and peripapillary area. (**c**, **d**) FAF showing large hypofluorescent area with hyperautofluorescent dots and ring surrounding the hypofluorescent zone. (**e**, **f**) The spectral domain OCT showing diffuse subretinal deposits of hyperreflective material, appearing as several focal dome-shaped elevations, at the perifoveal areas. At the subfoveal areas, there is a diffuse thickening corresponding very likely to fibrous metaplasia. Visual acuity is 0.3 in the right eye and 0.6 in the left

Paraclinic Testing and Their Use in Malattia Leventinese

Autofluorescence imaging allows the visualization of the complex RPE/photoreceptor outer segment health by taking advantage of the fluorescent properties of lipofuscin (von Rückmann et al. 1995). The increased AF associated with drusen in monogenic macular dystrophies has been reported (von Rückmann et al. 1998). In recent report in patients with a confirmed fibulin-3 mutation status, all increased foci of AF correlated to drusen, but some drusen displayed reduced or absent AF. Querques et al. (2013) observed increased and intense AF only in large drusen, but not in small, radial drusen. However the main highlight of autofluorescence imaging was to detect hyperfluorescent dots at the optic disc margin, confirming peripapillary drusen, which were not obvious on routine fundus examination (Michaelides et al. 2006; Zhang et al. 2014).

Time-domain and spectral domain optical coherence tomography (OCT) have provided insight into structural retinal changes in patients with autosomal dominant drusen due to *EFEMP1* mutation. A remarkable preservation of the neurosensory retina was observed, both in perimacular and in foveal areas (Souied et al. 2006). Later reports, using a SD OCT, provided a better understanding of the two types of drusen: large round drusen appeared as diffuse or focal deposition of hyperreflective material underneath the RPE—determining a diffuse RPE elevation or a focal dome-shaped elevation. The small drusen, described as located above the RPE, had a saw-tooth elevation appearance (Querques et al. 2013; Zweifel et al. 2012). The preservation of intact inner retina and preserved junction OS/IS being noted over small drusen, while the IS/OS junction was disrupted over large drusen (Querques et al. 2013).

To assess morphological and functional differences between the two types of drusen is given by reports of fluorescein angiography (FA) and indocyanine green angiography (ICG) features in Malattia Leventinese. On both FA and ICG, large round drusen are hypofluorescent in early phases, and turn into hyperfluorescent in late phase, of ICG frames. The small drusen hyperfluorescence in early phase and decrease their fluorescence toward the later phase (Guigui et al. 2011; Querques et al. 2013). Therefore, while small drusen share similitudes with cuticular drusen (Querques et al. 2011), the large drusen behave at FA and ICG more like age-related macular degeneration drusen with a late hyperfluorescence (Arnold et al. 1997).

Additional insight into detecting neovascular membrane in ML patient was recently described, using optical coherence tomography angiography, not otherwise detectable with traditional imaging (Corbelli et al. 2016; Serra et al. 2017)

Full-field ERGs, EOG, and multifocal ERG data are available. The full-field ERG showed normal rod b-wave responses, normal standard combined (mixed rod plus cone) response and reduced 30-Hz flicker responses in both eyes in a 42-year-old patient from the Japanese pedigree (Takeuchi et al. 2010). Similar findings were described by a British group (Haimovici et al. 2002) who found that the scotopic sensitivity was reduced and dark adaptation kinetics were prolonged over the macular deposits only, but were normal elsewhere in patients affected by Malattia Leventinese. A Swiss group (Gerber et al. 2003) described "low-normal" amplitudes of the b-wave of rod and cone response, suggesting discrete but widespread functional abnormalities, while the b-wave amplitudes were subnormal in more advance cases.

Molecular Genetics: Mapping

The first investigation was performed on five families (large American kindred with two affected branches and three kindreds from the Leventinese valley) with the ML phenotype with a total of 56 affected patients. They demonstrated linkage of ML to chromosome 2p. The maximum two-point lod score observed in all families combined was 10.5 and was obtained with the marker D2S378. To narrow the genetic interval containing the ML/DHRD gene, 63 members from a large nine generation DHRD British pedigree, originally described by O'Neill (2009) and Pearce (1968) were assessed for molecular genetic linkage study (Gregory et al. 1996). Two-point analysis showed a significant linkage of the DHRD to nine markers on the short arm of chromosome 2, a region overlapping the one recently reported to be linked to ML. A maximum lod score of 7.29 was obtained at marker locus D2S2251. A combination of positional and candidate gene methods in 39 families from Switzerland, the USA, and Australia helped identifying a single non-conservative Arginine 345 to Tryptophan mutation (Arg345Trp) in the gene *EFEMP1* (EGF-containing fibrillin-like extracellular matrix protein 1) coding for fibulin-3 in all families studied, inclusive of both phenotypes, ML and DHRD. In this original study, the authors found that among all families studied, there was a complete sharing of alleles of intragenic *EFEMP1* polymorphisms (SNPs). The same haplotype, and the absence of de novo R345W mutation in different ethnicities was highly suggestive that the R345W mutation occurred only once in a common ancestor of every affected patient (Stone et al. 1999). This study also confirmed that ML and DHRD are the same disorder.

Several years later, a genetic study revealed a novel disease haplotype with R345W mutation in an Indian pedigree, suggesting an independent origin (Fu et al. 2007). A novel, different haplotype with the R345W mutation was identified in a Japanese pedigree (Takeuchi et al. 2010), suggesting that the disease might have occurred independently in a common Japanese founder.

Hypothesis on R345W Fibulin-3 Function and Histopathological Studies

A single mutation (R345W) in the gene *EFEMP1* (fibulin-3) is responsible for all the ML cases reported to date (Stone et al. 1999). *EFEMP1* gene consists of 12 exons and spans approximately 60 kb of genomic DNA (Blackburn et al. 2003). The fibulin-3 is a basement membrane glycoprotein, broadly expressed throughout the body (Kobayashi et al. 2007; Marmorstein et al. 2002). It is one of seven highly conserved members of the fibulin family of extracellular matrix (ECM) proteins (Zhang and Marmorstein 2010).

A normal fibulin-3 interacts with several other proteins: a basement membrane protein (extracellular matrix protein-1), tissue inhibitor of metalloproteinase-3 (TIMP-3), collagen XVIII/endostatin, hepatitis B virus-encoded X antigen and elastin monomer tropoelastin. These interactions likely contribute to the integrity of basement membrane zone. Fibulin-3 colocalizes with fine elastic fibers and is involved in the formation of the extracellular matrix (Zhang and Marmorstein 2010).

The R345W mutation does not seem to impair fibulin-3's but rather renders the protein resistant do degradation (Marmorstein et al. 2002). In both ML and AMD eyes, fibulin-3 accumulates along drusen or other basal deposits (Zhang and Marmorstein 2010). In recent report it has been suggested that fibulin-3 is a central player in the development of basal laminar deposit and deletion of *EFEMP1* in mouse eyes is protective against the development of basal laminar deposits (Stanton et al. 2017).

Immunohistochemistry analysis, using monoclonal and polyclonal antibodies, of seven human donor eyes showed that, in normal retina, fibulin-3 is predominantly present in photoreceptor inner and outer segment regions and the nerve fiber layer, but not in the RPE, Bruch's membrane or choroid (Marmorstein et al. 2002). In a donor eye from an 86-year-old Malattia Leventinese patient carrying a homozygote R345W mutation, fibulin-3 was found to accumulate beneath the RPE, overlying drusen and in Bruch's membrane, in addition to its presence in the interphotoreceptor matrix and the nerve fiber layer (Marmorstein et al. 2002).

A recent morphologic and histochemical analysis of drusen in a Malattia Leventinese donor and seven age-related macular degeneration (AMD) donors showed that drusen from both diseases shared many major constituents. However, drusen from the ML donor had a unique onion-skin-like lamination and possessed collagen type IV, which was absent in age-related drusen (Sohn et al. 2015).

Clinical Management/Treatment

As for many genetic retinal diseases, there is no specific treatment. However, ML has a close phenotypic similarity to AMD, where laser photocoagulation has been shown to lead to drusen reabsorption and has been tried as prophylactic treatment (Cleasby et al. 1979; Gass 1973; Gross-Jendroska et al. 1998; Wetzig 1994). A meta-analysis of nine randomized controlled trials of laser treatment of AMD drusen confirmed that laser photocoagulation leads to drusen disappearance, but no evidence was found that it reduces vision loss, the risk of developing CNV or geographic atrophy (Parodi et al. 2009). A recent study assessed the efficacy of laser photocoagulation as therapeutic approach for patients with ML and showed encouraging results. One eye of 11 patients with genetically confirmed Malattia Leventinese was treated, and those treated eyes gained an average of 4.9 letters, while untreated eyes lost an average of 0.8 letters, over a 12 months period of the study. Some patients showed a significant improvement in retinal sensitivity in treated eyes. The mean drusen thickness increased in untreated eyes, but not in the treated eyes (Lenassi et al. 2013).

In later stages of the disease, subretinal neovascular membrane can occur and lead to severe vision loss (Michaelides et al. 2006; Sohn et al. 2011; Takeuchi et al. 2010; Zhang et al. 2014). Because of phenotypic similarities to the CNV in age-related macular degeneration, some reports determined the effects of anti-VEGF (bevacizumab) intravitreal injections in two patients with ML. In both patients, the treatment leads to resolution of intraretinal fluid and improvement in visual acuity (Sohn et al. 2011).

References

Arnold JJ, Quaranta M, Soubrane G, Sarks SH, Coscas G. Indocyanine green angiography of drusen. Am J Ophthalmol. 1997;124:344–56.

Blackburn J, Tarttelin EE, Gregory-Evans CY, Moosajee M, Gregory-Evans K. Transcriptional regulation and expression of the dominant drusen gene FBLN3 (EFEMP1) in mammalian retina. Invest Ophthalmol Vis Sci. 2003;44:4613–21.

Cleasby GW, Nakanishi AS, Norris JL. Prophylactic photocoagulation of the fellow eye in exudative senile maculopathy. A preliminary report. Mod Probl Ophthalmol. 1979;20:141–7.

Corbelli E, Corvi F, Carnevali A, Querques L, Zucchiatti I, Bandello F, Querques G. Optical coherence tomography angiography demonstration of Choroidal neovascularization in Malattia Leventinese. Ophthalmic Surg Lasers Imaging Retina. 2016;47:602–4. https://doi.org/10.3928/23258160-20160601-17.

Doyne RW. Peculiar condition of choroiditis occurring in several members of the same family. Trans Ophthalmol Soc UK. 1899;19:71.

Dusek J, Streicher T, Schmidt K. Hereditäre Drusen der Bruchschen Membran. II. Untersuchung von Semidünnschnitten und elektronenmikroskopischen Ergebnissen. Klinische Monatsblatter fur Augenheilkunde. 1982;181:79–83.

Evans K, Gregory CY, Wijesuriya SD, Kermani S, Jay MR, Plant C, Bird AC. Assessment of the phenotypic range seen in Doyne honeycomb retinal dystrophy. Arch Ophthalmol. 1997;115:904–10.

Forni S, Babel J. Etude clinique et histologique de la malattia leventinese. Affection appartenant au groupe des dégénérescences hyalines du pôle postérieur. Ophthalmologica. 1962;143:313–22.

Fu L, et al. The R345W mutation in EFEMP1 is pathogenic and causes AMD-like deposits in mice. Hum Mol Genet. 2007;16:2411–22. https://doi.org/10.1093/hmg/ddm198.

Gass JD. Drusen and disciform macular detachment and degeneration. Arch Ophthalmol. 1973;90:206–17.

Gass JDM. Dominantly inherited radial basal laminar drusen (malattia leventinese, Doyne's honeycomb macular dystrophy). In: Gass' atlas of macular diseases, 5th edn. New York: Elsevier; 2012. p. 292–5.

Gerber DM, Munier FL, Niemeyer G. Cross-sectional study of visual acuity and electroretinogram in two types of dominant drusen. Invest Ophthalmol Vis Sci. 2003;44:493–6.

Gregory CY, et al. The gene responsible for autosomal dominant Doyne's honeycomb retinal dystrophy (DHRD) maps to chromosome 2p16. Hum Mol Genet. 1996;5:1055–9.

Gross-Jendroska M, Owens SL, Flaxel CJ, Guymer RH, Bird AC. Prophylactic laser treatment to fellow eyes of unilateral retinal pigment epithelial tears. Am J Ophthalmol. 1998;126:77–81.

Guigui B, Leveziel N, Martinet V, Massamba N, Sterkers M, Coscas G, Souied EH. Angiography features of early onset drusen. Br J Ophthalmol. 2011;95:238–44. https://doi.org/10.1136/bjo.2009.178400.

Haimovici R, Wroblewski J, Piguet B, Fitzke FW, Holder GE, Arden GB, Bird AC. Symptomatic abnormalities of dark adaptation in patients with EFEMP1 retinal dystrophy (Malattia Leventinese/Doyne honeycomb retinal dystrophy). Eye (Lond). 2002;16:7–15. https://doi.org/10.1038/sj.eye.6700018.

Héon E, et al. Linkage of autosomal dominant radial drusen (malattia leventinese) to chromosome 2p16-21. Arch Ophthalmol. 1996;114:193–8.

Kobayashi N, et al. A comparative analysis of the fibulin protein family. Biochemical characterization, binding interactions, and tissue localization. J Biol Chem. 2007;282:11805–16. https://doi.org/10.1074/jbc.M611029200.

Lenassi E, Troeger E, Wilke R, Tufail A, Hawlina M, Jeffery G, Webster AR. Laser clearance of drusen deposit in patients with autosomal dominant drusen (p.Arg345Trp in EFEMP1). Am J Ophthalmol. 2013;155:190–8. https://doi.org/10.1016/j.ajo.2012.07.003.

Marmorstein LY, et al. Aberrant accumulation of EFEMP1 underlies drusen formation in Malattia Leventinese and age-related macular degeneration. Proc Natl Acad Sci U S A. 2002;99:13067–72. https://doi.org/10.1073/pnas.202491599.

Matsumoto M, Traboulsi EI. Dominant radial drusen and Arg345Trp EFEMP1 mutation. Am J Ophthalmol. 2001;131:810–2.

Michaelides M, et al. Maculopathy due to the R345W substitution in fibulin-3: distinct clinical features, disease variability, and extent of retinal dysfunction. Invest Ophthalmol Vis Sci. 2006;47:3085–97. https://doi.org/10.1167/iovs.05-1600.

O'Neill MJF. Doyne honeycomb retinal dystrophy; DHRD. 2009. http://omim.org/entry/126600?search=126600&highlight=126600. Accessed 16 Mar 2015.

Pager CK, Sarin LK, Federman JL, Eagle R, Hageman G, Rosenow J, Donoso LA. Malattia leventinese presenting with subretinal neovascular membrane and hemorrhage. Am J Ophthalmol. 2001;131:517–8.

Parodi MB, Virgili G, Evans JR. Laser treatment of drusen to prevent progression to advanced age-related macular degeneration. Cochrane Database Syst Rev. 2009;(3):CD006537. https://doi.org/10.1002/14651858.CD006537.pub2.

Pearce WG. Doyne's honeycomb retinal degeneration. Clinical and genetic features. Br J Ophthalmol. 1968;52:73–8.

Piguet B, Haimovici R, Bird AC. Dominantly inherited drusen represent more than one disorder: a historical review. Eye (Lond). 1995;9:34–41. https://doi.org/10.1038/eye.1995.5.

Querques G, Guigui B, Leveziel N, Querques L, Coscas G, Soubrane G, Souied EH. Insights into pathology of cuticular drusen from integrated confocal scanning laser ophthalmoscopy imaging and corresponding spectral domain optical coherence tomography. Graefe's Arch Clin Exp. 2011;249:1617–25. https://doi.org/10.1007/s00417-011-1702-0.

Querques G, Guigui B, Leveziel N, Querques L, Bandello F, Souied EH. Multimodal morphological and functional characterization of Malattia Leventinese. Graefe's Arch Clin Exp Ophthalmol. 2013;251:705–14. https://doi.org/10.1007/s00417-012-2106-5.

Scarpatetti A, Forni S, Niemeyer G. Die Netzhautfunktion bei Malattia leventinese (dominant drusen). Klinische Monatsblatter fur Augenheilkunde. 1978;172:590–7.

Serra R, Coscas F, Messaoudi N, Srour M, Souied E. Choroidal neovascularization in Malattia Leventinese diagnosed using optical coherence tomography angiography. Am J Ophthalmol. 2017;176:108–17. https://doi.org/10.1016/j.ajo.2016.12.027.

Sohn EH, Patel PJ, MacLaren RE, Adatia FA, Pal B, Webster AR, Tufail A. Responsiveness of choroidal neovascular membranes in patients with R345W mutation in fibulin 3 (Doyne honeycomb retinal dystrophy) to anti-vascular endothelial growth factor therapy. Arch Ophthalmol. 2011;129:1626–8. https://doi.org/10.1001/archophthalmol.2011.338.

Sohn EH, Wang K, Thompson S, Riker MJ, Hoffmann JM, Stone EM, Mullins RF. Comparison of drusen and modifying genes in autosomal dominant radial drusen and age-related macular degeneration. Retina (Philadelphia, Pa). 2015;35:48–57. https://doi.org/10.1097/iae.0000000000000263.

Souied EH, Leveziel N, Letien V, Darmon J, Coscas G, Soubrane G. Optical coherent tomography features of malattia leventinese. Am J Ophthalmol. 2006;141:404–7. https://doi.org/10.1016/j.ajo.2005.09.001.

Stanton JB, Marmorstein AD, Zhang Y, Marmorstein LY. Deletion of Efemp1 is protective against the development of sub-RPE deposits in mouse eyes. Invest Ophthalmol Vis Sci. 2017;58:1455–61. https://doi.org/10.1167/iovs.16-20955.

Stone EM, et al. A single EFEMP1 mutation associated with both Malattia Leventinese and Doyne honeycomb retinal dystrophy. Nat Genet. 1999;22:199–202. https://doi.org/10.1038/9722.

Streicher T, Krcmery K. Das fluoreszenzangiographische Bild der hereditären Drusen. Klinische Monatsblatter fur Augenheilkunde. 1976;169:22–30.

Takeuchi T, Hayashi T, Bedell M, Zhang K, Yamada H, Tsuneoka H. A novel haplotype with the R345W mutation in the EFEMP1 gene associated with autosomal dominant drusen in a Japanese family. Invest Ophthalmol Vis Sci. 2010;51:1643–50. https://doi.org/10.1167/iovs.09-4497.

Vogt A. Die Ophthalmoskopie im rotfreien Licht. In: Graefe A, Saemisch T, editors. Handbuch der gesammten Augenheilkunde. Untersuchungsmethoden. 3rd ed. Berlin: Verlag von Wilhelm Engelman; 1925. p. 1–118.

von Rückmann A, Fitzke FW, Bird AC. Distribution of fundus autofluorescence with a scanning laser ophthalmoscope. Br J Ophthalmol. 1995;79:407–12.

von Rückmann A, Schmidt KG, Fitzke FW, Bird AC, Jacobi KW. Fundus-Autofluoreszenz bei Patienten mit vererbten Makuladystrophien, Malattia leventinese, familiar dominanten und altersbedingten Drusen. Klinische Monatsblatter fur Augenheilkunde. 1998;213:81–6. https://doi.org/10.1055/s-2008-1034951.

Waardenburg PJ. On recognizability of latent conductors of universal albinism and of ocular albinism. Ophthalmologica. 1948;115:126.

Wetzig PC. Photocoagulation of drusen-related macular degeneration: a long-term outcome. Trans Am Ophthalmol Soc. 1994;92:299–303; discussion 303–296.

Zech JC, Zaouche S, Mourier F, Placuchu H, Grange JD, Trepsat C. Macular dystrophy of malattia leventinese. A 25 year follow up. Br J Ophthalmol. 1999;83:1195–6.

Zhang Y, Marmorstein LY. Focus on molecules: fibulin-3 (EFEMP1). Exp Eye Res. 2010;90:374–5. https://doi.org/10.1016/j.exer.2009.09.018.

Zhang T, et al. Malattia leventinese/Doyne honeycomb retinal dystrophy in a Chinese family with mutation of the EFEMP1 gene. Retina (Philadelphia, Pa). 2014;34:2462–71. https://doi.org/10.1097/iae.0000000000000259.

Zweifel SA, Maygar I, Berger W, Tschuor P, Becker M, Michels S. Multimodal imaging of autosomal dominant drusen. Klinische Monatsblatter fur Augenheilkunde. 2012;229:399–402. https://doi.org/10.1055/s-0031-1299404.

Bietti's Crystalline Dystrophy

10

Eugene Yu-Chuan Kang and Nan-Kai Wang

Introduction

Bietti's crystalline dystrophy (BCD, MIM 210370), an autosomal recessive retinal degeneration, most commonly affects the Asian population, especially Japanese and Chinese people (Kaiser-Kupfer et al. 1994; Hu 1983; Lin et al. 2005). BCD causes progressive nyctalopia and visual field loss from the second to fourth decade of life and is usually followed by severe visual loss in the fifth to sixth decade of life (Kaiser-Kupfer et al. 1994). Also known as Bietti's crystalline corneoretinal dystrophy, BCD was first described by an Italian ophthalmologist Bietti in 1937 (Bietti 1937). Bietti reported three cases with crystalline deposits in the retina and sparkling yellow-white spots in the limbal cornea. Those patients were subsequently followed by Bagolini and Ioli-Spada (Bagolini and Ioli-Spada 1968). The disease was initially defined as Bietti tapetoretinal degeneration with marginal corneal dystrophy and was categorized as a crystalline retinopathy in 1977 by Welch (Welch 1977). A mutated gene located on 4q35, *CYP4V2*, was identified in 2004 (Li et al. 2004), and since then, more than 50 studies have reported several novel mutations on this locus.

E. Y.-C. Kang
Department of Ophthalmology, Chang Gung Memorial Hospital, Linkou Medical Center, Taoyuan, Taiwan

College of Medicine, Chang Gung University, Taoyuan, Taiwan

N.-K. Wang (✉)
Department of Ophthalmology, Chang Gung Memorial Hospital, Linkou Medical Center, Taoyuan, Taiwan

College of Medicine, Chang Gung University, Taoyuan, Taiwan

Department of Ophthalmology, Edward S. Harkness Eye Institute, Columbia University, New York, USA

Genetics and Pathogenesis

BCD, a genetic disorder with an autosomal recessive inheritance (Jiao et al. 2000; Li et al. 2004), appears to be associated with abnormal lipid metabolism (Lee et al. 2001). Approximately half of patients with BCD carry compound heterozygous mutations (Xiao et al. 2011). The mutated *CYP4V2* gene, which can be expressed on human retina and retinal pigment epithelium (RPE) (Li et al. 2004), are related to the pathogenesis of BCD. Although there is yet an incomplete understanding of the pathogenesis, it is believed that impaired binding, elongation, or desaturation of fatty acid are the causes for this disease (Lee et al. 2001).

Impairment of fatty acid metabolism has been found to play an important role in BCD (Lee et al. 2001), and it also has a systemic influence in the human body (Wilson et al. 1989). Histopathologic studies showed panchorioretinal atrophy with complex lipid inclusions in choroidal fibroblasts (Kaiser-Kupfer et al. 1994). It is possible that this is the cause of progressive atrophy of the choriocapillaris and RPE layer, which then affects the visual presentation in BCD (Halford et al. 2014). Lower than normal conversion of fatty acid precursors into n-3 polyunsaturated fatty acid has been found (Lee et al. 2001). This characteristic was caused by a dysfunction of microsomal omega hydroxylase, which degrades lipids with mitochondrial and peroxisomal beta-oxidation enzymes, and the protein is encoded by the *CYP4V2* gene in the human body (Nakano et al. 2009; Kelly et al. 2011). Hence, mutation of *CYP4V2* is liable in this metabolic pathway.

CYP4V2 gene, which belongs to the cytochrome P450 gene family, is an 11-exon sequence and produces a 525-amino acid protein through protein synthesis. *CYP4V2* gene is a distinct gene in the *CYP4* family, because it only shares 35% of its sequence with other members in the family (Kelly et al. 2011). In BCD, the mutations of *CYP4V2* gene include missense and nonsense mutations, which were reported to be more prevalent in the Asian population (Xiao et al. 2011; Lai

G. Cheung (ed.), *Hereditary Chorioretinal Disorders*, Retina Atlas, https://doi.org/10.1007/978-981-15-0414-3_10

et al. 2007). According to one study, the prevalence was reported as 0.5–0.6% in the Chinese population (Hu 1983), which may be the reason for more cases reported from patients with Asian descent (Lai et al. 2007; Gekka et al. 2005; Jin et al. 2006; Lin et al. 2005; Shan et al. 2005; Wada et al. 2005; Yokoi et al. 2010; Xiao et al. 2011). After the first identification of *CYP4V2* gene mutation in BCD, more novel mutations associated with *CYP4V2* gene have been reported (Wada et al. 2005; Lin et al. 2005; Lee et al. 2005; Shan et al. 2005), and the severity of the disease is positively correlated with the number of mutations a patient has (Halford et al. 2014). Some genotypes related to more severe phenotypes were also identified (Ng et al. 2016). Age did not affect the severity of the disease even though BCD is believed to be a progressive disease (Lee et al. 2005). Embracing characteristics of metabolic disorders, environmental factors such as person's diet and lifestyle have been proved to affect the disease presentation (Lee et al. 2005). However, the specific correlation between its genotype and phenotype has not yet been clearly defined.

Clinical Features

Bietti's crystalline dystrophy has a clinical picture of numerous crystal deposits in the fundus. The most common lesion site is on or in the RPE–Bruch's membrane complex (Halford et al. 2014). Although corneal limbal crystals were found in the first few cases, it was not commonly reported in the following cases (Hayasaka and Okuyama 1984; Kaiser-Kupfer et al. 1994; Grizzard et al. 1978). Yuzawa et al. noted that corneal deposits may only be observed in the advanced stage, meaning that corneal crystalline deposits are not required for a diagnosis of BCD (Yuzawa et al. 1986). Halford et al. found that atrophy of RPE and Bruch's membrane was associated with the disappearance of the crystal deposits (Halford et al. 2014). The degeneration of the retina and sclerosis of the choroidal vessels may ultimately result in progressive visual disturbance (Lee et al. 2001), and the severity is positively correlated with the thinning of the retina (Lai et al. 2007).

The presenting symptoms and disease progression of BCD vary in individuals despite being similar in age and having similar gene mutations (Lee et al. 2005; Lin et al. 2005; Xiao et al. 2011). In most cases, patients presenting with visual problems are between the second and third decade of life, and the most common symptoms are decreased visual acuity, constriction of visual field, and nyctalopia (Lee et al. 2005). Following progressive atrophy and degeneration of RPE and choroidal vessels, patients experience profound visual impairment and become legally blind during the late stages. However, considerable variation in disease presentation and progression has been reported (Ng et al. 2016).

Color Fundus and Optos Images

The classic feature of color fundus images in BCD is retinal crystalline deposits. At an advanced stage, the crystals decrease and even disappear, and diffused RPE dystrophy and sclerotic choroidal vessels are seen (Figs. 10.1, 10.2, 10.3, 10.4, 10.5, 10.6, 10.7, and 10.8). Newly developed Optos images can offer a wider view of the retina, although the crystals may be more ambiguous (Figs. 10.2, 10.5, and 10.9).

Fundus Autofluorescence (FAF)

As FAF becomes more commonly used in fundus examinations, its role in the diagnosis of BCD has become even more important. Hypo-AF is representative of RPE cell loss, and its feature corresponds to defect lesions in optical coherence tomography (OCT) (Halford et al. 2014) (Figs. 10.2, 10.3, 10.6, 10.7, 10.8, and 10.9). FAF can also be used for detecting disease progression (Figs. 10.7 and 10.8). However, crystals in BCD cannot be found in FAF, since the crystals are suspected as collections of cholesterol esters (Wilson et al. 1989).

Near-Infrared (NIR) Imaging

Using NIR imaging, crystalline deposits and sclerotic choroidal vessels can be identified, and lesions found in other examinations can be coinvestigated (Figs. 10.3, 10.8, and 10.10). Although sclerotic choroidal vessels are rarely discussed in NIR imaging, it was found in the first three cases identified by Bietti (Bietti 1937).

Fluorescein Angiography (FA) and Indocyanine Green Angiography (ICGA)

Since RPE is the major disease site in BCD, changes in FA can be detected early in the disease (Wilson et al. 1989; Kaiser-Kupfer et al. 1994); these are observed as hyperfluorescent window defects (Fong et al. 2009) (Fig. 10.5). The hypofluorescent area can be seen in FA at the late stage of the disease (Fig. 10.8), and the area enlarges progressively in later stages. Yuzawa divides BCD into three stages based on clinical findings (Table 10.1) (Yuzawa et al. 1986). For ICGA, the lobular pattern of hypofluorescent lesions in the

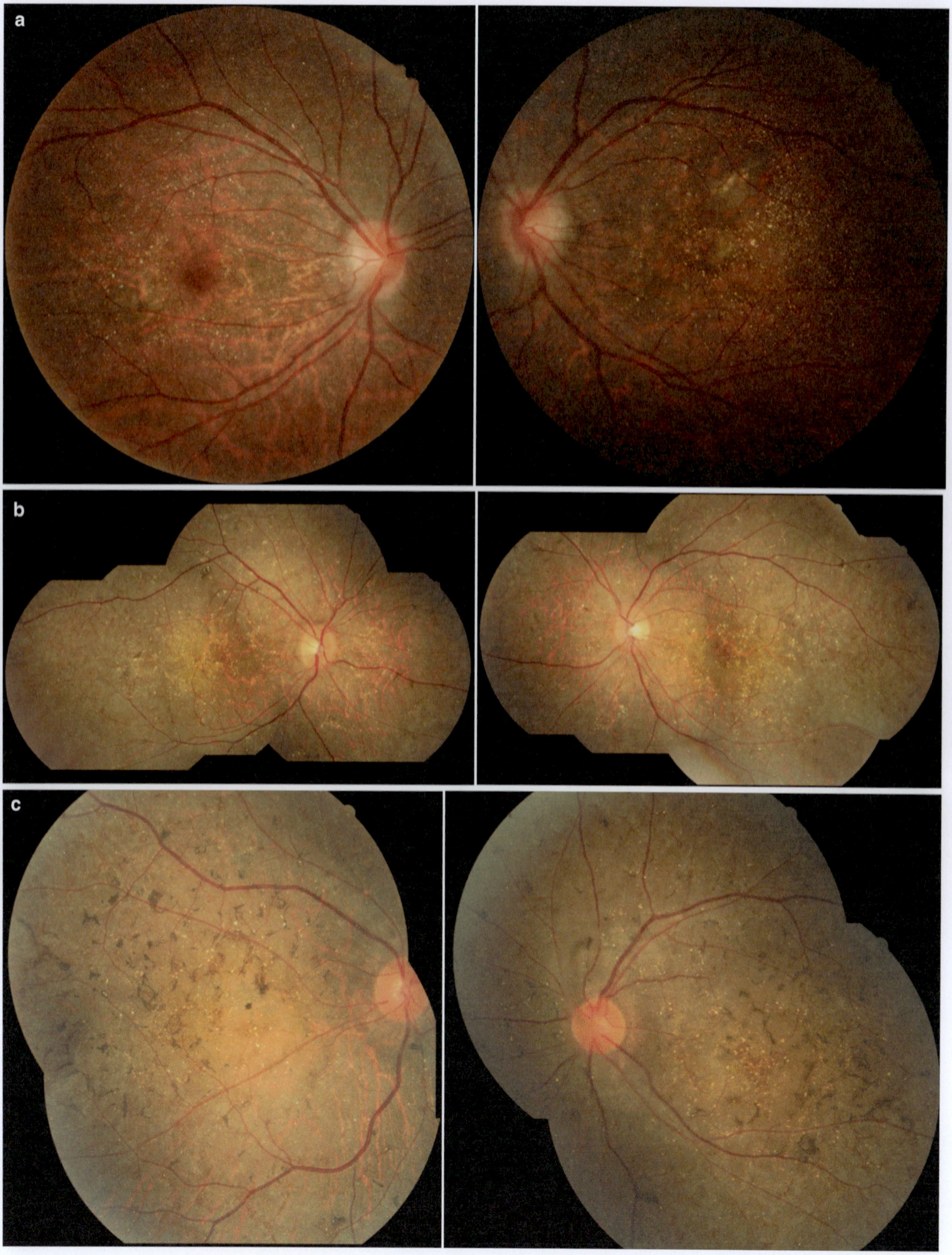

Fig. 10.1 Fundus features of BCD include multiple crystalline deposits in the initial stage (**a**, **b**, **c**). In the advanced stage, RPE dystrophy, disappearance of crystals, and sclerotic choroidal vessels may appear (**d**)

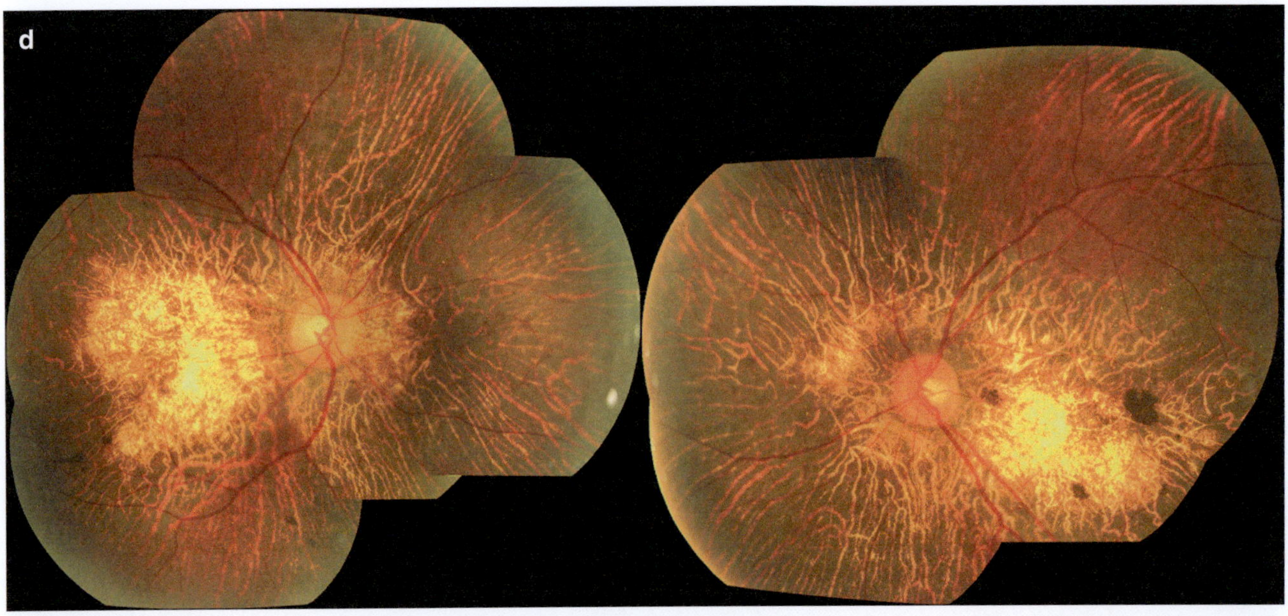

Fig. 10.1 (continued)

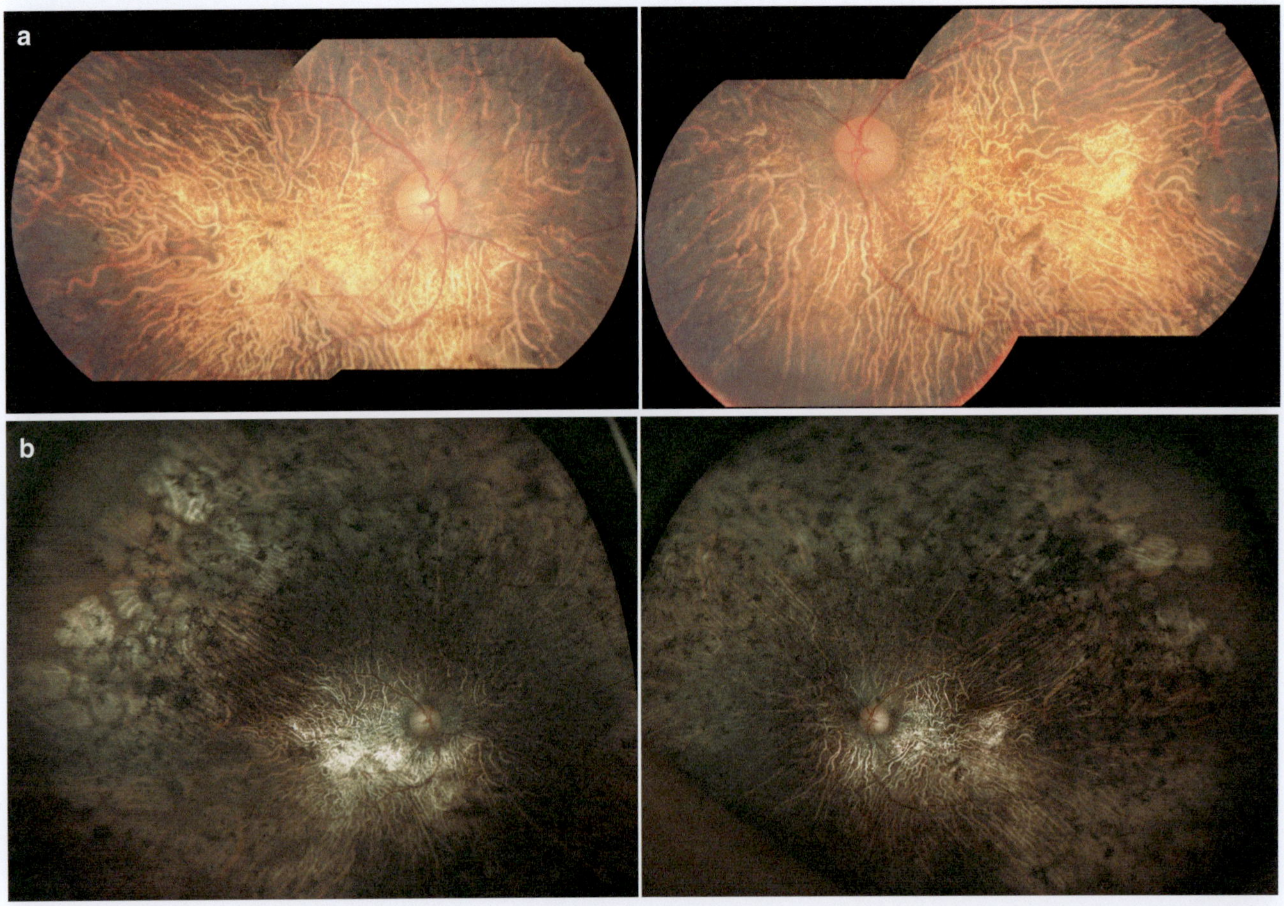

Fig. 10.2 A 57-year-old female with BCD has suffered from blurred vision that has progressively worsened for more than 20 years. (**a**) Her color fundus image showed RPE dystrophy, disappearance of crystals, and sclerotic choroidal vessels. (**b**) RPE dystrophy and sclerotic choroidal vessels were also obvious in Optos images. (**c**) FAF revealed lobular hypo-AF patches

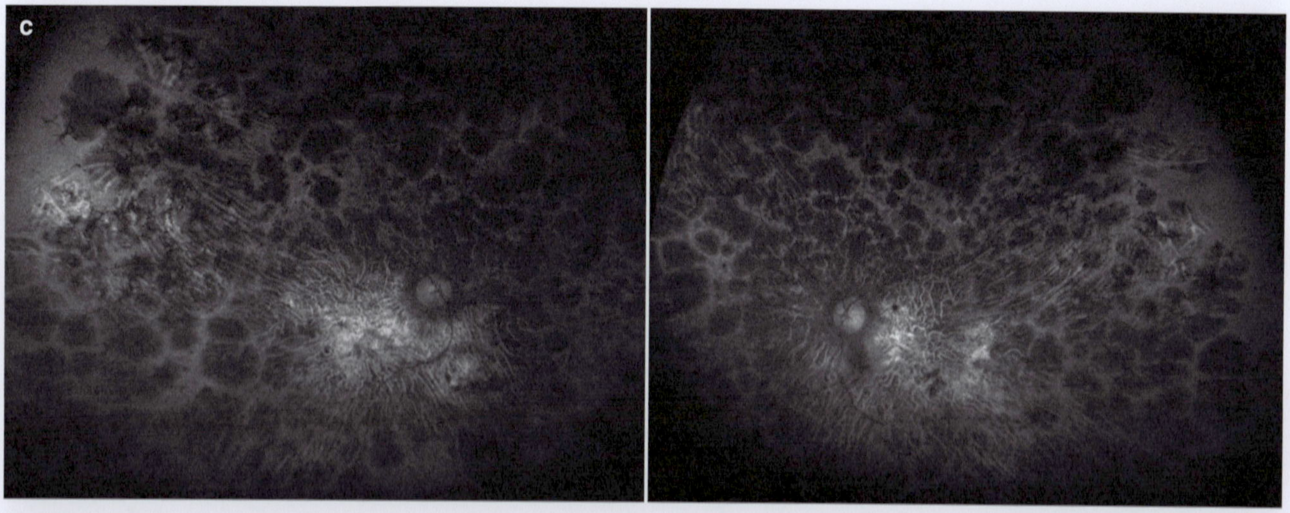

Fig. 10.2 (continued)

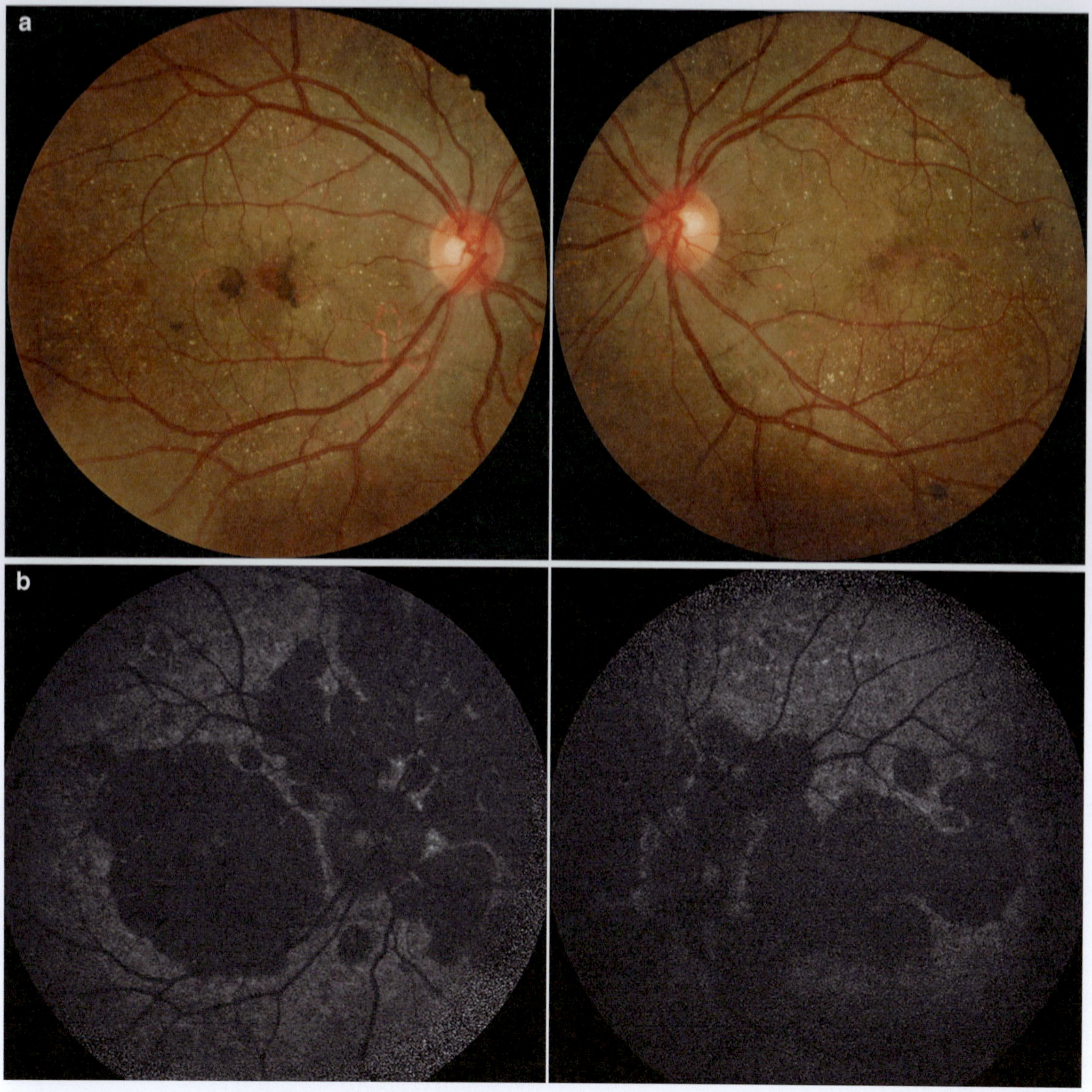

Fig. 10.3 A 35-year-old male with BCD has had blurred vision that has progressively worsened for many years. (**a**) His fundus image showed crystalline deposits. (**b**) FAF revealed many hypo-AF patches. (**c**) Crystalline deposits could be identified in NIR images. (**d**) OCT showed hyperreflective spots in all retinal layers and outer retinal tubulations (arrowhead)

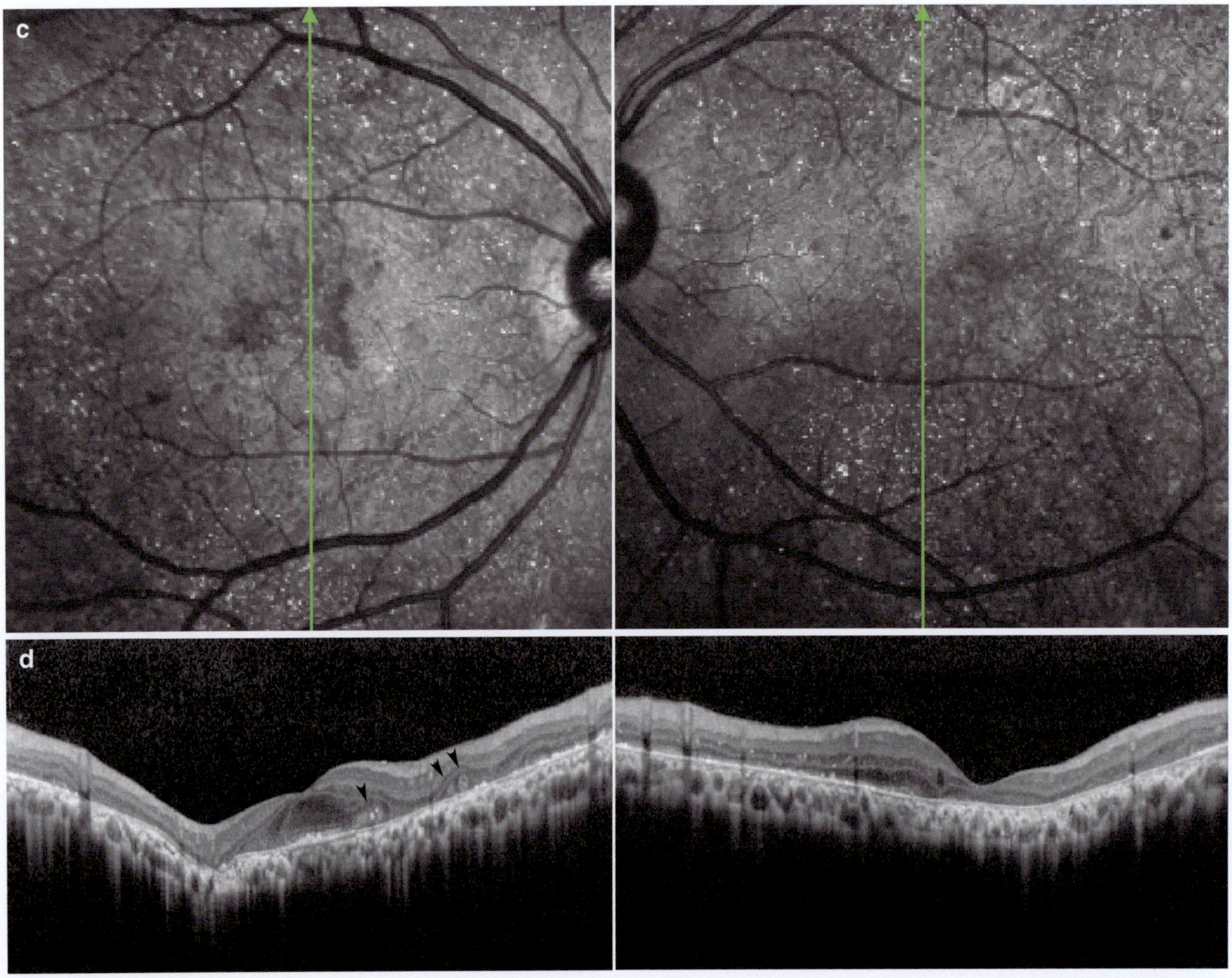

Fig. 10.3 (continued)

late phases has been described (Mataftsi et al. 2004), and the lesions are thought to be areas of choriocapillaris nonperfusion (Fong et al. 2009) (Fig. 10.5). In addition, FA can facilitate the localization of any vascular leakage, such as choroidal neovascularization (CNV) (Fuerst et al. 2016) (Fig. 10.11).

Electroretinogram (ERG)

Various features of ERG in BCD have been reported, including reduced amplitude, scotopic ERG, photopic ERG, and nonrecordable ERG (Lai et al. 2007; Wilson et al. 1989; Usui et al. 2001; Yanagi et al. 2004). The variation of ERG pattern is related to the different stage of the disease, so the relative preserved rod and cone response in ERG cannot exclude the diagnosis of BCD. The progression of ERG can sometimes be seen in BCD (Fig. 10.4).

Optical Coherence Tomography (OCT)

OCT enables the evaluation of the location of retinal crystals, which appear as hyperreflective spots. Hyperreflective spots have been found not only in RPE–Bruch's membrane but also throughout the neurosensory retina and choroid (Li et al. 2004; Rossi et al. 2013; Toto et al. 2013) (Figs. 10.3, 10.7, 10.8, 10.10, and 10.11). As the disease progresses, the RPE–Bruch's membrane complex starts to thin and the crystals start to disappear (Figs. 10.5 and 10.7). Meanwhile, OCT also shows the loss of the ellipsoid zone and the external limiting membrane, as well as the formation of tubulations in the outer retina (Halford et al. 2014) (Figs. 10.3, 10.6, 10.7, and 10.10). Although CNV is not common in BCD (Okialda et al. 2012), it is still crucial to carefully evaluate and manage the presence of CNV in patients with BCD so that further central vision loss in these patients can be prevented (Figs. 10.9 and 10.11).

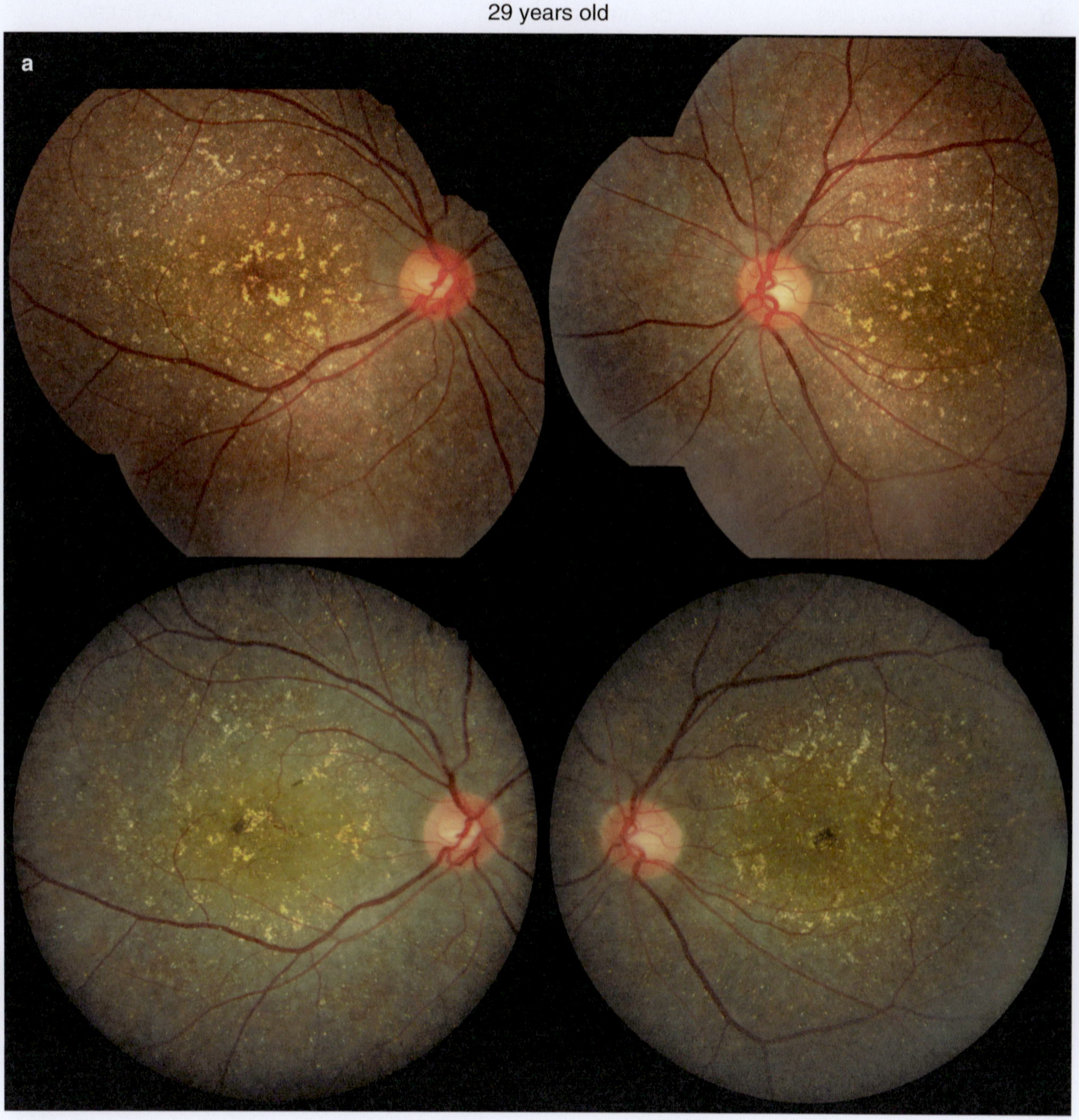

Fig. 10.4 A 29-year-old female has had impaired night vision since childhood. BCD was diagnosed after a complaint of blurry vision in her left eye for 1 month. Visual acuity was initially OD: 20/30 and OS: 20/400. After 5 years, her vision had deteriorated to OD: 20/100 and OS: 1/200. (**a**) The first color fundus images showed scattered crystalline deposits in the retina, and the follow-up color fundus images showed a greenish change in the retina and a decreased number of deposits. (**b**) The initial ERG showed delayed in rod responses, and progressed to rod-cone degeneration 5 years later

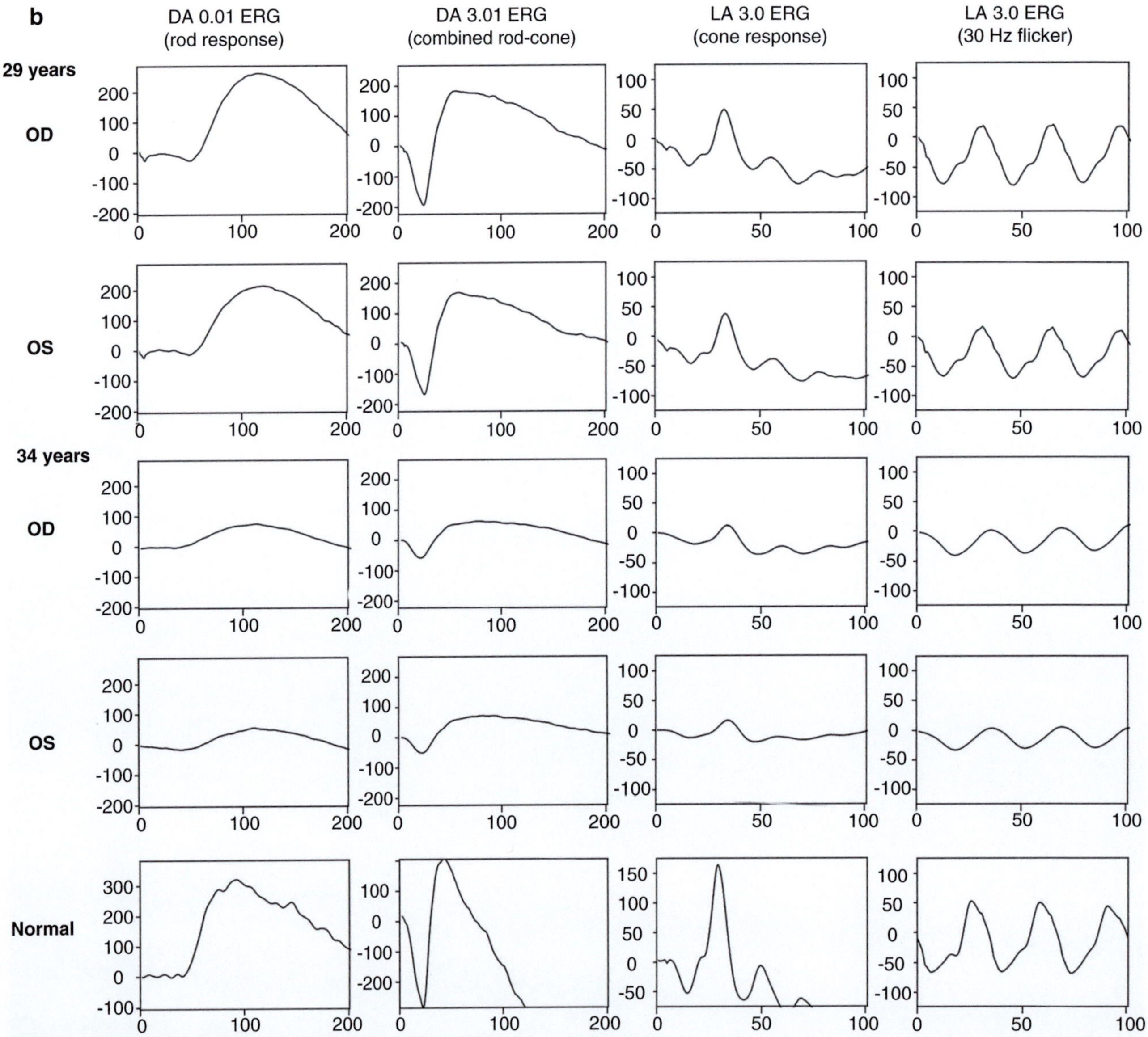

Fig. 10.4 (continued)

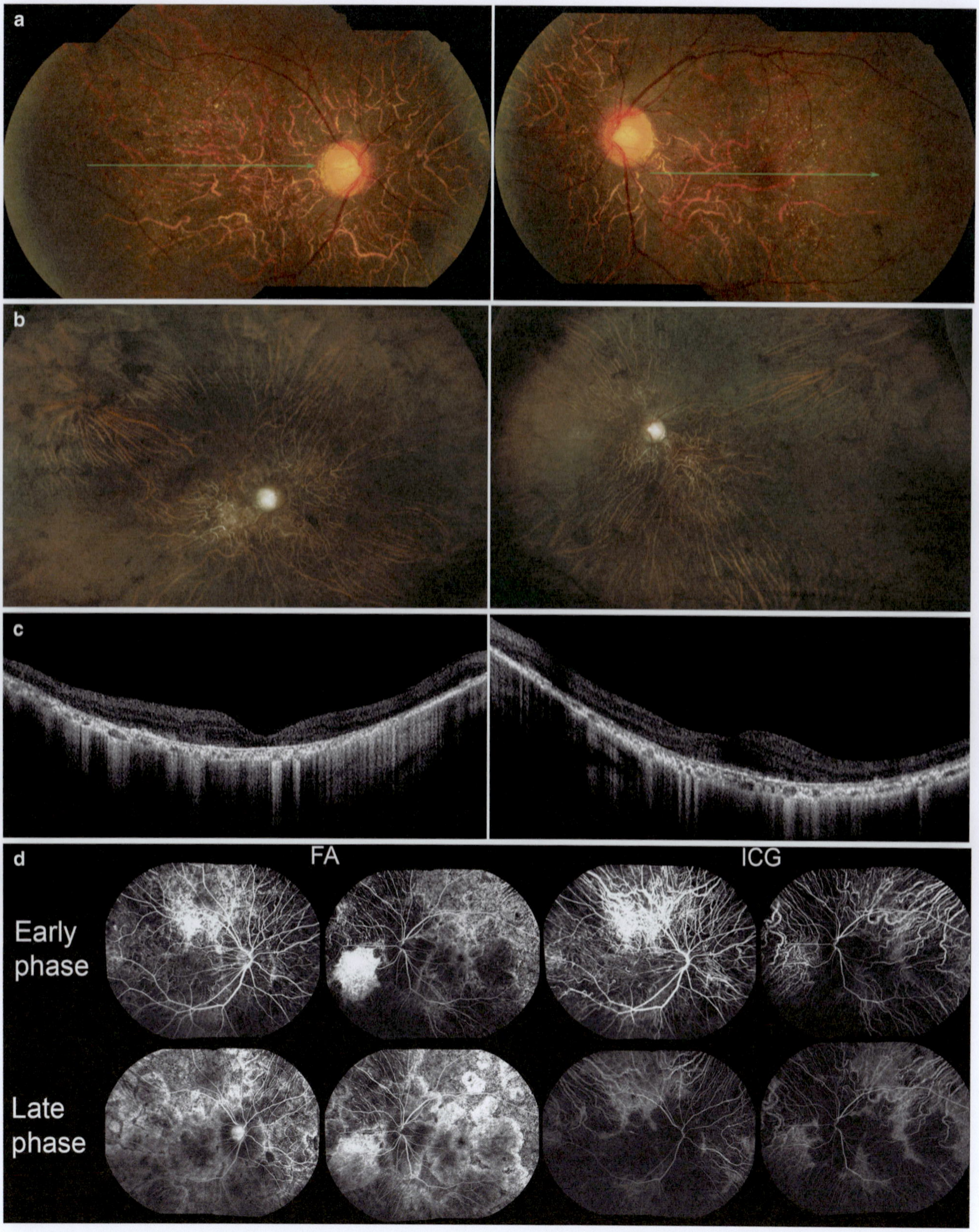

Fig. 10.5 A 55-year-old male had progressively blurred vision in his right eye, with impaired vision at night since childhood. His visual acuity was OD: 4/200 and OS: 20/20. (**a**) Color fundus images revealed a tessellated retina and scattered crystalline deposits. (**b**) The crystalline deposits are not prominent in the Optos image. (**c**) OCT of the right eye showed loss of the ellipsoid zone and thinning of the retina. The central retinal thickness was only 173 μm in the right eye and 285 μm in the left eye. (**d**) FA images showed window defect and ICGA images revealed poor perfusion of the choriocapillaris for both eyes. Although the vision of his left eye was not affected, abnormal FA/ICGA features were found

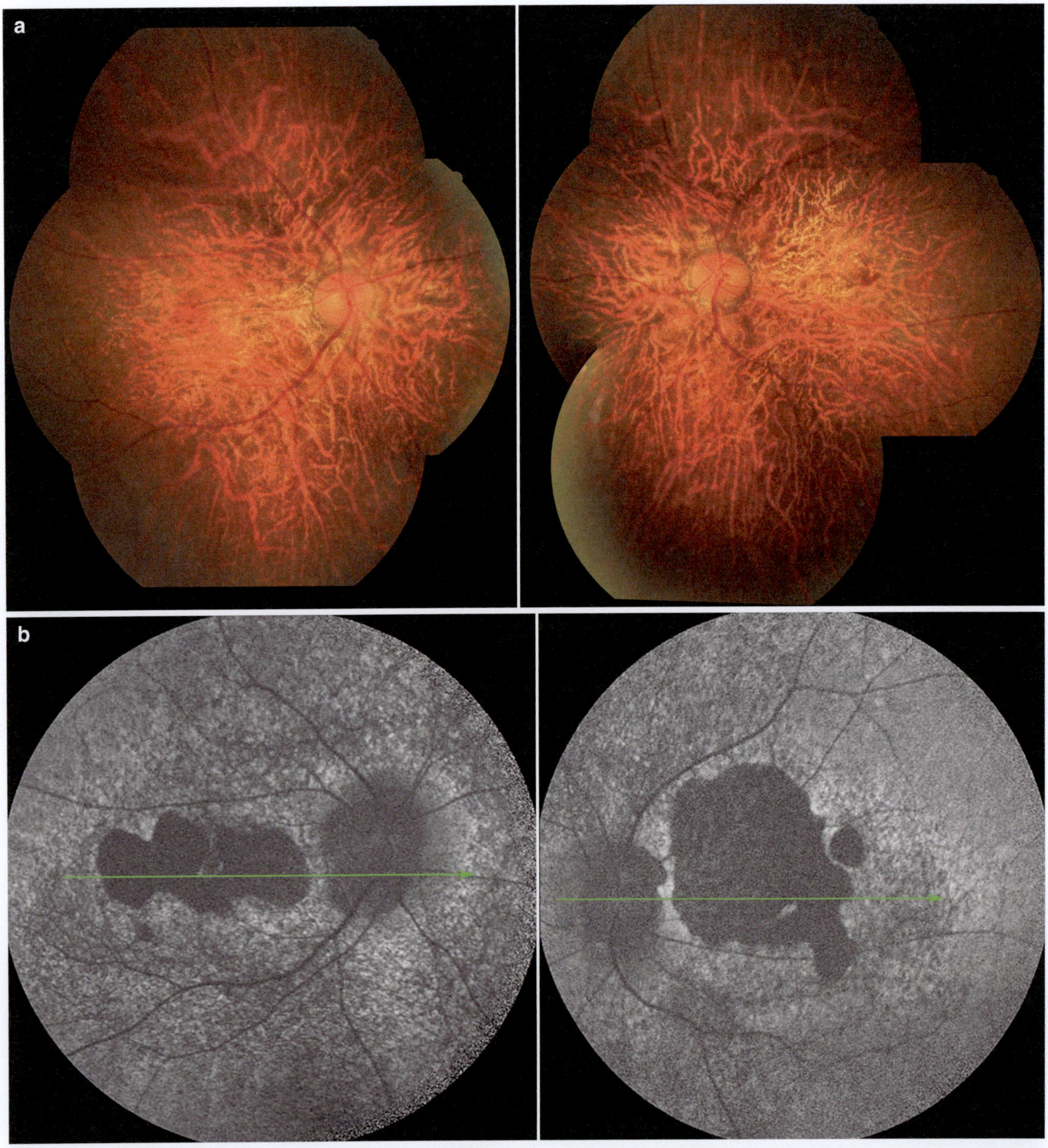

Fig. 10.6 A 57-year-old male has had progressively declining vision in his right eye and left eye for 14 and 5 years, respectively. He has also had progressively poor night vision for 2 years. His visual acuity was OD: 20/70 and OS: 20/100. (**a**) There were no obvious crystals in color fundus images. (**b**) Hypo-AF patches at the posterior pole of the retina in both eyes presented on FAF exam. (**c**) The swept-source OCT revealed outer retinal tubulations (black arrowheads) in the right eye

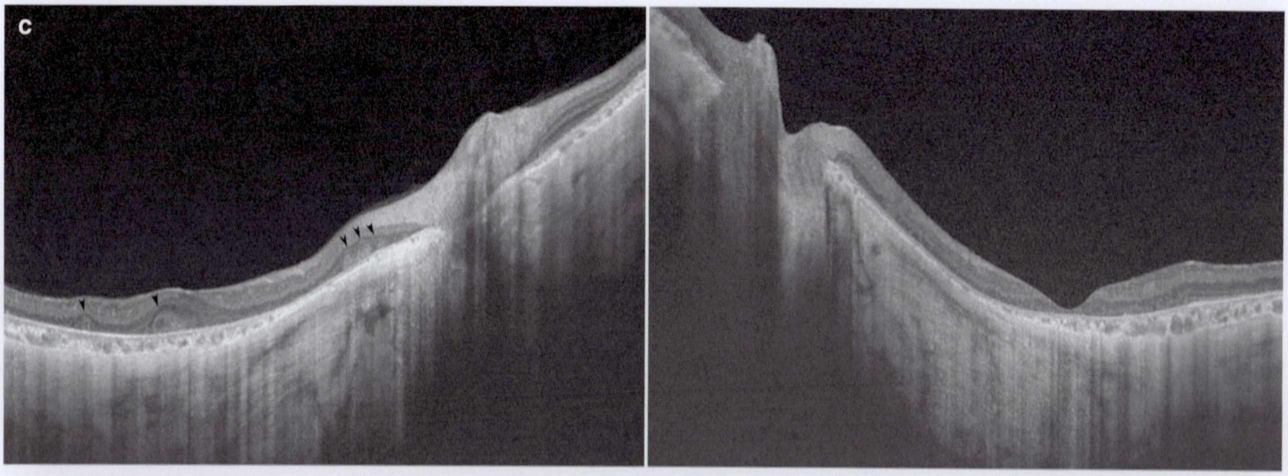

Fig.10.6 (continued)

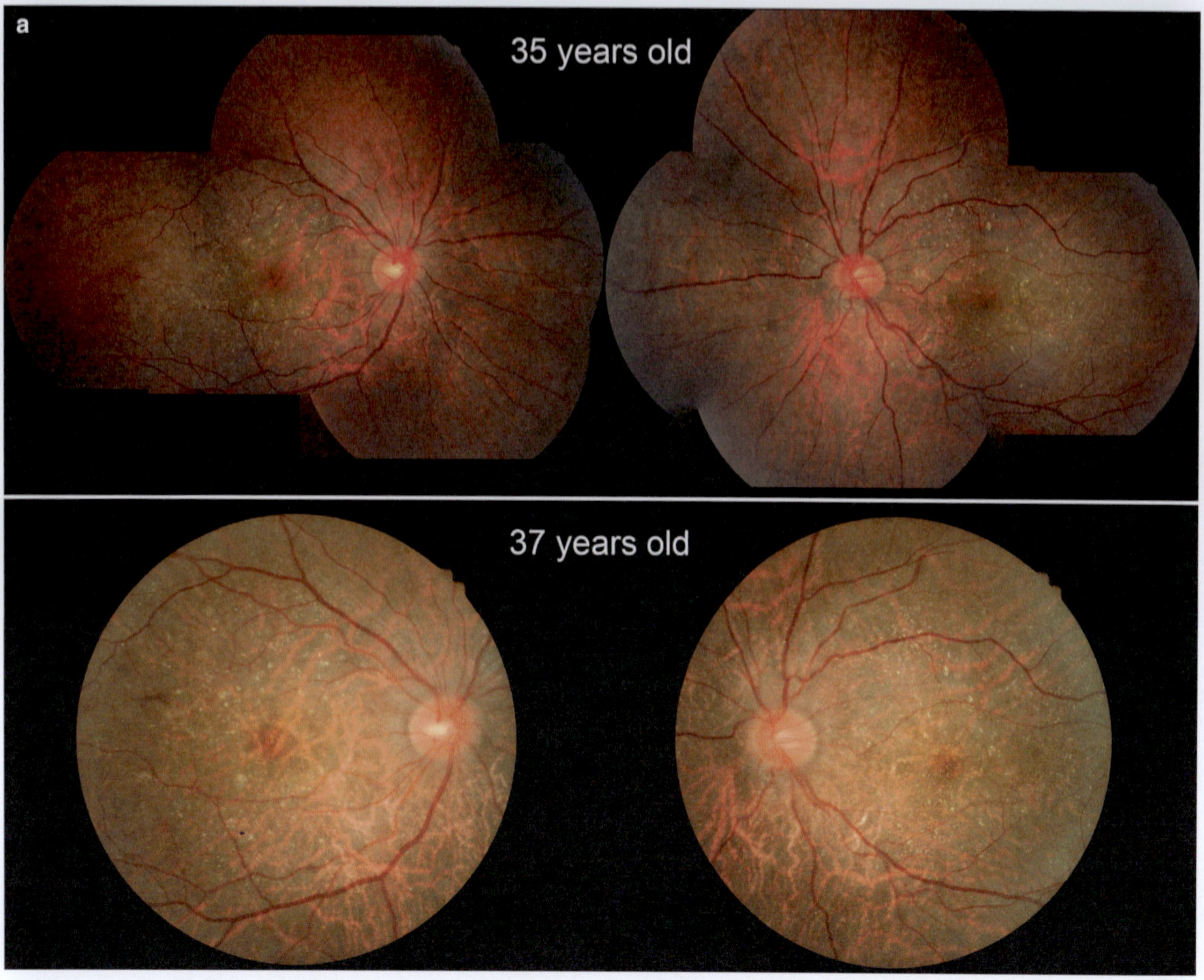

Fig. 10.7 A 35-year-old male with progressively blurred vision for 1 year was diagnosed with BCD. He denied any history of night blindness or color vision impairment. Initial best-corrected visual acuity was OD: 20/25 and OS: 20/30. After 2 years, there was no significant change in vision, but the features of the follow-up exams were different. (**a**) The initial fundus image showed scattered crystalline deposits, and RPE seemed thinner in follow-up fundus images. (**b**) The initial FAF showed a scattered hypo-AF area that extended from the posterior retina to the periphery, and the defect became larger. (**c**) OCT revealed some hyperreflective crystals in RPE and retinal layers in the initial exam. The follow-up OCT showed loss of the ellipsoid zone and some outer retinal tubulations

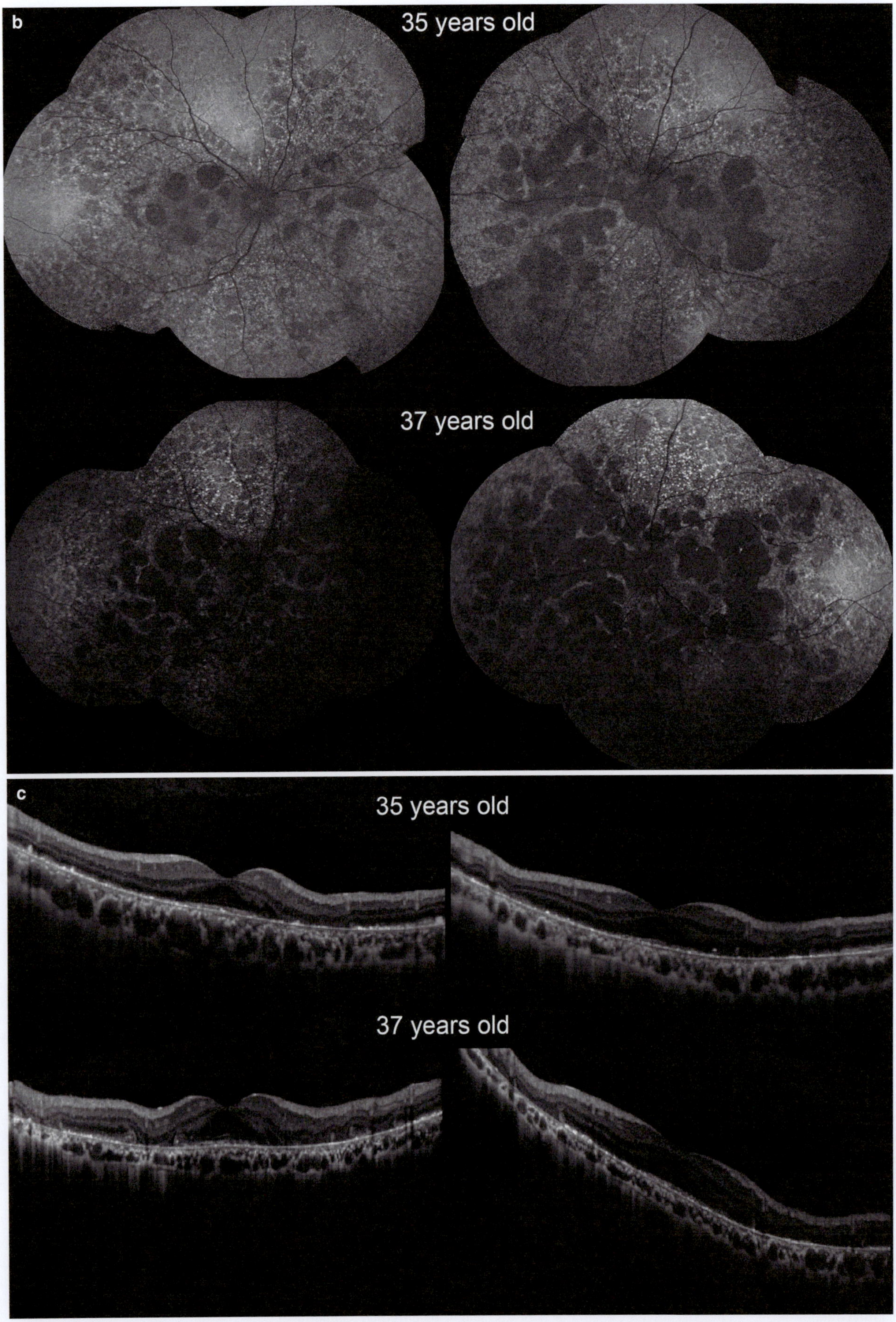

Fig. 10.7 (continued)

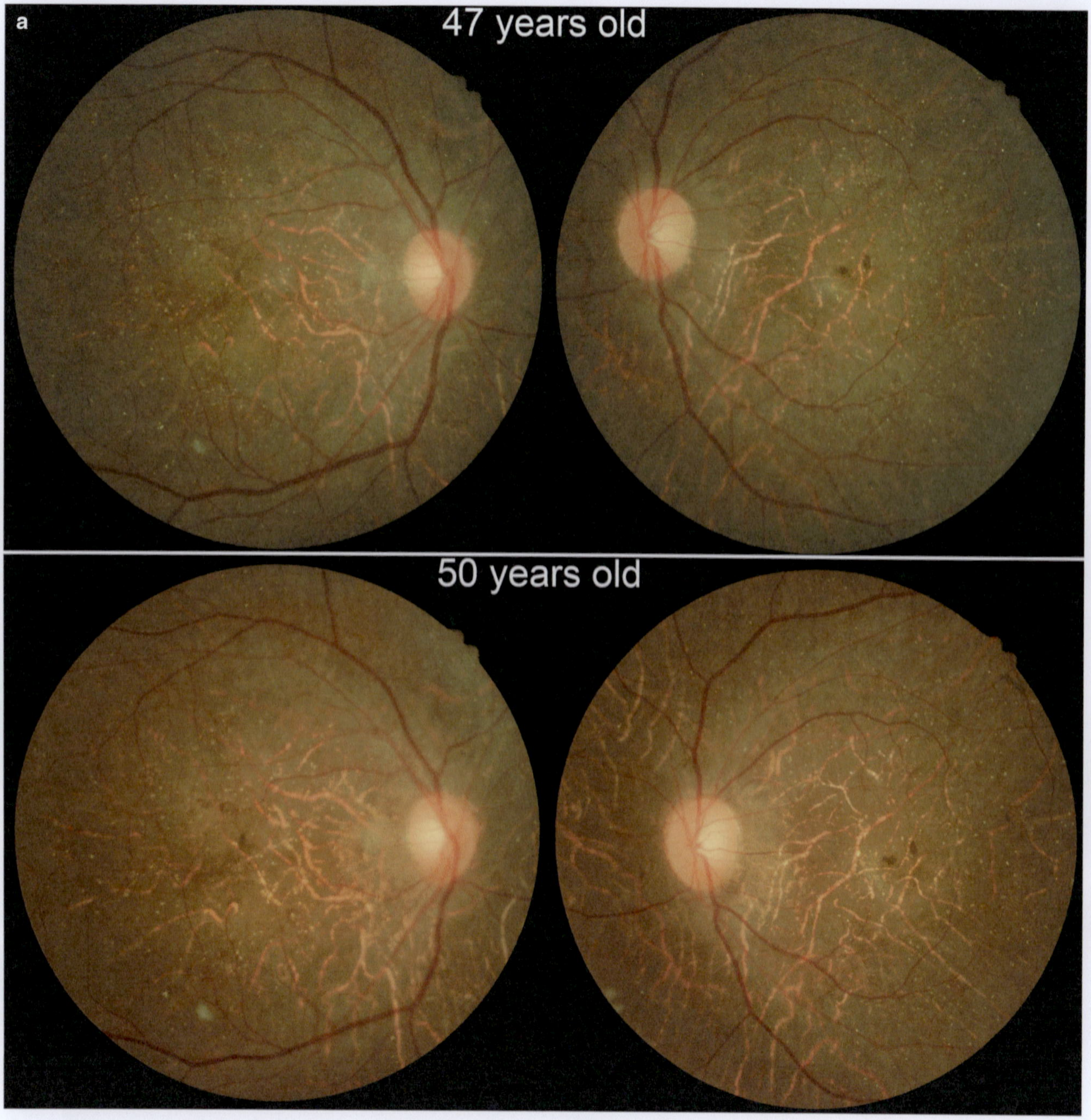

Fig. 10.8 A 47-year-old female had blurred vision for 2 years, and BCD was diagnosed. Her initial visual acuity was OD: 20/50 and OS: 4/200. After 3 years, her visual acuity became OD: 20/200 and OS: 1/200. (**a**) Her fundus images at age 47 and 50 years featured scattered crystals. (**b**) Sclerotic choroidal capillaries can also be seen in the NIR images. (**c**) The lobular hypo-FAF area became larger after 3 years. (**d**) OCT of her right eye revealed multiple outer retinal tubulations, loss of the ellipsoid zone in the macula, and some hyperreflective spots in all retinal layers. (**e**) The hypofluorescent area can be seen in FA at early and late phases

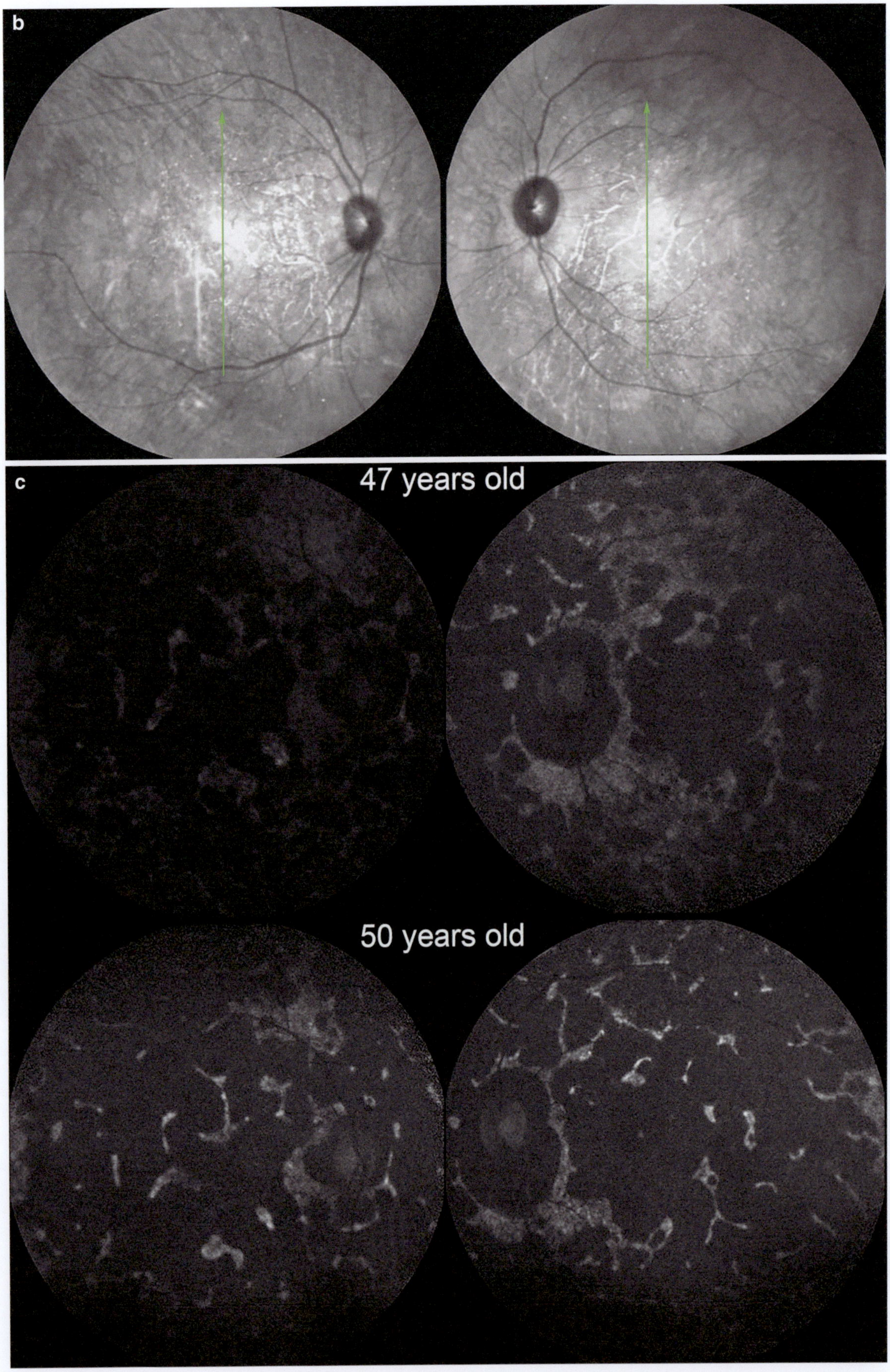

Fig. 10.8 (continued)

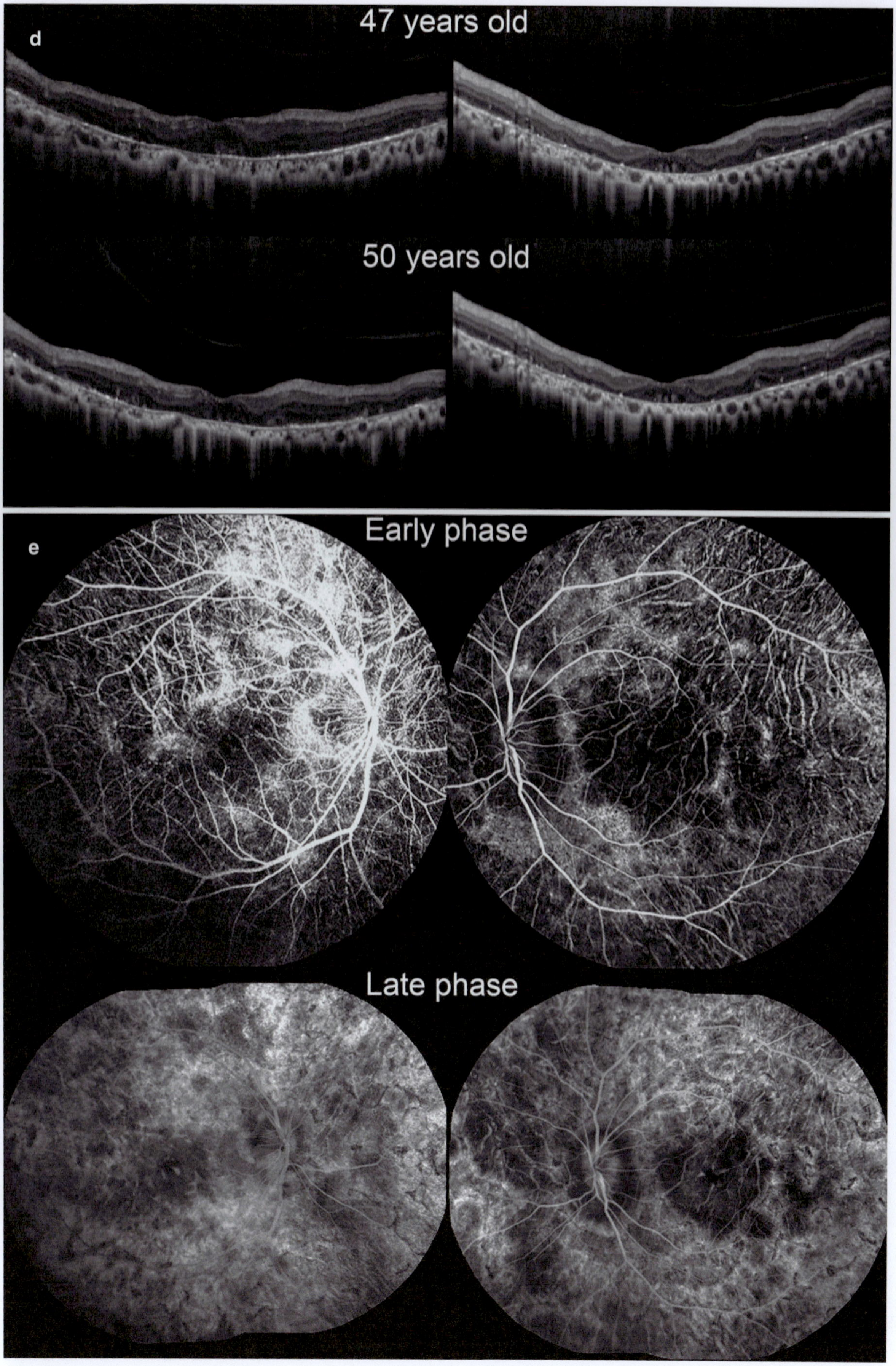

Fig. 10.8 (continued)

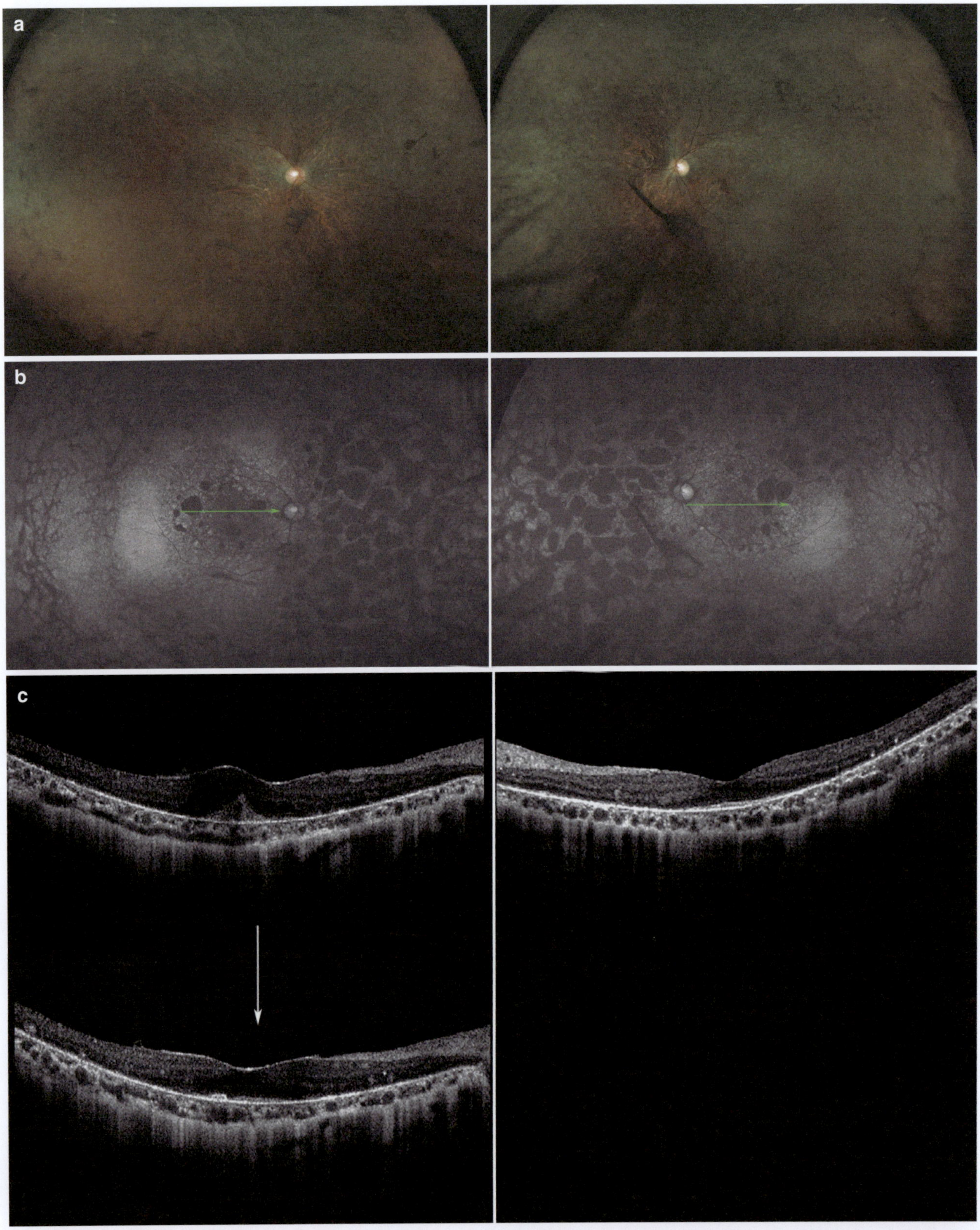

Fig. 10.9 A 42-year-old female had blurred right vision for 1 month and night blindness for 1 year. BCD was suspected based on her Optos image and FAF. (**a**) Some small crystal deposits can be found in the Optos image. (**b**) FAF images showed a reticular hypo-AF area at the peripheral retina and a round hypo-AF area around the macula. Initial visual acuity was OD: 20/50 and OS: 20/25. (**c**) Choroidal neovascularization (CNV) was suspected in her right eye OCT scan. The central retinal thickness was 353 μm. Intravitreal ranibizumab injection was performed twice, and after 2 months, visual acuity became OD: 20/25 and OS: 20/25. Follow-up OCT showed regressed CNV, and the central retinal thickness returned to 279 μm

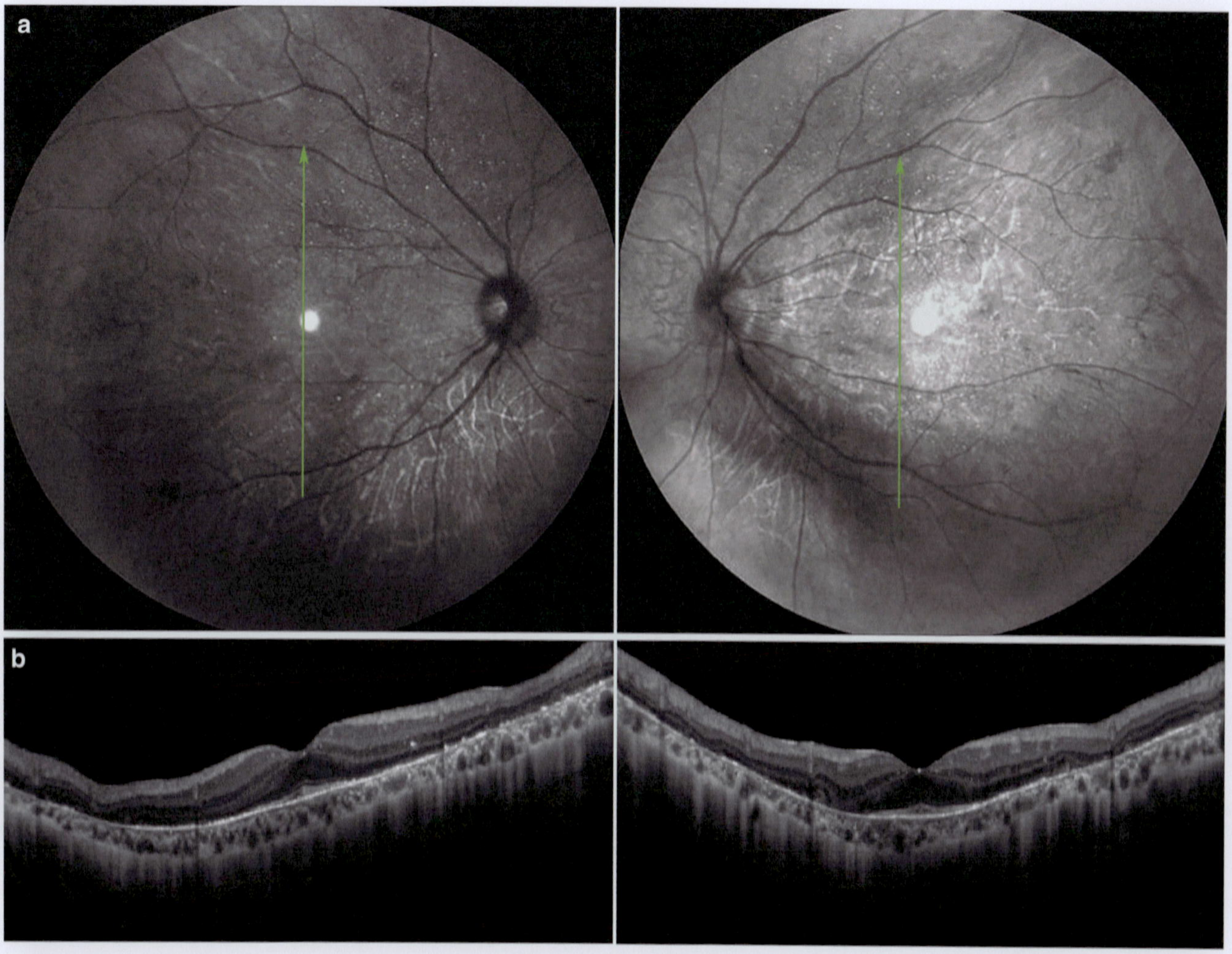

Fig. 10.10 A 40-year-old male had complained of impaired night vision for several months. His best-corrected visual acuity was 20/20 in both eyes. (**a**) NIR imaging revealed multiple crystals in the retina. (**b**) OCT showed a preserved ellipsoid zone in the macula and hyperreflective spots

Table 10.1 Staging for Bietti's crystalline dystrophy (Yuzawa et al. 1986)

Stage	Features
1	RPE atrophy with uniform, fine, white, crystalline deposits are observed at the macular area
2	RPE atrophy extends beyond the posterior pole. Choriocapillaris atrophy in addition to RPE atrophy appears noticeably at the posterior pole
3	RPE–choriocapillaris atrophy is observed throughout the fundus

RPE retinal pigment epithelium

Differential Diagnosis

Some diseases that present with crystalline deposits in the retina need to be differentiated from BCD. The differential diagnosis of retinal crystalline deposits collated by Nadim et al. is classified into systemic disorders, drug-induced disorders, primary ocular disorders, and embolic diseases (Nadim et al. 2002) (Table 10.2). However, patients at the late stage of BCD may be presented with diffused RPE dystrophy without obvious crystalline deposit, which may not be easy to differentiate from other retinal degenerative diseases such as retinitis pigmentosa and choroideremia. Genetic testing may help in this clinical situation.

Management

For patients with an initial diagnosis of BCD, a number of examinations can be performed to evaluate the baseline status, including fundus photography, FAF, ERG, visual field exam, OCT, and genetic consultation. Even though medical or surgical management for BCD does not currently exist, ophthalmologists should be aware of coexisting problems such as CNV, which can be treated with intravitreal anti-vascular endothelial growth factor injection instead of laser photocoagulation (Fuerst et al. 2016; Okialda et al. 2012) (Figs. 10.9 and 10.11).

Table 10.2 Differential diagnosis of retinal crystals (Nadim et al. 2002)

Disorder	Fundus features
1. Systemic disorder	
(a) Oxalosis	
• Primary hyperoxaluria	Yellow crystals along retinal arterioles Hyperpigmented spot with hypopigmentation Plaque of RPE hypertrophy in the macula
• Methoxyflurane anesthesia	Fundus albipunctatus-like image
(b) Cystinosis (infantile form)	Deep yellow crystals all over the posterior pole Diffuse pigmentary changes without crystals
(c) Hyperornithinemia	Crystals over velvet-like pigmentation in the macula and periphery
(d) Sjögren–Larsson syndrome	Superficial yellow white dots in the fovea and parafovea, excluding the foveola Mottled hypopigmentation in the macula
2. Drug-induced	
(a) Tamoxifen	White crystals mostly concentrated temporal to the macula
(b) Canthaxanthine	Golden yellow crystals in an oval configuration around the fovea
(c) Talc	White glistening crystals inside the perifoveal arterioles
(d) Nitrofurantoin	Superficial and deep crystals in a circinate pattern in the posterior pole
3. Primary ocular disorders	
(a) Calcified macular drusen	Deep yellow-white crystals in the macula
(b) Idiopathic parafoveal telangiectasis	Superficial golden yellow crystals concentrated in the parafovea
(c) Bietti's crystalline dystrophy	Superficial deep yellow-white crystals all over the posterior pole
(d) Longstanding retinal detachment	Superficial yellowish crystals in the area of detached retina
4. Embolic diseases	
(a) Calcium emboli	White crystals inside affected retinal arteriole(s)
(b) Cholesterol emboli	Yellow crystals inside affected retinal arteriole(s)

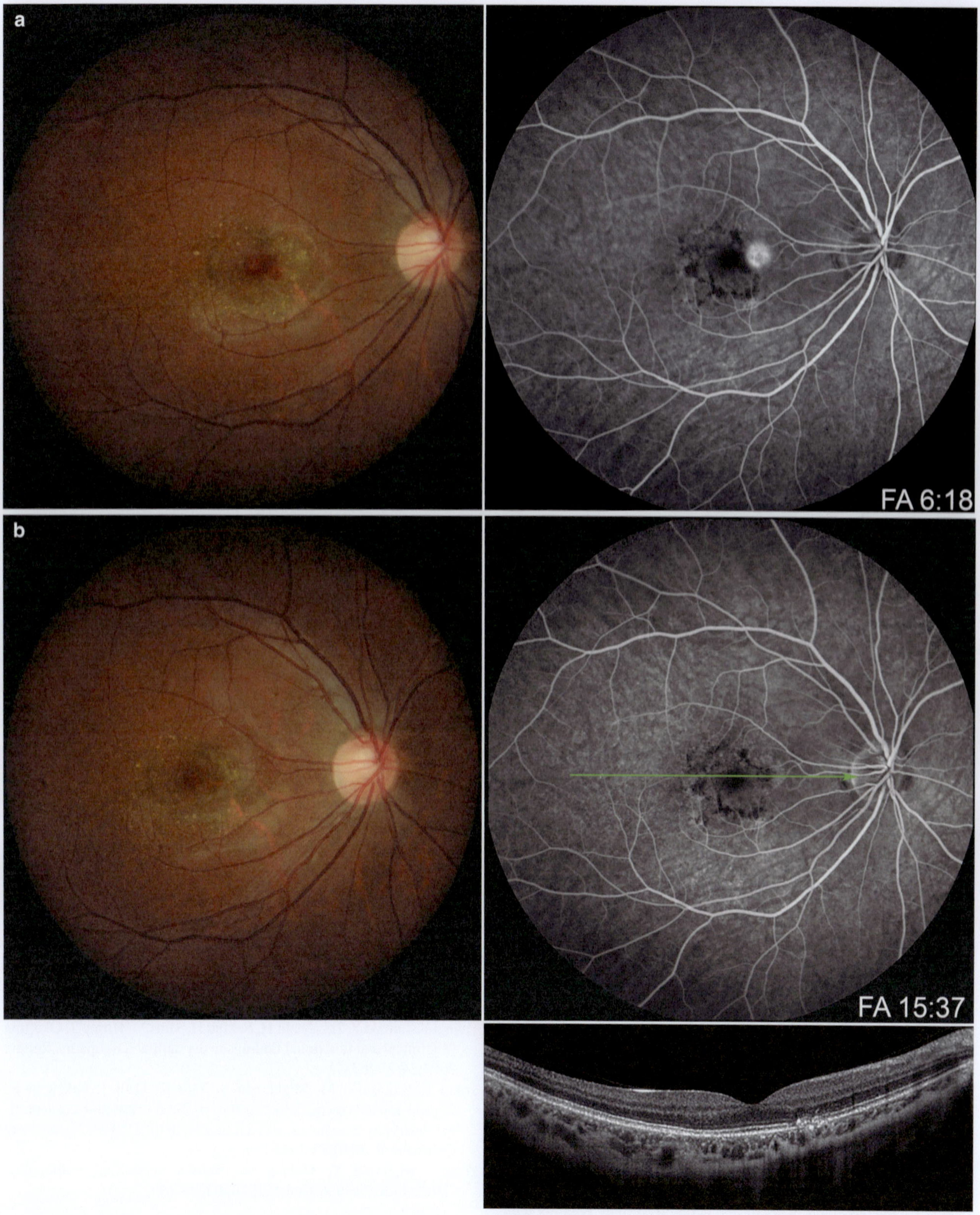

Fig. 10.11 A 26-year-old female diagnosed with BCD had suffered from blurred right vision for a few months. (**a**) Crystalline deposits and a hemorrhage at the macula were found in her color fundus image of the right eye. FA showed CNV at the nasal superior side of the fovea with active leakage and hypofluorescent spots around the fovea. Intravitreal bevacizumab injection was performed, and the CNV regressed after 1 month. (**b**) The follow-up color fundus image showed the disappearance of the hemorrhage, FA showed no leakage, and OCT showed no subretinal fluid

Acknowledgments N. K. Wang is supported by the Taiwan Ministry of Science and Technology MOST 106-2314-B-182A-041 and the Chang Gung Memorial Hospital CMRPG3F1241-3F1242.

References

Bagolini B, Ioli-Spada G. Bietti's tapetoretinal degeneration with marginal corneal dystrophy. Am J Ophthalmol. 1968;65(1):53–60.

Bietti G. Ueber familiares Vorkommen von "Retinitis punctata albescens" (verbunden mit "Dystrophis marginalis cristallinea cornea"), Glitzern, des Glaskorpers und anderen degenerativen Augenveranderungen. Klin Monatsbl Augenheilkd. 1937;99:737–56.

Fong AM, Koh A, Lee K, Ang CL. Bietti's crystalline dystrophy in Asians: clinical, angiographic and electrophysiological characteristics. Int Ophthalmol. 2009;29(6):459–70.

Fuerst NM, Serrano L, Han G, Morgan JI, Maguire AM, Leroy BP, Kim BJ, Aleman TS. Detailed functional and structural phenotype of Bietti crystalline dystrophy associated with mutations in CYP4V2 complicated by choroidal neovascularization. Ophthalmic Genet. 2016;37(4):445–52.

Gekka T, Hayashi T, Takeuchi T, Goto-Omoto S, Kitahara K. CYP4V2 mutations in two Japanese patients with Bietti's crystalline dystrophy. Ophthalmic Res. 2005;37(5):262–9.

Grizzard WS, Deutman AF, Nijhuis F, de Kerk AA. Crystalline retinopathy. Am J Ophthalmol. 1978;86(1):81–8.

Halford S, Liew G, Mackay DS, Sergouniotis PI, Holt R, Broadgate S, Volpi EV, Ocaka L, Robson AG, Holder GE, Moore AT, Michaelides M, Webster AR. Detailed phenotypic and genotypic characterization of Bietti crystalline dystrophy. Ophthalmology. 2014;121(6):1174–84.

Hayasaka S, Okuyama S. Crystalline retinopathy. Retina. 1984;4(3):177–81.

Hu D-M. Ophthalmic genetics in China. Ophthalmic Paediatr Genet. 1983;2(1):39–45.

Jiao X, Munier FL, Iwata F, Hayakawa M, Kanai A, Lee J, Schorderet DF, Chen MS, Kaiser-Kupfer M, Hejtmancik JF. Genetic linkage of Bietti crystalline corneoretinal dystrophy to chromosome 4q35. Am J Hum Genet. 2000;67(5):1309–13.

Jin ZB, Ito S, Saito Y, Inoue Y, Yanagi Y, Nao-i N. Clinical and molecular findings in three Japanese patients with crystalline retinopathy. Jpn J Ophthalmol. 2006;50(5):426–31.

Kaiser-Kupfer MI, Chan CC, Markello TC, Crawford MA, Caruso RC, Csaky KG, Guo J, Gahl WA. Clinical biochemical and pathologic correlations in Bietti's crystalline dystrophy. Am J Ophthalmol. 1994;118(5):569–82.

Kelly EJ, Nakano M, Rohatgi P, Yarov-Yarovoy V, Rettie AE. Finding homes for orphan cytochrome P450s: CYP4V2 and CYP4F22 in disease states. Mol Interv. 2011;11(2):124–32.

Lai TY, Ng TK, Tam PO, Yam GH, Ngai JW, Chan WM, Liu DT, Lam DS, Pang CP. Genotype phenotype analysis of Bietti's crystalline dystrophy in patients with CYP4V2 mutations. Invest Ophthalmol Vis Sci. 2007;48(11):5212–20.

Lee J, Jiao X, Hejtmancik JF, Kaiser-Kupfer M, Gahl WA, Markello TC, Guo J, Chader GJ. The metabolism of fatty acids in human Bietti crystalline dystrophy. Invest Ophthalmol Vis Sci. 2001;42(8):1707–14.

Lee KY, Koh AH, Aung T, Yong VH, Yeung K, Ang CL, Vithana EN. Characterization of Bietti crystalline dystrophy patients with CYP4V2 mutations. Invest Ophthalmol Vis Sci. 2005;46(10):3812–6.

Li A, Jiao X, Munier FL, Schorderet DF, Yao W, Iwata F, Hayakawa M, Kanai A, Shy Chen M, Alan Lewis R, Heckenlively J, Weleber RG, Traboulsi EI, Zhang Q, Xiao X, Kaiser-Kupfer M, Sergeev YV, Hejtmancik JF. Bietti crystalline corneoretinal dystrophy is caused by mutations in the novel gene CYP4V2. Am J Hum Genet. 2004;74(5):817–26.

Lin J, Nishiguchi KM, Nakamura M, Dryja TP, Berson EL, Miyake Y. Recessive mutations in the CYP4V2 gene in east Asian and middle eastern patients with Bietti crystalline corneoretinal dystrophy. J Med Genet. 2005;42(6):e38.

Mataftsi A, Zografos L, Milla E, Secretan M, Munier FL. Bietti's crystalline corneoretinal dystrophy: a cross-sectional study. Retina. 2004;24(3):416–26.

Nadim F, Walid H, Adib J. The differential diagnosis of crystals in the retina. Int Ophthalmol. 2002;24:113–21.

Nakano M, Kelly EJ, Rettie AE. Expression and characterization of CYP4V2 as a fatty acid omega-hydroxylase. Drug Metab Dispos. 2009;37(11):2119–22.

Ng DS, Lai TY, Ng TK, Pang CP. Genetics of Bietti crystalline dystrophy. Asia Pac J Ophthalmol. 2016;5(4):245–52.

Okialda KA, Stover NB, Weleber RG, Kelly EJ. Bietti crystalline dystrophy. In: Pagon RA, Adam MP, Ardinger HH, et al., editors. GeneReviews®. Seattle, WA: University of Washington; 2012.

Rossi S, Testa F, Li A, Yaylacioglu F, Gesualdo C, Hejtmancik JF, Simonelli F. Clinical and genetic features in Italian Bietti crystalline dystrophy patients. Br J Ophthalmol. 2013;97(2):174–9.

Shan M, Dong B, Zhao X, Wang J, Li G, Yang Y, Li Y. Novel mutations in the CYP4V2 gene associated with Bietti crystalline corneoretinal dystrophy. Mol Vis. 2005;11:738–43.

Toto L, Carpineto P, Parodi MB, Di Antonio L, Mastropasqua A, Mastropasqua L. Spectral domain optical coherence tomography and in vivo confocal microscopy imaging of a case of Bietti's crystalline dystrophy. Clin Exp Optom. 2013;96(1):39–45.

Usui T, Tanimoto N, Takagi M, Hasegawa S, Abe H. Rod and cone a-waves in three cases of Bietti crystalline chorioretinal dystrophy. Am J Ophthalmol. 2001;132(3):395–402.

Wada Y, Itabashi T, Sato H, Kawamura M, Tada A, Tamai M. Screening for mutations in CYP4V2 gene in Japanese patients with Bietti's crystalline corneoretinal dystrophy. Am J Ophthalmol. 2005;139(5):894–9.

Welch RB. Bietti's tapetoretinal degeneration with marginal corneal dystrophy crystalline retinopathy. Trans Am Ophthalmol Soc. 1977;75:164–79.

Wilson DJ, Weleber RG, Klein ML, Welch RB, Green WR. Bietti's crystalline dystrophy. A clinicopathologic correlative study. Arch Ophthalmol. 1989;107(2):213–21.

Xiao X, Mai G, Li S, Guo X, Zhang Q. Identification of CYP4V2 mutation in 21 families and overview of mutation spectrum in Bietti crystalline corneoretinal dystrophy. Biochem Biophys Res Commun. 2011;409(2):181–6.

Yanagi Y, Tamaki Y, Takahashi H, Sekine H, Mori M, Hirato T, Okajima O. Clinical and functional findings in crystalline retinopathy. Retina. 2004;24(2):267–74.

Yokoi Y, Nakazawa M, Mizukoshi S, Sato K, Usui T, Takeuchi K. Crystal deposits on the lens capsules in Bietti crystalline corneoretinal dystrophy associated with a mutation in the CYP4V2 gene. Acta Ophthalmol. 2010;88(5):607–9.

Yuzawa M, Mae Y, Matsui M. Bietti's crystalline retinopathy. Ophthalmic Paediatr Genet. 1986;7(1):9–20.

Albinism

11

Jessy Choi and Alexander Bossuyt

Abbreviations

CHS	Chédiak–Higashi syndrome
HPS	Hermansky–Pudlak syndrome
L-DOPA	L-3-4-dihydroxyphenylalanine
OA	Ocular albinism
OCA	Oculocutaneous albinism
UV	Ultraviolet

Introduction

In 1908, Archibald Garrod, an English physician, included albinism in his 'Inborn errors of metabolism'; proposing later in 1923 that albinism was a disorder of an enzyme involved in the synthesis or maintenance of the molecule melanin. Garrod's work was controversial at the time prior to the acceptance of Mendelian inheritance. However, it was later confirmed in oculocutaneous albinism OCA1A (see section 'Non-syndromic OCA') that the tyrosinase enzyme was found to be defective (Scriver 2008).

Albinism is a common term used to describe a range of congenital disorders characterised by a variable degree of hypopigmentation, associated with a partial or complete absence of the melanin pigment (Kinnear et al. 1985). The disease is traditionally classified according to the clinical phenotype in to two main categories: oculocutaneous albinism (OCA) in which the skin, eyes, and hair are affected and ocular albinism (OA) in which the eyes are affected alone. Within these broad categories, albinism is currently classified genetically, making the formerly used terms such as 'tyrosinase-positive' or 'tyrosinase-negative' redundant (Summers 2009). As well as the two broad categories, syndromic forms of albinism, occur infrequently. These include Hermansky–Pudlak syndrome (an autosomal recessive condition presenting with bleeding and OCA) (Hermansky and Pudlak 1959) and Chédiak–Higashi syndrome (an autosomal recessive condition presenting with immunodeficiency and OCA) (Sato 1955).

There is so far limited epidemiological data for all known forms of albinism, with the prevalence of 1 in 14,000 in Danish populations (Grønskov et al. 2009) and 1 in 10,000 in Northern Irish populations (Froggatt 1960), giving a rough idea of the prevalence in western populations. Several other studies also quote the figure of 1 in 17,000 for North American and European populations. Although albinism is relatively rare in the world, a relatively high prevalence has been reported in sub-Saharan African populations, with the figures of 1 in 4000 for Zimbabwe and 1 in 1400 in Tanzania. This has been partially attributed to consanguinity (Mártinez-García and Montoliu 2013; Cruz-Inigo et al. 2011). The prevalence for specific albinism genes has been researched in more detail, with the OCA1 gene being the most common and OCA4 being especially rare worldwide (see section 'Non-Syndromic OCA') (Suzuki and Tomita 2008). Ocular albinism has been found to be most commonly inherited in an X-linked pattern, and has an estimated prevalence of 1 in 60,000 (Martinez-Garcia et al. 2010).

Albinism is characterised by hypopigmentation of the irides (Fig. 11.1), leading to different degrees of iris transillumination (Fig. 11.2). The reduced pigmentation of the retinal pigment epithelium makes the underlying choroidal circulation more visible and is typically described as fundal hypopigmentation (Fig. 11.3). The lack of melanin leads to underdevelopment of the fovea (Figs. 11.4 and 11.5) and optic disc (Fig. 11.6). In OCA, there is hypopigmentation of the skin and hair, in addition to ocular findings. Other clinical findings include nystagmus, reduced or absent stereopsis, strabismus and refractive errors (Dorey et al. 2003).

J. Choi (✉)
Department of Ophthalmology, Royal Hallamshire Hospital, Sheffield, UK
e-mail: jessy.choi@nhs.net

A. Bossuyt
University of Nottingham, Nottingham, UK

G. Cheung (ed.), *Hereditary Chorioretinal Disorders*, Retina Atlas, https://doi.org/10.1007/978-981-15-0414-3_11

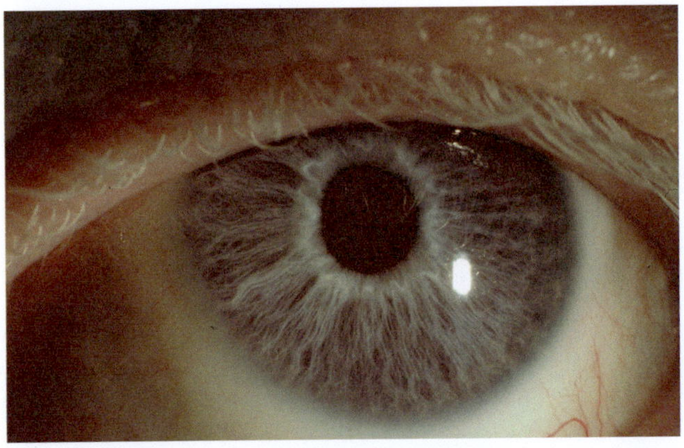

Fig. 11.1 Slit lamp colour photograph of OCA demonstrating the hypopigmentation of the iris. Also note the hypopigmented eyelashes

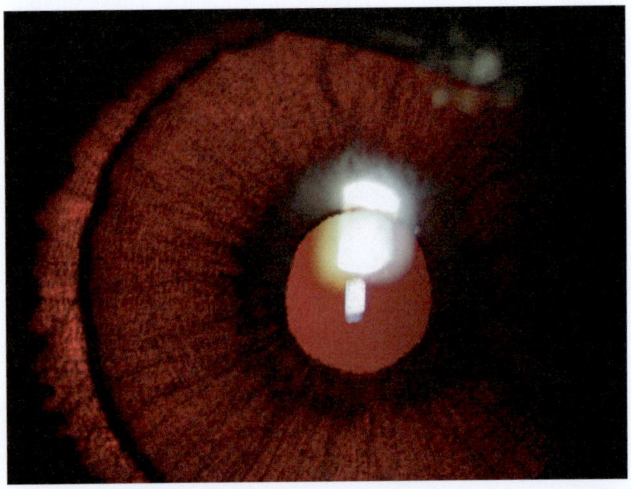

Fig. 11.2 Iris transillumination of the eye from Fig. 11.1

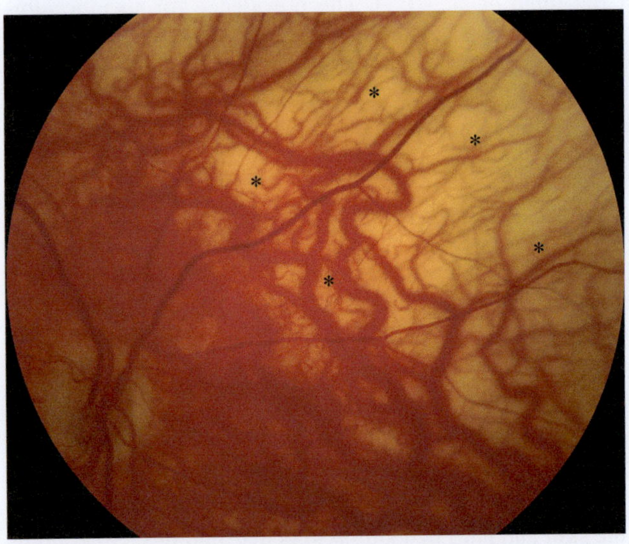

Fig. 11.3 Colour fundus photograph demonstrating fundal hypopigmentation. Note the visible choroidal vessels as indicated by *

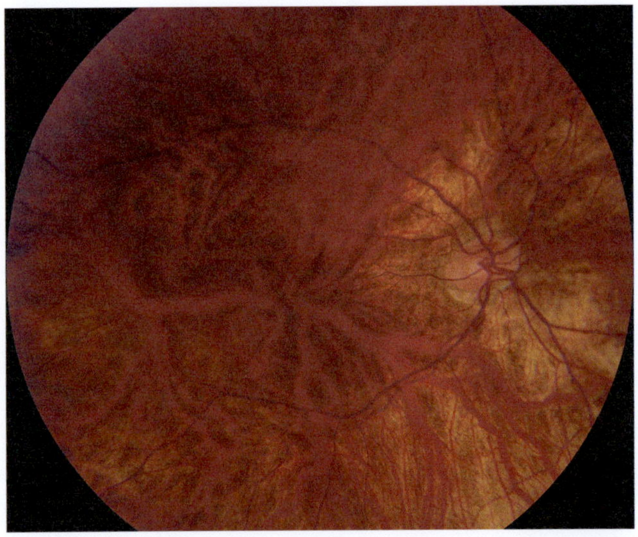

Fig. 11.4 Colour fundus photograph of the right eye demonstrating a typical appearance of foveal hypoplasia

Etiopathogenesis

The etiopathogenesis of albinism is directly related to the specific gene that is affected. All forms of albinism share a reduction or absence of melanin, resulting in the phenotype of hypopigmentation (Levin and Stroh 2011).

Melanin plays an important role in the development of the retina. Without melanin, the fovea does not develop properly, and retinal–brain neuronal connections are altered. The optic nerves, chiasm and optic tracts of individuals with albinism have been consistently found to have smaller diameters. This can be attributed to a reduction in central retinal ganglion cells and foveal hypoplasia (Fig. 11.5) (Welton et al. 2017). Due to the reduction in the diameter of optic neuronal tracts, the lateral geniculate nuclei have been found to be significantly reduced in size in those with albinism. In unaffected individuals, 50% of retinal ganglion cells typically decussate in the optic chiasm (nasal retinal fibres) and 50% remain ipsilateral (temporal retinal fibres). However, in albinism, 70–85% of fibres decussate with only 15–30% passing ipsilaterally. The misrouting of these fibres can lead to abnormal routing of fibres to the lateral geniculate nucleus (McKetton et al. 2014). The excessive decussation of the retinal nerve fibre can be detected with visual evoked potentials (VEP), a form of electrodiagnostic assessment (see section 'Ocular Albinism').

Oculocutaneous Albinism

Oculocutaneous albinism (OCA) is an autosomal recessive disorder due to an absence or reduction of melanin biosynthesis in melanocytes. Melanin synthesis and regulation

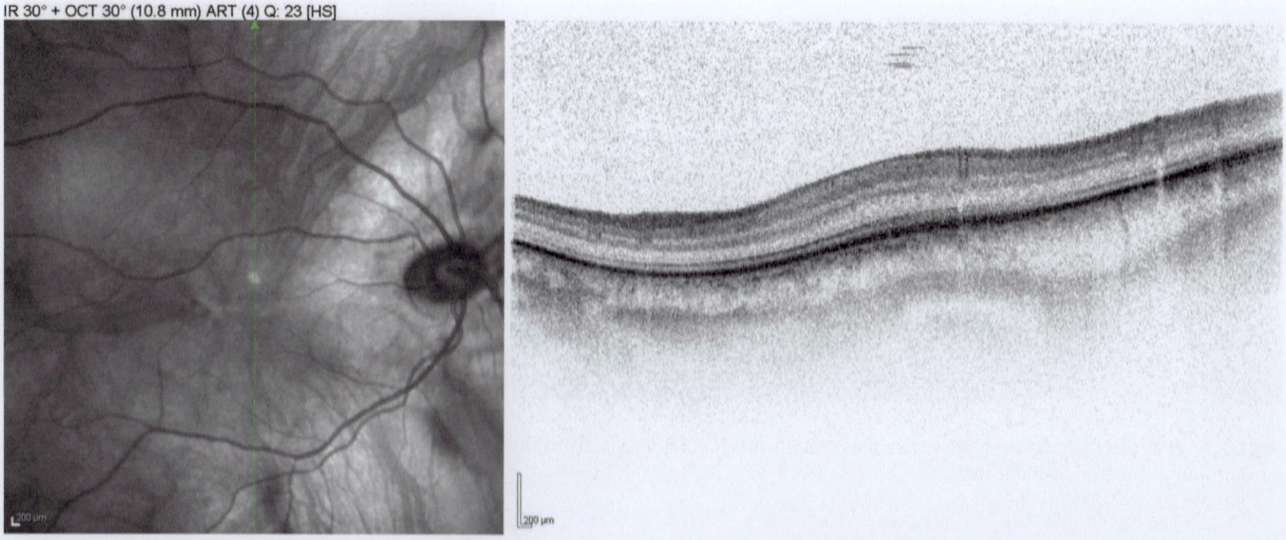

Fig. 11.5 Corresponding tracking laser tomography of the retina from Fig. 11.4 demonstrating the absence of foveal structure, consistent with foveal hypoplasia

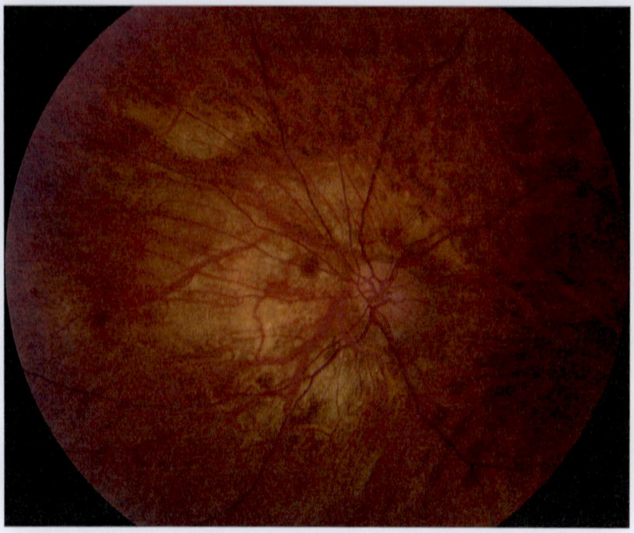

Fig. 11.6 Colour fundus photograph of the left eye demonstrating an underdeveloped optic nerve in a hypopigmented fundus

occurs in specialised cells called melanocytes derived from the ectoderm. Within the melanocytes, melanosome organelles produce melanin. Melanocytes are categorised as cutaneous (hair and skin) and extracutaneous (eye and cochlea); but deafness is rarely seen in OCA and has been described only once. Although the clinical phenotype can be quite similar, population studies have shown albinism to be a heterogeneous genetic disorder caused by multiple different genes. OCA gene disorders can be split into two categories: non-syndromic (*TYR*, *OCA2*, *TYRP1* and *SLC45A2*) and syndromic (*HPS1*, *AP3B1*, *HPS3*, *HPS4*, *HPS5*, *HPS6*, *HPSP7* and *LYST*) (Kamaraj and Purohit 2014). The clinical manifestations of all four non-syndromic forms of OCA are very similar, making it hard to differentiate between them from clinical examination. For proper identification, molecular analysis of the genes is required (Mártinez-García and Montoliu 2013).

Table 11.1 Genetic classification of oculocutaneous albinism

Albinism	Responsible gene	Gene location
OCA1	*TYR*	11q14-q21
OCA2	*OCA2*	15q
OCA3	*TYRP1*	9p23
OCA4	*SLC45A2*	5p

Non-syndromic OCA

OCA1 is the most severe form of OCA and is caused by mutations in the gene for the enzyme tyrosinase (*TYR*, see Table 11.1), an enzyme that catalyses the first two steps of melanin biosynthesis. Tyrosinase catalyses the conversion of tyrosine to L-3-4-dihydroxyphenylalanine (L-DOPA) and L-DOPA to DOPA quinone (Nicholson and Traboulsi 2012). Where there is a complete absence of tyrosinase activity, the term OCA1A is used. The classical phenotype can range from light blue to pink irides. Alternatively, the defect could be milder with reduced tyrosinase activity rather than absent activity. In these cases, the term OCA1B is used, sometimes referred to as 'yellow' albinism wherein phenotypes can show blue, green or brown irides (Fig. 11.7) (Gargiulo et al. 2011). OCA1 has been found to be most prevalent amongst Caucasians and accounts for about 50% of OCA cases worldwide (Simeonov et al. 2013).

OCA2, previously under the nomenclature 'brown OCA', is due to a mutation in the *OCA2* gene (see Table 11.1), which performs essential function in the modulation of melanosome pH. When *OCA2* is defective, the pH control

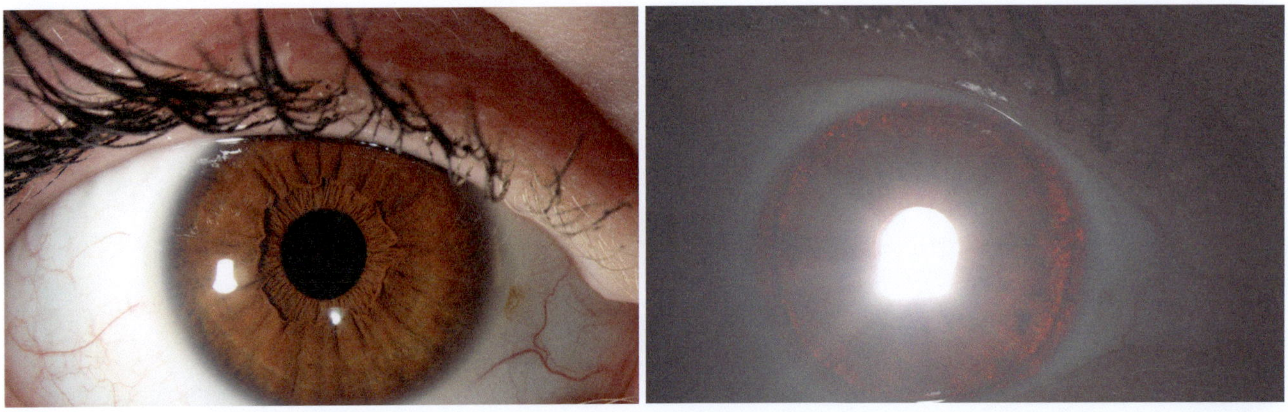

Fig. 11.7 *Left:* Slit lamp colour photograph of a patient with OCA1B. *Right:* Iris transillumination of the same eye. Note the dark eyelashes are a result from the use of cosmetic mascara

of melanosomes becomes defective, resulting in a reduction in tyrosinase activity (Bellono et al. 2014). It has also been proposed that *OCA2* plays an important role in modulating the processing and releasing of tyrosinase to melanosomes. When defective, it is logical to assume that tyrosinase is improperly released, and thus pigmentation is impaired (Toyofuku et al. 2002). *OCA2* has been found to be the most prevalent amongst African populations and accounts for around 30% of OCA worldwide (Simeonov et al. 2013).

OCA3 is caused by mutations in *TYRP1* (see Table 11.1) and can also be referred to as 'rufous OCA'. The gene *TYRP1* encodes the protein 'tyrosine related protein 1', which appears to be the most abundant melanosomal protein. Structurally, the TYRP1 protein is very similar to the enzyme tyrosinase and has been speculated to have tyrosinase-like activity (Kamaraj and Purohit 2013). The TYRP1 protein has been shown to have some tyrosine hydroxylase activity and no DOPA oxidase activity. It has been linked to melanosome structure as well as melanosome proliferation and death. TYRP1 is essential in tyrosinase activity. As such, when defective, tyrosinase activity is reduced and melanin production is also reduced (Kamaraj and Purohit 2014). OCA3 is very rare in Western and Asian populations, being most common in African populations (Gronskov et al. 2007).

OCA4 is caused by a mutation in the gene *SLC45A2* (see Table 11.1), also known as the membrane-associated transporter protein gene. The protein has similarities to plant sucrose transporters and is expressed in melanosomal cells (Gronskov et al. 2007). Mutations in *SLC45A2* have been proposed to cause misrouting of tyrosinase and TYRP1. Because tyrosine is misrouted, it cannot play its role in melanogenesis, and this results in hypopigmentation. Note the similarity to the role of the OCA2 protein in tyrosinase transport (Costin et al. 2003). OCA4 is one of the rarest forms of OCA but has an unusually high prevalence amongst Japanese populations (Kamaraj and Purohit 2014).

Table 11.2 Classification of Hermansky–Pudlak genes to subunits

Subunit	Gene(s)
BLOC-1	*HPS7, HPS8, HPS9*
BLOC-2	*HPS3, HPS5, HPS6*
BLOC-3	*HPS1, HPS4*
AP3	*HPS2*

Syndromic OCA

Hermansky–Pudlak syndrome (HPS) is the most common syndromic form of OCA, wherein multiple gene products are present. Each gene product has defects in subunits of either biogenesis of lysosome-related organelles complex (BLOC)-1, -2 or -3 or adaptor protein-3 (AP3). The genes involved in each of these complexes are listed in Table 11.2 (Huizing et al. 2008).

Whilst extremely rare worldwide, HPS is most commonly found in Puerto Rico. The BLOCs are heavily involved in the trafficking of melanosomes (El-Chemaly and Young 2016), which is a critical component of melanogenesis. If defective, hypopigmentation is an inevitable outcome. The genes behind HPS have not been well explored, but it is generally regarded that they are all involved in the regulation or trafficking of lysosome-related organelles. These organelles include melanosomes, lysosomes, and platelets. Defects in these processes result in the main features of the HPS syndrome—OCA and an increased bleeding tendency (see section 'Syndromic OCA') (Schneier and Fulton 2013).

Chédiak–Higashi syndrome (CHS) is caused by mutations in a single gene *LYST*, located at chromosome 1q42-43. The main feature of CHS is the presence of massive lysosomal inclusions in leukocytes, fibroblasts and melanocytes due to a microtubular defect. Studies have shown that lysosomal exocytosis can be defective in CHS (Rudramurthy and Lokanatha 2015). The most important ocular pathology in CHS is the enlargement of melanosomes in the retinal pigment epithelium, leading to abnormal eye pigmentation resulting in photophobia and decreased visual acuity (Ji et al. 2016).

Ocular Albinism

Mutations in the gene *GPR143* on the X chromosome (at Xp22.3-2.2) are responsible for most ocular albinism cases and are denoted OA1. This gene encodes a protein that controls melanosome number and size (Levin and Stroh 2011). The gene mainly affects functioning of a G-protein-coupled receptor involved in melanosome synthesis in retinal pigment epithelial cells and iris epithelium cells (Mártinez-García and Montoliu 2013). When *GPR143* is defective, melanosome synthesis is impaired, leading to impaired melanin synthesis. OA1 is a non-progressive condition and remains stable throughout life (Hu et al. 2011).

As ocular albinism is predominantly an X-linked recessive condition, these disorders tend to present more frequently amongst men. Males with X-linked genetic disorders pass the gene to all daughters, but cannot pass the defected X chromosome to their sons. Females who have one affected X chromosome are carriers of the gene and have the capability to pass on the gene. It is uncommon for a female to inherit two affected X chromosomes and become affected (Winsor 1988).

Clinical Characteristics

The ocular features of oculocutaneous albinism are identical to ocular albinism; thus, the main ophthalmic features will be covered in section 'Ocular Albinism'.

Oculocutaneous Albinism

It is important to be able to differentiate between syndromic and non-syndromic forms of OCA, so appropriate management and genetic counselling can be considered.

Non-syndromic OCA

Individuals born with OCA1A typically have white hair at birth and will fail to show any melanin pigment in the hair, skin, or eyes for their entire lifetime, whereas individuals born with OCA1B can develop pigmentation in their hair and lashes over time. OCA1B can also have temperature-sensitive variants wherein hypopigmentation of hairs only occurs on warmer parts of the body. Individuals born with OCA2 are usually born with red hair or blond hair; however, skin hypopigmentation remains. It is also important to be aware that OCA4 and OCA2 have very similar clinical phenotypes and can be hard to differentiate. OCA3 is associated with red hair or reddish brown skin in African populations. There is often very little visual impairment as the hypopigmentation is not severe enough to alter the development of the visual system (Summers 2009; Kamaraj and Purohit 2014).

Malignant melanoma in patients with albinism is exceedingly rare in populations living in cooler climates, with very few cases being presented in literature. However, in Africa, albinism is recognised as a risk factor for skin cancer. In African countries nearer to the equator, e.g. Nigeria, a large proportion of individuals with OCA under age 20 years have malignant or premalignant lesions (Levine et al. 1992; Kiprono et al. 2014; Lookingbill et al. 1995). This is due to the proximity to the equator where the ultraviolet (UV) light is at its strongest. In a review for malignant carcinomas in Africans with albinism, squamous cell carcinomas were found to be slightly more common than basal cell carcinomas.

Syndromic OCA

HPS shares many common symptoms with non-syndromic OCA1A, but it is vital for ophthalmologists to consider other systemic features as they are associated with higher morbidity and mortality rates. When diagnosing OCA, it is imperative to consider HPS as a differential diagnosis. The main symptom of HPS is excessive bleeding. This may present as ease of bruising, epistaxis, heavy menses and bleeding complications of childbirth. In addition to bleeding, pulmonary fibrosis has been found in adults, which can first present as wheezing in childhood. It is recommended to involve a haematologist and a geneticist if HPS is suspected. On diagnosis, genetic subtyping can be performed, but all HPS patients require counselling regarding bleeding tendency despite their subtype (Schneier and Fulton 2013). A restrictive lung disease can start in an individual's early 30s and progress to death within a decade (Brantly et al. 2000).

CHS also shares the common symptoms of non-syndromic OCA1A, but individuals are at risk for lymphoreticular malignancy, as well as presenting with a greyer sheen to the hair, grey patches on the skin and macromelanosomes on skin biopsy. Hepatosplenomegaly and progressive visual loss are common as the disease progresses. CHS can lead to an early death (Levin and Stroh 2011; Sayanagi et al. 2003).

Ocular Albinism

Ocular albinism shares all the ophthalmic features of oculocutaneous albinism, listed below:

- Iris transillumination (Figs. 11.8 and 11.9)—this is best performed in a dark room with a bright slit beam in the slit lamp. The iris is seen to be translucent. In severe

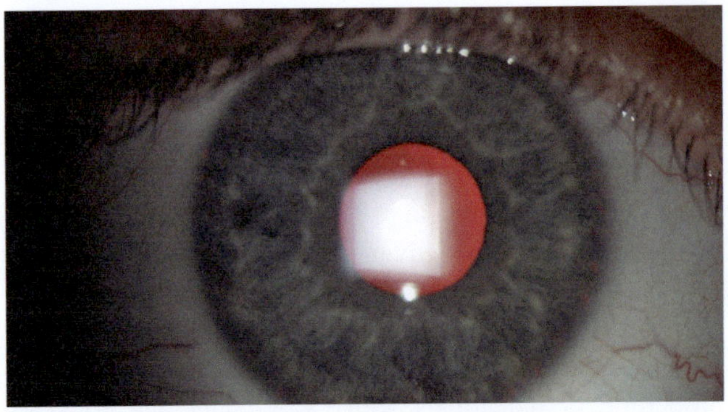

Fig. 11.8 Grade 1: Punctate iris transillumination

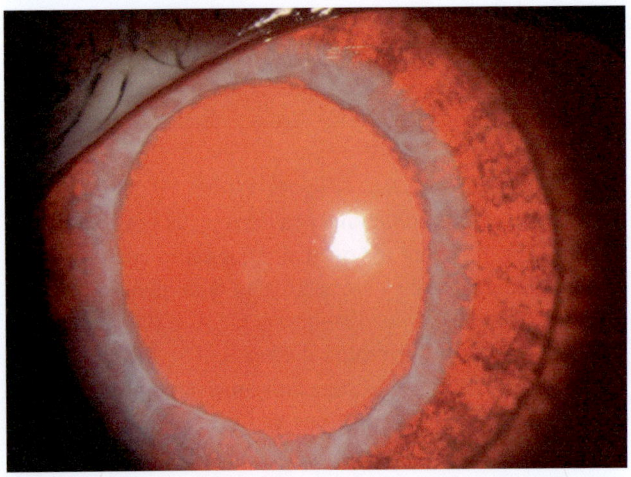

Fig. 11.9 Grade 4: Full iris transillumination

cases, the outline of the lens can be apparent. The less pigmented the iris, the greater the iris transillumination (Table 11.3).

- Foveal hypoplasia (Fig. 11.10)—severe forms often result in marked visual impairment. Those with 20/50 or better vision can show some foveal development.
- Fundal hypopigmentation (Fig. 11.11)—due to the absence or reduction of melanin in the retinal pigment epithelium. Choroidal vessels become more visible (Table 11.4).
- Reduced visual acuity and stereopsis—a result of foveal hypoplasia and abnormal development of the visual system.
- Strabismus and nystagmus are common—again, due to the abnormal development of the visual system.
- Refractive errors—with high hypermetropia more commonly found in OCA1A and astigmatism being the most common visually significant refractive error across all subtypes.

Visual evoked potentials (VEP) are useful in demonstrating excessive decussation of optic nerve fibres in the chiasm and tracts, especially if the clinical features are not clear

Table 11.3 Classification of iris transillumination

Grade	Features
Grade 1 (Fig. 11.8)	Punctate areas transillumination
Grade 2	Moderate iris pigment
Grade 3	Minimal iris pigment
Grade 4 (Fig. 11.9)	Full transillumination due to absence of pigment

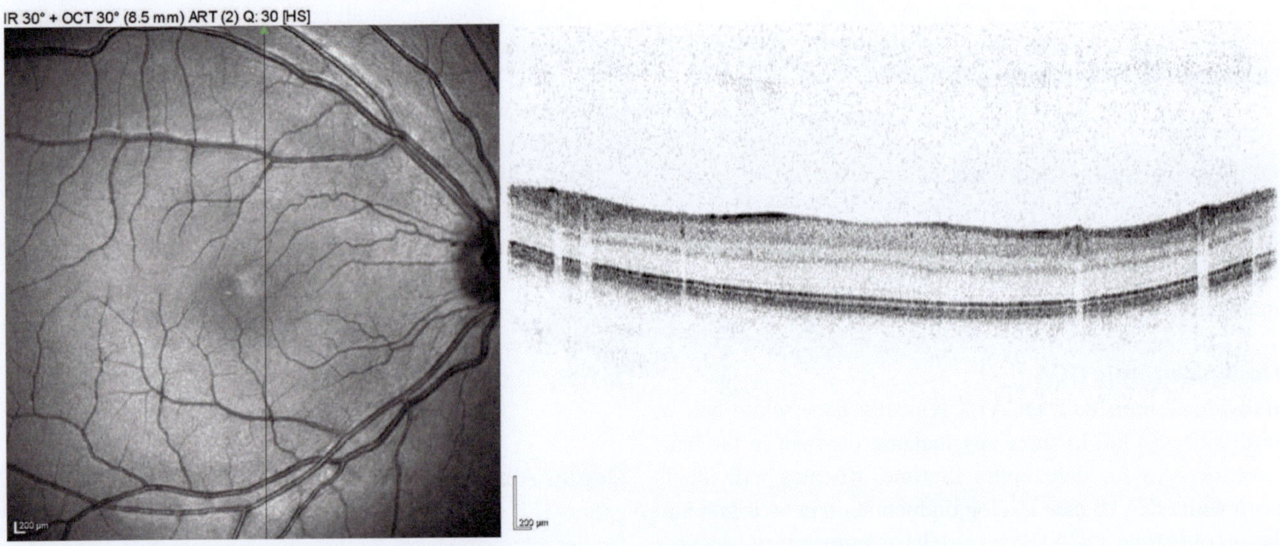

Fig. 11.10 Tracking laser tomography showing underdevelopment of the right fovea

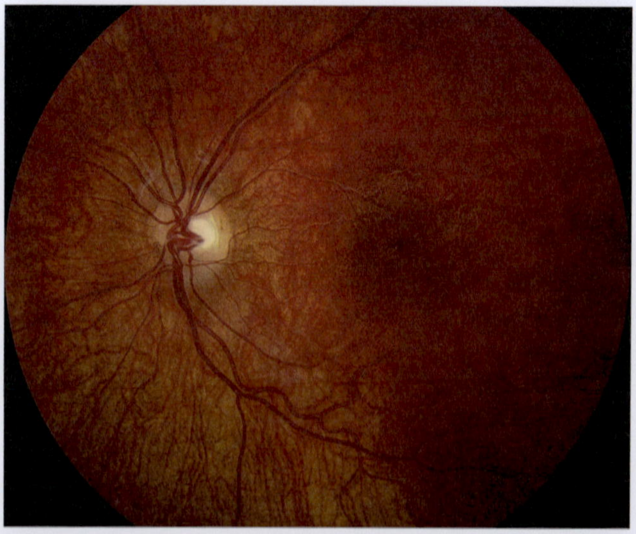

Fig. 11.11 Colour fundus photo showing fundal hypopigmentation with choroidal vessels easily seen

Table 11.4 Classification of macular hypopigmentation

Grade	Features
Grade 1	Choroidal vessels easily seen
Grade 2	Choroidal vessels less distinctly seen because of translucent retinal pigment epithelium
Grade 3	Opaque macula so choroidal vessels are not visible

enough to warrant a definite diagnosis (Dorey et al. 2003; Summers 2009; Izquierdo et al. 1995; Summers et al. 1988; Yahalom et al. 2012).

Management

There is currently no cure for albinism. Understanding and managing the condition are essential.

Ocular Management

Many babies with albinism may appear to have severely impaired vision, but their vision can improve after a few months, as a result of a form of delayed visual maturation (Illingworth 1961).

Spectacles can be used to correct significant refractive errors and help to maximise visual acuity. Tinted spectacles can be prescribed for use in bright environment to reduce symptoms of glare and thus improve the quality of vision (Rosenblum et al. 2000).

Amblyopia therapy can be considered when amblyopia is clearly demonstrated, with patching or pharmacological penalisation with 1% gutta atropine in the better-seeing eye (Bretas and Soriano 2016). However, monocular visual acuity is often more reduced than vision binocularly, due to an element of latent nystagmus (nystagmus oscillations increase in frequency and amplitude with monocular occlusion during a monocular vision check) (Papageorgiou et al. 2014). Therefore it can be a challenge to confirm true amblyopia in the presence of foveal hypoplasia.

Educational support is important for children with albinism and can be delivered by visual impairment support services in some countries e.g. the United Kingdom. These services include home visits at preschool ages to initiate visual sensory stimulation and later liaison with schools on educational needs such as larger font sizes and higher contrast learning materials. This can be made easier by electronic educational devices. Children with severe forms of visual impairment can benefit from learning braille, which can be introduced as young as 3 years old (Keil 2004). The Royal National Institute for Blind people in the UK is an excellent source of advice on this.

Surgical Correction for Nystagmus

Nystagmus is a condition that rarely benefits from surgical treatment to the extraocular muscles. However, under certain circumstances, extraocular muscle surgery may help a few patients with specific problems associated with nystagmus.

Head posture in nystagmus can sometimes be adopted to bring the vision into the 'null zone', a position of gaze in which the nystagmus is most dampened, hence an area with the best visual acuity. The Kestenbaum procedure is used to produce a deviation of the eyes horizontally, in the direction of the head turn and lead to reduction of an unacceptable eccentric horizontal head posture. The Kestenbaum procedure involves recession and resection of all four horizontal rectus muscles and is also called the '5, 6, 7, 8 procedure' i.e. for the correction of right head turn, the aim is to produce a slight restriction of left gaze eye movement, relieving the head turn, and to put the eye in primary position. This is achieved by performing a 6 mm right medial rectus recession and 7 mm right lateral rectus resection combined with a 5 mm left medial rectus resection and 8 mm left lateral rectus recession. Whereas, Anderson advocated resection of horizontal muscles and Goto advocated resections of the antagonistic muscles of each eye. Kestenbaum's method has proven to be most popular; however, follow-up research has been lacking (Sturm et al. 2014).

An alternative approach is 'four muscle tenotomy'. This involves each horizontal eye muscle being isolated and a 6–0 vicryl suture placed in the muscle, just posterior to its insertion. Each horizontal rectus muscle is detached and immediately reattached to the same insertion site. After a four muscle tenotomy, visual acuity has been shown to be improved and nystagmus intensity can be decreased. This procedure does not have significant complications. It is thought that the afferent signalling from the extraocular muscles are dampened by detaching and reattaching the muscles; however, further research is required to fully understand the long-term impact of the four muscle tenotomy in the treatment of nystagmus (Greven and Nelson 2014; Dubner et al. 2016).

Skin Management

Due to the higher risk of skin cancers in those with oculocutaneous albinism, use of hats and sunglasses have been recommended to those affected. Sunscreen can also be used to reduce the frequency of burns. This is especially important near to the equator where ultraviolet radiation is strongest (Kirkwood 2009; Lookingbill et al. 1995).

References

Bellono NW, Escobar IE, Lefkovith AJ, Marks MS, Oancea E. An intracellular anion channel critical for pigmentation. eLife. 2014;3:e04543. https://doi.org/10.7554/eLife.04543.

Brantly M, Avila NA, Shotelersuk V, Lucero C, Huizing M, Gahl WA. Pulmonary function and high-resolution CT findings in patients with an inherited form of pulmonary fibrosis, Hermansky-Pudlak syndrome, due to mutations in HPS-1. Chest. 2000;117(1):129–36. https://doi.org/10.1378/chest.117.1.129.

Bretas CCP, Soriano RN. Amblyopia: neural basis and therapeutic approaches. Arq Bras Oftalmol. 2016;79(5):346–51.

Costin G-E, Valencia JC, Vieira WD, Lamoreux ML, Hearing VJ. Tyrosinase processing and intracellular trafficking is disrupted in mouse primary melanocytes carrying the underwhite (uw) mutation. A model for oculocutaneous albinism (OCA) type 4. J Cell Sci. 2003;116(15):3203–12. https://doi.org/10.1242/jcs.00598.

Cruz-Inigo AE, Ladizinski B, Sethi A. Albinism in Africa: stigma, slaughter and awareness campaigns. Dermatol Clin. 2011;29(1):79–+. https://doi.org/10.1016/j.det.2010.08.015.

Dorey SE, Neveu MM, Burton LC, Sloper JJ, Holder GE. The clinical features of albinism and their correlation with visual evoked potentials. Br J Ophthalmol. 2003;87(6):767–72. https://doi.org/10.1136/bjo.87.6.767.

Dubner M, Nelson LB, Gunton KB, Lavrich J, Schnall B, Wasserman BN. Clinical evaluation of four-muscle tenotomy surgery for Nystagmus. J Pediatr Ophthalmol Strabismus. 2016;53(1):16–21. https://doi.org/10.3928/01913913-20160113-03.

El-Chemaly S, Young LR. Hermansky-Pudlak syndrome. Clin Chest Med. 2016;37(3):505–11. https://doi.org/10.1016/j.ccm.2016.04.012.

Froggatt P. Albinism in Northern Ireland. Ann Hum Genet. 1960;24(3):213–38. https://doi.org/10.1111/j.1469-1809.1960.tb01734.x.

Gargiulo A, Testa F, Rossi S, Di Iorio V, Fecarotta S, de Berardinis T, Iovine A, Magli A, Signorini S, Fazzi E, Galantuomo MS, Fossarello M, Montefusco S, Ciccodicola A, Neri A, Macaluso C, Simonelli F, Surace EM. Molecular and clinical characterization of albinism in a large cohort of Italian patients. Invest Ophthalmol Vis Sci. 2011;52(3):1281–9. https://doi.org/10.1167/iovs.10-6091.

Greven MA, Nelson LB. Four-muscle tenotomy surgery for nystagmus. Curr Opin Ophthalmol. 2014;25(5):400–5.

Gronskov K, Ek J, Brondum-Nielsen K. Oculocutaneous albinism. Orphanet J Rare Dis. 2007;2(8):b25. https://doi.org/10.1186/1750-1172-2-43.

Grønskov K, Ek J, Sand A, Scheller R, Bygum A, Brixen K, Brondum-Nielsen K, Rosenberg T. Birth prevalence and mutation Spectrum in Danish patients with autosomal recessive albinism. Invest Ophthalmol Amp Vis Sci. 2009;50(3):1058–64. https://doi.org/10.1167/iovs.08-2639.

Hermansky F, Pudlak P. Albinism associated with hemorrhagic diathesis and unusual pigmented reticular cells in the bone marrow: report of two cases with Histochemical studies. Blood. 1959;14(2):162–9.

Hu J, Liang D, Xue J, Liu J, Wu L. A novel GPR143 splicing mutation in a Chinese family with X-linked congenital nystagmus. Mol Vis. 2011;17:715–22.

Huizing M, Helip-Wooley A, Westbroek W, Gunay-Aygun M, Gahl WA. Disorders of lysosome-related organelle biogenesis: clinical and molecular genetics. Annu Rev Genomics Hum Genet. 2008;9:359–86. https://doi.org/10.1146/annurev.genom.9.081307.164303.

Illingworth RS. Delayed visual maturation. Arch Dis Child. 1961;36(188):407–9.

Izquierdo NJ, Townsend W, Hussels IE. Ocular findings in the Hermansky-Pudlak syndrome. Trans Am Ophthalmol Soc. 1995;93:191–202.

Ji X, Chang B, Naggert JK, Nishina PM. Lysosomal trafficking regulator (LYST). In: Bowes Rickman C, LaVail MM, Anderson RE, Grimm C, Hollyfield J, Ash J, editors. Retinal degenerative diseases: mechanisms and experimental therapy. Cham: Springer; 2016. p. 745–50. https://doi.org/10.1007/978-3-319-17121-0_99.

Kamaraj B, Purohit R. In silico screening and molecular dynamics simulation of disease-associated nsSNP in TYRP1 gene and its structural consequences in OCA3. Biomed Res Int. 2013;2013:13. https://doi.org/10.1155/2013/697051.

Kamaraj B, Purohit R. Mutational analysis of oculocutaneous albinism: a compact review. Biomed Res Int. 2014;2014:10. https://doi.org/10.1155/2014/905472.

Keil S. Teaching braille to children. Br J Vis Impair. 2004;22(1):13–6. https://doi.org/10.1177/026461960402200103.

Kinnear PE, Jay B, Witkop CJ. Albinism. Surv Ophthalmol. 1985;30(2):75–101. https://doi.org/10.1016/0039-6257(85)90077-3.

Kiprono SK, Chaula BM, Beltraminelli H. Histological review of skin cancers in African albinos: a 10-year retrospective review. BMC Cancer. 2014;14:157. https://doi.org/10.1186/1471-2407-14-157.

Kirkwood B. Albinism and its implications with vision. Insight. 2009;34(2):13–6.

Levin AV, Stroh E. Albinism for the busy clinician. J Am Assoc Pediatr Ophthalmol Strabismus. 2011;15(1):59–66. https://doi.org/10.1016/j.jaapos.2010.10.012.

Levine EA, Ronan SG, Shirali SS, Gupta TKD, Karakousis CP. Malignant melanoma in a child with oculocutaneous albinism. J Surg Oncol. 1992;51(2):138–42. https://doi.org/10.1002/jso.2930510215.

Lookingbill DP, Lookingbill GL, Leppard B. Actinic damage and skin cancer in albinos in northern Tanzania: findings in 164 patients enrolled in an outreach skin care program. J Am Acad Dermatol. 1995;32(4):653–8. https://doi.org/10.1016/0190-9622(95)90352-6.

Mártinez-García M, Montoliu L. Albinism in Europe. J Dermatol. 2013;40(5):319–24. https://doi.org/10.1111/1346-8138.12170.

Martinez-Garcia M, Riveiro-Alvarez R, Villaverde-Montero C, Cantalapiedra D, Garcia-Sandoval B, Ayuso C, Trujillo-Tiebas MJ. Identification of a novel deletion in the OA1 gene: report of the first Spanish family with X-linked ocular albinism. Clin Exp Ophthalmol. 2010;38(5):489–95. https://doi.org/10.1111/j.1442-9071.2010.02282.x.

McKetton L, Kelly KR, Schneider KA. Abnormal lateral geniculate nucleus and optic chiasm in human albinism. J Comp Neurol. 2014;522(11):2680–7. https://doi.org/10.1002/cne.23565.

Nicholson PB, Traboulsi IE. Albinism. In: Wright KW, Strube YNJ, editors. Pediatric ophthalmology and strabismus. 3rd ed. New York: Oxford University Press; 2012. p. 1148–9.

Papageorgiou E, McLean RJ, Gottlob I. Nystagmus in childhood. Pediatr Neonatol. 2014;55(5):341–51. https://doi.org/10.1016/j.pedneo.2014.02.007.

Rosenblum YZ, Zak PP, Ostrovsky MA, Smolyaninova IL, Bora EV, Dyadina UV, Trofimova NN, Aliyev AGD. Spectral filters in low-vision correction. Ophthalmic Physiol Opt. 2000;20(4):335–41. https://doi.org/10.1046/j.1475-1313.2000.00545.x.

Rudramurthy P, Lokanatha H. Chediak-Higashi syndrome: a case series from Karnataka, India. Indian J Dermatol. 2015;60(5):524. https://doi.org/10.4103/0019-5154.159662.

Sato A. Chédiak and Higashi's disease. Probable identity of "a new leucocytal anomaly (Chédiak)" and "congenital gigantism of peroxidase granules (Higashi)". Tohoku J Exp Med. 1955;61(2–3):201–10. https://doi.org/10.1620/tjem.61.201.

Sayanagi K, Fujikado T, Onodera T, Tano Y. Chediak-Higashi syndrome with progressive visual loss. Jpn J Ophthalmol. 2003;47(3):304–6. https://doi.org/10.1016/S0021-5155(03)00018-2.

Schneier AJ, Fulton AB. The Hermansky-Pudlak syndrome: clinical features and imperatives from an ophthalmic perspective. Semin Ophthalmol. 2013;28(5–6):387–91. https://doi.org/10.3109/08820538.2013.825280.

Scriver CR. Garrod's Croonian Lectures (1908) and the charter 'Inborn errors of metabolism': albinism, alkaptonuria, cystinuria, and pentosuria at age 100 in 2008. J Inherit Metab Dis. 2008;31(5):580. https://doi.org/10.1007/s10545-008-0984-9.

Simeonov DR, Wang X, Wang C, Sergeev Y, Dolinska M, Bower M, Fischer R, Winer D, Dubrovsky G, Balog JZ, Huizing M, Hart R, Zein WM, Gahl WA, Brooks BP, Adams DR. DNA variations in oculocutaneous albinism: an updated mutation list and current outstanding issues in molecular diagnostics. Hum Mutat. 2013;34(6):827–35. https://doi.org/10.1002/humu.22315.

Sturm V, Hejcmanova M, Landau K. Effects of extraocular muscle surgery in children with monocular blindness and bilateral nystagmus. BMC Ophthalmol. 2014;14(1):137. https://doi.org/10.1186/1471-2415-14-137.

Summers CG. Albinism: classification, clinical characteristics, and recent findings. Optom Vis Sci. 2009;86(6):659–62.

Summers GC, Knobloch WH, Witkop CJ Jr, King RA. Hermansky-Pudlak syndrome. Ophthalmology. 1988;95(4):545–54. https://doi.org/10.1016/S0161-6420(88)33152-0.

Suzuki T, Tomita Y. Recent advances in genetic analyses of oculocutaneous albinism types 2 and 4. J Dermatol Sci. 2008;51(1):1–9. https://doi.org/10.1016/j.jdermsci.2007.12.008.

Toyofuku K, Valencia JC, Kushimoto T, Costin G-E, Virador VM, Vieira WD, Ferrans VJ, Hearing VJ. The etiology of oculocutaneous albinism (OCA) type II: the pink protein modulates the processing and transport of Tyrosinase. Pigment Cell Res. 2002;15(3):217–24. https://doi.org/10.1034/j.1600-0749.2002.02007.x.

Welton T, Ather S, Proudlock FA, Gottlob I, Dineen RA. Altered whole-brain connectivity in albinism. Hum Brain Mapp. 2017;38(2):740–52. https://doi.org/10.1002/hbm.23414.

Winsor E. Mendelian genetics. Can Fam Physician. 1988;34:859–62.

Yahalom C, Tzur V, Blumenfeld A, Greifner G, Eli D, Rosenmann A, Glanzer S, Anteby I. Refractive profile in oculocutaneous albinism and its correlation with final visual outcome. Br J Ophthalmol. 2012;96(4):537–9. https://doi.org/10.1136/bjophthalmol-2011-300072.

MIX
Papier aus verantwortungsvollen Quellen
Paper from responsible sources
FSC® C105338

If you have any concerns about our products,
you can contact us on
ProductSafety@springernature.com

In case Publisher is established outside the EU,
the EU authorized representative is:
Springer Nature Customer Service Center GmbH
Europaplatz 3, 69115 Heidelberg, Germany

Printed by Libri Plureos GmbH
in Hamburg, Germany